RABIES IN THE STREETS

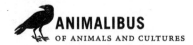

ANIMALIBUS
OF ANIMALS AND CULTURES

Nigel Rothfels, *General Editor*

ADVISORY BOARD:
Steve Baker (University of Central Lancashire)
Garry Marvin (Roehampton University)
Susan McHugh (University of New England)
Kari Weil (Wesleyan University)

Books in the Animalibus series share a fascination with the status and the role of animals in human life. Crossing the humanities and the social sciences to include work in history, anthropology, social and cultural geography, environmental studies, and literary and art criticism, these books ask what thinking about nonhuman animals can teach us about human cultures, about what it means to be human, and about how that meaning might shift across times and places.

OTHER TITLES IN THE SERIES:

Rachel Poliquin, *The Breathless Zoo: Taxidermy and the Cultures of Longing*

Joan B. Landes, Paula Young Lee, and Paul Youngquist, eds., *Gorgeous Beasts: Animal Bodies in Historical Perspective*

Liv Emma Thorsen, Karen A. Rader, and Adam Dodd, eds., *Animals on Display: The Creaturely in Museums, Zoos, and Natural History*

Ann-Janine Morey, *Picturing Dogs, Seeing Ourselves: Vintage American Photographs*

Mary Sanders Pollock, *Storytelling Apes: Primatology Narratives Past and Future*

Ingrid H. Tague, *Animal Companions: Pets and Social Change in Eighteenth-Century Britain*

Dick Blau and Nigel Rothfels, *Elephant House*

Marcus Baynes-Rock, *Among the Bone Eaters: Encounters with Hyenas in Harar*

Monica Mattfeld, *Becoming Centaur: Eighteenth-Century Masculinity and English Horsemanship*

Heather Swan, *Where Honeybees Thrive: Stories from the Field*

Karen Raber and Monica Mattfeld, eds., *Performing Animals: History, Agency, Theater*

J. Keri Cronin, *Art for Animals: Visual Culture and Animal Advocacy, 1870–1914*

Elizabeth Marshall Thomas, *The Hidden Life of Life: A Walk Through the Reaches of Time*

Elizabeth Young, *Pet Projects: Animal Fiction and Taxidermy in the Nineteenth-Century Archive*

Marcus Baynes-Rock, *Crocodile Undone: The Domestication of Australia's Fauna*

RABIES IN THE STREETS

Interspecies Camaraderie in Urban India

DEBORAH NADAL

THE PENNSYLVANIA STATE UNIVERSITY PRESS

UNIVERSITY PARK, PENNSYLVANIA

Library of Congress Cataloging-in-Publication Data

Names: Nadal, Deborah, 1985– author.
Title: Rabies in the streets : interspecies camaraderie
    in urban India / Deborah Nadal.
Other titles: Animalibus
Description: University Park, Pennsylvania : The
    Pennsylvania State University Press, [2020] |
    Series: Animalibus: of animals and cultures |
    includes bibliographical references and index
Summary: "Explores the relationship between
    people, street animals, and rabies in urban
    India. Incorporates epidemiological goals within
    anthropological frameworks to investigate the
    ways in which people come into contact with
    animals and create favorable conditions for the
    rabies virus to flourish"—Provided by publisher.
Identifiers: LCCN 2019059672 | ISBN 9780271085951
    (hardback)
Subjects: Rabies—India. | Rabies in animals—India.
    | Urban animals—India. | Human-animal
    relationships—India.
Classification: LCC RA644.R3 N33 2020 | DDC
    636.089/69530954—dc23
LC record available at https://lccn.loc.gov/2019059672

Published by The Pennsylvania
State University Press,
University Park, PA 16802-1003

The Pennsylvania State University Press is a member
of the Association of University Presses.

It is the policy of The Pennsylvania State University
Press to use acid-free paper. Publications on
uncoated stock satisfy the minimum requirements
of American National Standard for Information
Sciences—Permanence of Paper for Printed Library
Material, ANSI Z39.48–1992.

To my childhood dream
of becoming a veterinarian

CONTENTS

ACKNOWLEDGMENTS

I honestly do not know whether I would ever have thought of working on rabies had I not met the bull who, on a quiet evening in May 2012, invited himself to my dinner on the fringe of the Thar Desert, in Rajasthan. My deepest thanks go to him.

In India, this work has allowed me to cross paths with an incredibly wide range of people, each of whom has made a unique contribution to this book, whether directly or indirectly. Unfortunately, I cannot mention them all—in many cases, I do not even know their names. Yet I remember their faces very well, and I hope I will have the chance to meet them again to thank them in person. In any case, I need explicitly to thank Pradeep, Dhruv, Mala, Jack, Arina, Saleeq, Erika, Father Edwin, Kirti, Devi, Iqbal, and Sapna.

I am grateful to the dogs, cows, and monkeys who let me observe, touch, handle, feed, wash, and follow them. This book owes so much to them. I hope they would agree with what I have written about them, were they able to read.

At Ca' Foscari University of Venice and the University of Verona, my special thanks go to Glauco, for his caring attitude, to Stefano, for his contagious enthusiasm, to Franca, for her passion for anthropology, and to Anna, for her encouragement.

The writing of this book has been possible mainly thanks to the Hunt Postdoctoral Fellowship that I received from the Wenner-Gren Foundation. I am so grateful to the people at Wenner-Gren for believing in this project.

Thanks to everyone at Penn State University Press, who helped me turn my manuscript into this book. Special thanks to Kendra for her professionalism, to Alex for her technical assistance, to Suzanne for taking such precious care of the manuscript, to Regina for choosing my pictures from the field for the cover, and to Laura and Brian for moving the book smoothly through the final stages of production. I also want to thank Nigel, the series editor, for his support. Writing this book and seeing it through to production has been a labor of love.

No words are enough to thank the three most important persons in my life: my husband, for holding together the pieces of me better than I could ever do; my two-year-old daughter, for loving dogs so much that she easily accepted my long stays in India to work for them; and my sister, for being my safe harbor.

ABBREVIATIONS

ABC	animal birth control
APCRI	Association for Prevention and Control of Rabies in India
ARV	anti-rabies vaccination
AWBI	Animal Welfare Board of India
AWO	animal-welfare organization
CCV	cell culture vaccine
CWG	Commonwealth Games
FIAPO	Federation of Indian Animal Protection Organizations
GARC	Global Alliance for Rabies Control
HIS	Help In Suffering
MCD	Municipal Corporation of Delhi
NDMC	New Delhi Municipal Council
NGO	nongovernmental organization
NTV	nerve tissue vaccine
OIE	Office International des Épizooties (World Organization for Animal Health)
PEP	post-exposure prophylaxis
RWA	resident welfare association
WHO	World Health Organization

INTRODUCTION

Viral Connections

Whenever I went to the Sarai Kale Khan slum, in the heart of Delhi, I never saw Neelam attending the informal lessons given there by the social worker. She was too old to attend school, she would tell me later. Neelam was twelve when we met, and for the past five years she had been working as a plastic collector in the nearby Nizamuddin railway station. Our first chat occurred while she was sorting her collected stuff, next to the one-room house where her family of six lived. Neelam could not remember the incident that left a protruding scar on her thin left calf. It was just one among the many that resulted from her job. What she did remember vividly was what had happened to her cousin Charita, who died in their native village in Maharashtra six weeks after being bitten by a dog. Neelam still could not understand how Charita was suddenly unable to recognize her family or know where she was. She remembered Charita staring at her with empty eyes, looking at her own house as if she had never seen it before. Then, Neelam told me, Charita started throwing things; she was particularly terrified by glasses of water. Neelam's mother, Nidhi, nods in agreement while her daughter speaks. Nidhi's only consolation regarding her niece's death is that at least she did not have to suffer puppies growing in her stomach. This, Nidhi has heard from her neighbors in Delhi, is the unfortunate fate of many dog bite victims.

This book is about how and why Charita, the dog who bit her, and the rabies virus came to be in close enough proximity that a lethal infection was triggered. It is also about monkeys and cattle, for rabies is a multispecies issue in India and, like dogs, these animals have now become part of the Indian urban society and ecosystem, strengthening important ecological, spiritual, symbolic, and economic ties with the history and landscape of Indian cities and towns, particularly Delhi and Jaipur, where I did most of the research for this book. In other words, this study investigates the worlds that people and these three animal species have more or less consciously built for one another and, much to their regret, for the rabies virus as well. Following Alex M. Nading's reasoning about entanglement, in the context of this book it is useful to see life not simply as a vitality to be secured but as "the unfolding, often incidental attachments and affinities, antagonisms and animosities that bring people, nonhuman animals, and materials into each other's worlds" (2012, 574). One of the results of this collective world building is increased mutual vulnerability. This book deals with rabies-driven human torment and death, but it is also about the "silenced non-human dimension of health" (Nading 2014b, 205). As Donna Haraway famously wrote, in a multispecies world, "becoming is always becoming with" (2008, 244). In the case of rabies—a disease that kills across species—suffering is always suffering with.

Rabies is a cruel disease, and not just because its victims think that they will have to bear an agonizing, unnatural pregnancy. It is the deadliest disease on earth, fatal in over 99% of cases. It has no effective cure once its clinical signs appear. Given that it is a neuro-invasive disease that affects the brain, it has devastating effects on the behavior of its victims, making them unrecognizable to their friends and family (whatever their species). No single test is available to diagnose rabies infection before the onset of symptoms. Its unpredictable and sometimes very long incubation period makes the course of the illness potentially more devastating than death itself. Finally, rabies deeply unsettles the relationship between human and nonhuman animals, no matter what side you view it from.

Rabies is technically defined as a zoonosis—that is, a disease that is naturally transmissible to humans from animals. The main characteristic of any zoonosis is that its infectivity completely disregards the boundary lines between species, which are regularly crossed by viruses in their role as transboundary tricksters. At present, it is estimated that 60% of existing human infectious diseases are of animal origin, as are 75% of emerging human diseases (WHO 2014, 1). In three-fourths of the world's countries where rabies is rife, mammals are at particular risk, although there are many variants of the rabies virus, each maintained in a particular reservoir animal in which the virus typically lives and from which it moves both within and between species to infect. Dogs are the main reservoirs for rabies and, because of their proximity to humans, the most common vectors of the disease to people.

Rabies causes similar physical suffering and death in all the species it affects. Yet given the state of underreporting in many countries, estimating how many animals across the world suffer from rabies at any given time remains particularly difficult. Consequently, the topic of animal *well-being*—which I and others (Rock and Degeling 2016, 70) prefer to the term *welfare*, which is more commonly used in veterinary medicine, as if "a state of *being* or *doing well* in life" (OED, emphasis added) could not apply to animals—is largely ignored. Paradoxically, this is the case even if rabies is, strictly speaking, a disease of animals rather than of humans, who rarely transmit it but are generally dead-end hosts. Dogs, so close to humans yet so overlooked when it comes to rabies, are the species that suffers the most from this situation, to the extent that the Global Alliance for Rabies Control (GARC) considers them "rabies' forgotten victims," not only because they suffer and die from the disease in far greater numbers than people do, but also because people kill them out of fear and loathing. In fact, up to ten million dogs a year, or 27,397 a day, may be culled across the world in attempts to control rabies (GARC n.d.).

Now that rabies is formally recognized as a shared health issue of humans and animals, the Office International des Épizooties (OIE, or World Organization for Animal Health), the World Health Organization (WHO), the UN Food and Agriculture Organization (FAO), and GARC have joined forces to mount a sustained effort to control it under the banner of the One Health Initiative. In December 2015, these agencies gave themselves fifteen years to bring the annual number of human rabies deaths to zero from the current 59,000 (WHO 2017, 77). At present, someone dies from rabies every nine minutes, predominantly in the rural and economically disadvantaged and marginalized areas of Asia and Africa (WHO 2018b, 5). This collaborative initiative marks the first time that the human and animal health sectors have come together to pursue a common strategy to combat this disease. Although the elimination of rabies in humans is the ultimate target of this project (its complete eradication being far beyond current capacities, given the broad range of rabies vectors), its success will depend heavily on the drastic reduction of the disease in animals. In fact, only a solid commitment to reducing rabies in both humans and animals can hope to make a significant difference in the multispecies fight against rabies. In practical terms, given that more than 95% of all human deaths (and most spillovers—Grover et al. 2018) result from transmission via dog bite, controlling this disease in dogs is the only means of undermining its infectious cycle. As I argue in chapter 3, dog vaccination—not dog culling—is the way to go. However counterintuitive it may seem, decades of scientific research have demonstrated that culling dogs is not only useless but also counterproductive, as vaccinated dogs are the most effective barrier against rabies. This is why we should look at them as "co-participants rather than vessels of disease" (Brown and Kelly 2014, 286): they die of rabies like us, they fight rabies with us.

This approach to rabies is grounded not only on an ethical foundation, as it humanely relieves both humans and animals from the threat of this disease, but also on a concrete, practical one. Rabies causes an annual worldwide direct economic loss of US$8.6 billion (Hampson et al. 2015, 12) and an indirect, aggregate loss of US$120 billion (Anderson and Shwiff 2013, 449). By comparison, the 2014 Ebola epidemic was responsible for 11,316 deaths and US$2.2 billion in economic losses. The largest portion of the economic cost of rabies is due to premature deaths (55%), followed by the direct costs of post-bite vaccination (20%), lost income and loss of labor within households while seeking treatment (15%), and additional costs to communities from livestock losses (6%). Only 1.5% of the US$8.6 billion can be attributed to the cost of dog vaccinations by veterinarians. Every year, about fifteen million people worldwide receive post-exposure prophylaxis (PEP), but even if this prevents hundreds of thousands of rabies deaths annually, this emergency strategy is costly. What is worse, this financial and psychological cost is largely paid by the world's poorest people, thus perpetuating their poverty. In fact, a post-bite treatment course can cost up to US$40 in Africa and US$49 in Asia (Knobel et al. 2005, 365), where the average daily income is only a few dollars. The irony is that just 10% of the current budget for emergency treatment of bite wounds would probably be enough to vaccinate all the unvaccinated dogs in the world, thus virtually eliminating canine rabies worldwide (WHO 2015, 150). By contrast, the US$2.7 billion spent worldwide for PEP each year (or 31% of the aforementioned US$8.6 billion in direct economic costs) is wasted, as it is administered on an ungrounded precautionary basis, rather than only in cases where there is good reason to suspect genuine infection (Lavan et al. 2017, 1670).

The basis of the new joint policy of OIE, WHO, FAO, and GARC is the One Health framework. The integration of human, animal, and environmental health has a long history, but it remained somehow limited to theory until 2008, when this paradigm was formally structured and launched specifically to tackle the complexity of zoonoses. Rabies has turned out to be the zoonosis that most perfectly fits into the One Health strategy (Rupprecht, Kuzmin, and Meslin 2017, 3). The joint policy agenda maintains not only that human, animal, and environmental health are deeply intertwined but also that the fight against the diseases that affect them requires interdisciplinary and intersectoral cooperation. In other words, major opportunities exist to protect public health if policies are aimed at preventing and controlling pathogens at the human-animal-environment interface instead of dealing with these three sectors as unconnected entities. Understandably, this approach is particularly useful when it comes to zoonoses, as they can easily fall into the "no-man's-land" between public health, environmental management, and veterinary medicine.

Although appropriate tools and proven strategies for controlling rabies and making it 100% preventable already exist on paper, this disease receives marginal attention at the practical level. In fact, rabies is one of the neglected zoonotic diseases that WHO has identified within the class of "neglected tropical diseases" (NTDs). NTDs are a group of communicable pathologies common in tropical and subtropical conditions that affect more than one billion so-called abandoned victims. These diseases have an impact mainly on poor and marginalized populations in low-resource settings—people who live without adequate sanitation and in close contact with infectious vectors and animals, people whose feeble political voices are often unheard. While several NTDs with a somewhat smaller impact receive far greater attention than rabies (Rupprecht, Kuzmin, and Meslin 2017, 3), WHO (2013b, 1) currently lists it as one of the priorities. According to Cathleen A. Hanlon et al. (2001, 2273), rabies is the most important viral zoonosis from a global perspective. The objective of reaching zero human deaths by 2030 would contribute to fulfilling the UN's Sustainable Development Goals, particularly goal 3.3, an end to NTD epidemics.

Neglect when it comes to addressing rabies is largely explained by the fact that in developing countries this disease predominantly affects dogs, who have trifling economic value compared to livestock and receive minimal attention from the veterinary sector, at least in rural areas. What is not minimal, though, is the psychological trauma that rabies and animal bites cause in individuals, families, and communities, which unfortunately is also ignored. Apart from damaging the human-animal bond, the fear of bites and rabies in rabies-endemic countries may limit people's movement outdoors, with all of the negative consequences that can result. Therefore, as Katie Hampson et al. (2015, 14) point out, this anxiety should be given more attention and precise quantification. Moreover, dog-mediated rabies affects not only people but also their livestock, which are often the economic backbone of developing countries like India. In killing livestock, rabies has a strong impact on food availability (i.e., milk and meat), on nonconsumable products (i.e., leather and manure), and on the power of livestock for transportation and plowing. Darryn L. Knobel et al. (2005, 363) estimate 11,500 livestock losses annually due to rabies in Africa and 21,150 in Asia, at a cost of US$150 and US$500, respectively, per head of cattle.

Although rabies is a global concern, it is particularly linked to India. The term *rabies* comes from the Latin, which is in turn related to the Sanskrit word *rabhas*, which the Monier-Williams dictionary translates as "violence," "impetuosity," "zeal," "ardor," "force," or "energy." Rabies is one of the oldest diseases known to humankind. The first detailed medical account of it appeared in the *Sushruta Samhita*, a Sanskrit text on human medicine composed in northern India in the third century C.E. Centuries later, in 1911, at the Kasauli Pasteur Institute, Sir David Semple developed the sheep-brain vaccine, which was used to fight rabies until modern cell culture vaccines were made available in the early 1980s. Despite this historical connection to rabies, today India still pays the highest toll globally in terms of human deaths, almost 21,000 annually (Garg 2014, 16). It has been calculated that someone in India is bitten by an animal every two seconds, and someone dies of rabies every twenty minutes. Thus WHO currently considers India not only a high-risk country but a widely acknowledged global hotspot for this disease.

Nevertheless, rabies remains neglected in India. Formally speaking, it is not a notifiable disease, meaning that Indian law does not require that occurrences be reported to the national epidemiological tracking system or to international organizations such as OIE or WHO. Consequently, the number of rabies deaths in India has so far emerged only from estimates (Taylor et al. 2017, 133), mainly thanks to the health centers that keep registers of rabies cases and communicate them to the appropriate authorities in a systematic manner. However, these data inevitably leave out the people who do not seek proper medical advice and who die at home. Furthermore, because of the long incubation period, rabies victims may miss the link between exposure and illness, thus preventing hospitals from registering their history of animal bite. When it comes to medical staff, the paralytic form of rabies is often misdiagnosed (e.g., it is confused with Guillain-Barré syndrome), contributing to the underreporting of the disease. There is also confusion about whether the available data are based on actual rabies deaths or, more generally, on the PEP administered to patients who have been exposed to animal bites. In addition, if the same patient visits different hospitals in search of vaccination, doubts arise as to how many times the case is registered. Finally, the fact that India is challenged by several competing health priorities is another reason for the widespread negligence regarding this disease. Only 4% of the global research on rabies was dedicated to understanding the disease in India between 2001 and 2011 (Abbas and Kakkar 2013a, 560).

Although this book deals with rabies in the challenging Indian context, highlighting the peculiarities of the relationship between this country and rabies, it also provides hints for understanding this disease more generally. And it looks not only at rabies but also at animal bites, which are a widespread public health issue at the global level (Gilchrist et al. 2008, 296). Unlike many other zoonoses, exposure to rabies occurs through direct, individual contact with the infected animal, in most cases through a bite that lacerates skin and tears flesh. If the absence of data on rabies hides the actual number of deaths it causes, it also inevitably fails to account for the many more animal bites that may or may not eventually cause rabies. And even if the incidence of rabies is a major concern in affected communities, animal bites alone may cause physical suffering, debilitating private and public expenditure, and psychological stress, and they are thus worth studying in their own right.

The fieldwork on which this book is based was carried out in the cities of Delhi and Jaipur. Although rabies is most deadly in the rural areas of India, several factors explain my choice of urban settings. First of all, like rural areas, urban slums are vulnerable to this disease because of the convergence of risk factors such as social marginalization, financial constraints, and poor education. A study conducted in some rural and urban slums of Delhi in 2016 reported a higher incidence of dog bites than found in the nationwide survey conventionally used as a point of reference by researchers on rabies in India (Sharma et al. 2016, 118). Furthermore, given that the urban population (of a combined eighty-seven Indian cities) may reach 255 million by 2030 (NIUA 2011), zoonotic infections, including rabies, will soon threaten a growing number of the urban poor (PHFI and WHO 2008, 8). In addition, when it comes to the proximity of humans and animals, and hence the possibility for pathogen transmission, urban India is often not too different from rural India. In villages and towns, animal farming is generally unorganized, with 70% of the Indian livestock market owned by 67% of small and marginal farmers, and meat and milk production is relevant not just in rural but also in urban India. As Ajay Gandhi and Lotte Hoek observe, "Animals remain an inextricable element of the South Asian city" (2012, 9), despite attempts to cleanse and segregate the urban space, which are described in the following chapters. Finally, the first experiments with rabies-control measures in India began in its major cities, Jaipur being among the forerunners. Because of its role as the capital city and its international exposure, Delhi is another ideal location for this research.

Like data on rabies in dogs, information on rabies in cattle and macaques is predictably very spotty, when it exists at all. Nevertheless, rabies in livestock is attracting growing interest at the global level, mainly because of its economic impact. Similarly, the role of primates in relation to rabies and bites is of urgent importance, given the increased opportunities for humans to interact with these animals in temples, parks, and tourist spots around the world. Moreover, rabies in primates and other wildlife presents the risk of species spillover, which must be closely monitored for its potential epidemiological impact (Singh and Gajadhar 2014, 74). Incidentally, in January 2017, evidence of infection with rabies in bats was found for the first time in India, prompting health authorities to adopt a more holistic view of this zoonosis and to revise national guidelines for rabies management (Anand 2017).

Yet as I learned from Indian wildlife advocates and conservationists (e.g., Vanak, Belsare, and Gompper 2007), this revised approach to rabies in wildlife should put the domestic dog at the heart of the discussion. Not only are dogs the most abundant reservoir of rabies, but especially in rural India (and in many African countries) they live and interact with local wildlife so closely—often even inside protected areas—that they can introduce rabies into these populations quite easily. This results in the decline of wildlife populations, which is particularly dangerous in the case of species on the verge of extinction, and in more rabid attacks on humans, which not only cause additional human deaths but also influence the attitudes of people toward wildlife (e.g., wolves—Isloor et al. 2014), and consequently toward wildlife policies and conservation (Gompper 2013b). Given the focus of this book on urban India, this issue is marginal to the discussion here. But however India eventually approaches its problem with rabies, it cannot avoid considering the impact of the dog population (and, consequently, dog population management and dog ownership policies) on wildlife. The case of a rabid dog biting an adult tiger in the Panna Tiger Reserve, one of the key sites of India's tiger protection project, speaks for itself (Neha 2013). India needs to pursue a balanced strategy that goes beyond the domestic sphere—and its members, such as our canine "best friends"—that we humans value so much, and take other species into account as well.

In a milestone of medical anthropology, Peter J. Brown, Marcia C. Inhorn, and Daniel J. Smith clearly state that diseases cannot be explained as "things in themselves" (1996, 183). When it comes to one of the most aggressive infectious diseases known to humankind, it is clear that diseased beings, whether human or animal, cannot be considered "bodies in themselves." Even clearer is that these bodies have not become infected for purely biological reasons. In fact, rabies is endemic in India for reasons that are as much social, cultural, economic, political, and religious as they are biological. This book aims to reconstruct the broad and complex web of factors that bring people into contact with animals and create favorable conditions and pathways for the rabies virus to infect, kill, and thrive. As Alex M. Nading stresses, "Bodily biologies are linked in some meaningful way to extrabodily ecologies" (2014a, 5). What I aim to explore here is the extrabodily ecology of rabies.

I want to investigate the context in which rabies lives on the streets of Delhi and Jaipur, for it is crucial that we reconstruct the intricate dynamics of rabies transmission. In fact, like any living organism, the rabies virus evolves not only in response to its own internal circumstances but also in response to the environment into which it is inserted and with which it must cope. "Organisms are constructed in development, not simply 'programmed' to develop by genes. Living things do not evolve to fit into preexisting environments, but coconstruct and coevolve with their environments, in the process changing the structure of ecosystems" (Laland et al. 2015, 162). The environment in which they develop is, of course, composed of much more than mere physical elements grouped together. It is a space made of entwined human-animal-environment relations, which include the possibilities that people and animals more or less consciously offer to the rabies virus to spread, along with the human attempts to contain it. Within this mesh of relations, the rabies virus is a social being like the other human and animal beings around it, though its agency is clearly ontologically different. This co-construction of relations continuously alters the virus's world, making rabies ecology far less knowable and stable than public health policy tends to understand or acknowledge. In fact, as Natalie Porter concludes in her study of avian influenza, infectious, multispecies, multidimensional diseases must be looked at as "constantly changing" (2012, 118).

The need for the multifactorial, inclusive, and integrative perspective that I propose here has also been advocated by the Public Health Foundation of India. Its "Roadmap for Combating Zoonoses in India" openly declares that the major mistake in recent strategies of rabies management in India has been reliance on an overly mechanistic, linear, simplistic, and disconnected approach at the expense of a much more useful "big picture" approach (PHFI and WHO 2008, 8). In fact, most research on rabies carried out in India (87%) has focused on genetics and biology, giving minimal attention to the other components of the disease (Kakkar et al. 2012, 3). This kind of research struggles for biomedical solutions that cannot solve a complex systemic challenge like rabies on their own. Ironically, given that rabies potentially affects many species, Indian research on rabies has focused primarily on the rabies virus (58%) and humans (34%), largely ignoring dogs (6%) and almost never taking a multiple-animal approach (1%) (Kakkar et al. 2012, 3). In more general terms, original studies in the wide field of public health (including epidemiology, health policy, and systems research) are limited in India (Dandona et al. 2004, 1).

When we do pursue a big-picture approach, rabies can reveal a lot about the society in which it is embedded. In fact, the ecology of rabies is what Richard Levins and Richard Lewontin (1985) describe as "dialectical"—that is, as emerging from a specific historical, economic, and political context. For me, understanding this disease has entailed comprehending India itself. Within my broader interest in the contextual aspects of rabies, I have focused particularly on sociocultural drivers, largely because of my background in anthropology. But this approach is also in line with the latest recommendations of WHO and OIE. At a conference titled "Global Elimination of Dog-Mediated Human Rabies" in December 2015, the first of five key pillars of rabies elimination was identified as sociocultural. "The socio-cultural context influences rabies perceptions and dog-keeping practices of at-risk populations," the conference report stated. "Understanding the context guides approaches to motivate behavioural change and plan feasible delivery of services" (WHO and OIE 2015, 14). Determining what rabies means to people and how they see the animals they live with is the first step to comprehending this disease and the world around it. Understanding how rabies is perceived also reveals a lot about how it can eventually be managed, at both an individual and a collective level. If we remove rabies from its sociocultural context, this zoonosis can easily be kept at bay: it has a low basic reproduction number (which is used to measure the transmission potential of a disease), and high-quality vaccines exist for both humans and animals. Clearly, something more—something different—is causing rabies to be the public health threat that it is. As Meike Wolf points out (2015, 6), the role of culture must be considered simply because it is an integral part of diseases, bodies, and biologies.

That said, as will become clearer in chapter 6, I do not simplistically place all, or even many, of the dynamics of rabies inside "culture," as if this were a bottomless container. As Charles Briggs and Clara Mantini-Briggs (2016, 232) teach us in their account of a rabies epidemic in Venezuela, health inequalities due to structural factors are often turned into a "cultural pathology" that is all too easy to blame. An often cited example of this tendency is the reliance on local systems of medicine and traditional healers, which biomedicine conveniently prefers to describe as barriers to health and health-related institutional efforts rather than as consequences—not causes—of sick health systems or, more simply, of the common denominator of neglected tropical diseases: poverty. Ironically, for these diseases of poverty—as NTDs are often called—there is still insufficient research on how the underlying context of poverty (i.e., structural inequalities in access to health services, infrastructure, education, and political power) influences the effectiveness and outcome of NTD-control strategies (Bardosh 2014, 2).

Meeting a Quasi–Life Form

Understanding rabies demands a certain familiarity not only with the life forms affected by it but especially with the quasi–life form (following Lowe 2010, 626) that spreads this disease around. Rabies is caused by a plethora of different lyssaviruses, negative-strand RNA virus species of the genus *Lyssavirus*, family Rhabdoviridae, order Mononegavirales. However, the prototypical rabies virus, the RABV, is the main causative agent of classic rabies in animals and humans. Bullet-shaped, it moves from the entry point in the body along the nerves to the spinal cord and thence the brain, where it eventually causes acute encephalitis. Infection occurs when the virus enters the body through transdermal inoculation (a bite or, if the claws are covered with saliva, a scratch) or direct contact between infected saliva (e.g., through a lick) and mucous membranes (e.g., eyeballs or mouth) or abraded skin. Milk and meat from a rabid animal are unsafe if drunk, eaten, or handled raw, but cooking them at a temperature above 60 degrees Celsius (140 degrees Fahrenheit) will kill the virus. Human-to-human transmission by bite (or kiss, in the case of abraded skin in the recipient) is theoretically possible but has never been confirmed, while there have been unfortunate events of transmission by the transplantation of infected organs.

Immediately after infection, the rabies virus enters an eclipse phase during which it replicates in the muscle cells close to the site of infection without stimulating any immune response. This incubation period in humans is highly variable—from two weeks to, more rarely, some years—depending on the distance from the wound to the central nervous system, the amount of virus inoculated, and the virus strain. Animals like dogs and cats usually show signs of the disease between two and eight weeks, while in cattle it may take up to four months. When the virus reaches the brain, the clinical signs of rabies invariably appear. The infective period for dogs, cats, and ferrets is considered to start ten days before the onset of the first evident clinical signs, constituting an insidious threat to anyone encountering seemingly healthy animals in this period of time. When the virus is eventually shed in the saliva, the infection cycle of rabies is complete and the lyssavirus is ready to move on to another victim, relying on the aggressive behavior and abnormal production of saliva it causes in the current host.

All animals exhibit certain neurological signs as a result of rabies, which may differ slightly from species to species. In the prodromal stage, minor behavioral changes might occur, such as unprovoked aggressiveness in tame animals, daytime activities in nocturnal animals, and no fear of humans in wild animals. Symptoms may also include vomiting, fever, and dilation of the pupils. In the case of furious rabies, the first stage is generally followed by a period of severe restlessness and aggressiveness, marked by repetitive movements, running for no apparent reason, and unprovoked attacks. Violent convulsions eventually lead to death. In the case of paralytic, or dumb, rabies, animals are unable to swallow due to the paralysis of face and throat muscles, and thus show abnormal vocalizations and the typical sign of foaming saliva around the mouth. However, contrary to common belief, rabid dogs are not hydrophobic (scared of choking on water owing to the virus's inhibition of the operation of throat muscles). Paralysis usually begins in the hind legs and, once extended to the rest of the body, leads to death.

Many of these symptoms also occur in humans. The prodromal phase of human rabies is marked by generic signs such as weakness, fever, headache, loss of appetite, nausea, myalgia (muscle pain), asthenia (reduction of muscle power), anorexia, insomnia, and abnormal sensations of tingling or burning at the wound site. The second and last phase, when the rabies virus starts "suppressing the rational and stimulating the animal" (Wasik and Murphy 2012, 3), is characterized by more specific neurological symptoms, in the case of both furious and dumb rabies. In furious rabies, symptoms include uncontrolled hyperactivity, confusion, hallucinations, combativeness, tachycardia, meningism, disorientation, hypersensitivity to stimuli, hyperesthesia, muscle spasms (when they affect the mouth, they cause excessive salivation), and paralysis of the vocal chords (which causes voice alterations). These phases of extreme excitement are often interspersed with lucid intervals, during which patients may fully understand their appalling predicament. Hydrophobia—the sensation of drowning stimulated by the mere sight of a glass of water—appears in about half of cases. In the case of dumb rabies (about 30% of human cases), the course of the disease is longer, usually less dramatic, and includes lethargy, gradual paralysis of breathing and swallowing muscles, coma, and eventually a fatal cardiorespiratory arrest. It is not by chance that the virus owes its name to the Greek word *lyssa*, which means "frenzy" and "madness."

No single test is available to diagnose rabies in humans before the onset of its symptoms, and unless the rabies-specific signs of hydrophobia or aerophobia (fear of drafts or fresh air) are present, a clinical diagnosis may be difficult to establish (Rupprecht, Kuzmin, and Meslin 2017, 8). Moreover, laboratory diagnosis in live human patients is usually reliable only in the case of positive results. Thus postmortem analysis of brain tissue or skin/hair follicles remains the preferred method of detecting this disease (WHO 2018b, 23–34). When the symptoms of rabies become evident, even the most intensive supportive care is usually futile, and there are no specific drugs or therapies that can save the patient's life. In 2005, Jeanna Giese became the first person to survive rabies thanks to the Milwaukee protocol. This procedure involves inducing a coma to protect the brain while the body fights off the rabies virus. Since then, only a tiny handful of people with early symptoms of rabies have managed to survive despite neurological deficits, thanks to this procedure (or similar intensive medical care), which, however, is understandably impractical for most rabies-endemic areas. Both humans and animals rarely survive more than ten days from the onset of symptoms.

The only chance of survival after the bite of a rabid animal but before the onset of symptoms is immediate and accurate post-exposure prophylaxis. Thoroughly washing and flushing the wound with soap and running water for fifteen minutes is effective in dramatically reducing the number of viral particles deposited in it. If available, alcohol/ethanol, sodium hypochlorite, and povidone-iodine are also recommended to chemically remove the infected saliva. Covering the wound with dressings or bandages or stitching it shut should be avoided whenever possible. Victims should promptly be taken to a doctor, who should treat the case according to the epidemiology of rabies in the area and as per the national and WHO guidelines. WHO (2013b, 57) identifies three categories of risk based on the type of exposure to an animal suspected or confirmed to be rabid, or an animal unavailable for testing. Category 1 includes touching or feeding animals, licks on intact skin, contact of intact skin with secretions or excretions of a rabid animal or human case. No PEP is needed if a reliable case history is available. Category 2 includes nibbling of uncovered skin and minor scratches or abrasions without bleeding. In this case, the vaccine must be administered immediately in three or four doses according to the latest vaccination regimens recommended by WHO (2018a, 208). Treatment can be stopped if the animal remains healthy throughout the observation period or is proved to be negative for rabies by a reliable laboratory. For dogs, cats, and domestic ferrets, WHO (2018b, 156) recommends observation for ten days, while for other domestic and wild species it suggests a more conservative fourteen-day clinical investigation, or euthanasia if the severity of the situation requires it. Category 3 includes single or multiple transdermal bites or scratches, licks on broken skin, contamination of mucous membrane with saliva, and exposure to bats. In addition to the vaccine treatment (which can be stopped in the case of a nonrabid animal), one dose of rabies immunoglobulin (RIG) must be injected as soon as possible—but only once in a lifetime and no later than seven days after the first dose of vaccine—in and around the wound site. RIG is a biological product that provides immediate antibodies until the patient's own immune system can respond to the virus. PEP vaccination (via intramuscular or intradermal route) should be given in the deltoid muscle or, in small children, into the upper thigh. PEP is highly successful in preventing the disease if administered within about a week of exposure.

Indian Deaths

In many of the developing countries stricken by rabies, data on human deaths, access to vaccines, and occurrence in animal populations are limited, outdated, probably unreliable, and thus much disputed. In Africa, for example, the actual number of human deaths may be underreported one hundredfold (Scott et al. 2017, 2). In India, by contrast, the NGO the Voice of Stray Dogs maintains on its website that the human death toll of 20,000 per year used by WHO and "imported" by the Association for Prevention and Control of Rabies in India (APCRI) is inflated by a factor of nearly one hundred, if compared with the "authentic rabies deaths figures" provided in July 2012 by the Central Bureau of Health Intelligence (under the Ministry of Health and Family Welfare), according to which Indian hospitals reported an average of 292 rabies deaths per year in the period from 2004 to 2010. At the same time, the National Centre for Disease Control (under the same Ministry of Health and Family Welfare) reports the 20,000 figure on the page of its website devoted to the National Rabies Control Programme. In 2018 the *WHO Expert Consultation on Rabies* report put together estimates from five different sources and gave the number of Indian deaths as ranging from 12,700 to 20,847 (WHO 2018b, 7). In the World Animal Health Information System managed by OIE, the data about rabies provided by India are limited and erratic.

Newspapers and other media follow this rollercoaster of numbers closely, creating further confusion when dealing simultaneously with rabies deaths and animal bites, though of course animal bites do not always transmit rabies. Given this numerical uncertainty in India, and in many other countries, WHO concludes that national data on rabies are more likely to indicate the presence of the disease than to document its full extent. While I do not deny the utility of high-quality surveillance data—primarily to break the circle of neglect that surrounds rabies and to allow authorities to prioritize diseases in an accurate and sensible way—I fully align myself with WHO's clear and wise claim, and thus choose not to indulge further in an inconclusive debate here over the number of bites and rabies cases. Because rabies is totally preventable through vaccination, every death is one too many. Given the horrendous course of this disease—YouTube is full of heartbreaking videos of people and animals succumbing to rabies—each experience of agony is unacceptable. Leaving aside the actual number of rabies cases, the mere presence of the disease in a multispecies community is enough to damage the human-animal bond that, in turn, is a triggering factor for rabies.

According to WHO data, nearly 35% of all human rabies deaths occur in India. The Public Health Foundation of India's "Roadmap for Combating Zoonoses" suggests that what makes India particularly vulnerable to rabies, and more generally to zoonotic diseases, is its status as a developing country with a huge human population. This puts pressure on local habitats and on the human-animal interface, and the problem is exacerbated by particular cultural beliefs and practices regarding the human-animal relationship (e.g., dog ownership practices). This situation is aggravated by many other serious health challenges that crowd out the threat of rabies and discourage a well-planned, long-term strategy for its prevention and control. The result, the Public Health Foundation of India concludes, is insufficient technical capacity, a lack of research-based policymaking, and irregular surveillance and response. To make matters worse, considering the size of India, few medical institutions have the laboratory facilities necessary to detect rabies. Adagonda Sherikar and V. S. Waskar (2005, 700) highlight such additional obstacles as the consumption of unpasteurized milk, illicit animal slaughter, inappropriate waste disposal, and illegal trade in animals and animal products. The situation is further complicated by the vastness of the country and the decentralized, three-tier system of national, state, and local government (GARC and RIA 2012, preface), and by a weak interdisciplinary disease-management approach on the part of the human, domestic animal, wildlife, and environmental sectors. All of these factors contribute to putting rabies on the list of priority diseases in the "Roadmap for Combating Zoonoses" (Sekar et al. 2011, 4). A study by Arun Kurian et al. (2014, 359) ranks rabies first among the twenty-two zoonoses affecting India. Currently, India spends about two billion rupees (US$28 million) each year on PEP, with a loss of thirty-eight man-hours for every post-bite treatment (Vanak 2017).

The latest survey on rabies in India, carried out in 2017 by the APCRI (2018, 10) and sponsored by WHO, found that slightly more than two-thirds of rabies victims are males, and that 68% of victims live in rural or semi-urban areas. They are often the breadwinners, and their deaths may have severe consequences for the financial situation of their families. In 31% of rabies cases, the victim is under fourteen years of age. In an APCRI study of 2004, dogs were the biting animals in 96% of cases of rabies (17); in the 2018 APCRI study, dogs accounted for 74% of cases (49). The 2018 study found that the second-most-common biting animal is the cat, but Himangshu Dutta (2012, 760) claims that the number of rabies cases caused by monkey bites has been constantly increasing over the years, especially in northern India. At a conference titled "Rabies Post-Exposure Prophylaxis: Recommendations and Practices" in Delhi in March 2013, the municipal health officer N. K. Yadav stated that 5% of all bite cases treated in Delhi by Maharishi Valmiki Infectious Diseases Hospital between 2006 and 2011 were caused by monkeys. A survey of Delhi slum dwellers showed that monkeys are perceived, after dogs, as the second-most dangerous animals when it comes to the risk of catching rabies (Sharma et al. 2016, 117). Concern with primate-mediated rabies in India is increasing also within the international medical community, as monkey bites account for 31% of injuries necessitating PEP in international tourists returning from countries where rabies is endemic (Gautret et al. 2014, 4).

With reference to (dog-mediated) rabies in cattle, official statistics of the Ministry of Agriculture (2016, 159) report ninety-four deaths in 2015–16 for the entire country, but it is likely that these numbers are incomplete. In fact, Stephanie Shwiff, Katie Hampson, and Aaron Anderson (2013, 354) claim that rabies disproportionately affects Asia when it comes to cattle deaths. Cases of cattle bites to humans and consequent cattle-mediated rabies are rare (or unlikely to be reported), but they do occur. To mention just one, in February 2017 a cow attacked about twenty people in a village in Tamil Nadu and, while kept under observation for suspected rabies, she died some days later. After the disease was confirmed, all her victims underwent anti-rabies treatment (Oppili 2017). This event demonstrates that the possibility that rabies may be behind abnormal cattle behavior should always be considered. Concerns about the consumption of infected milk are more frequent. For example, in January 2017 the *Times of India* (2017b) reported that eighty people in Aurangabad district fell ill after consuming the milk of two cows who had allegedly been bitten by rabid dogs. The article mentioned nausea and vomiting as the only symptoms reported by the patients, who were treated immediately, and did not clarify the final diagnosis, but it stressed the risk posed by milk in relation to rabies. This by-product is particularly risky because of the central role of cow's milk in Hindu rituals, especially because in order to make *prasad* (religious offerings to the deities, including sanctified food occasionally consumed by devotees), it can be used raw.

In his survey of cases of animal rabies in the period 1949 to 1967, B. K. Kathuria (1970, 2) reported high rates of the disease in cattle, sometimes higher than in dogs. Moreover, as B. C. Ramanna, Guddeti S. Reddy, and Villuppanoor A. Srinivasan observe (1991, 285), and as I discuss in chapter 5, while many developed countries recommend the destruction of livestock exposed to the bite of a rabid animal, this policy is difficult to implement in India because of harsh socioeconomic conditions and the religious veneration of cows. Thus it is essential to stress that cattle may catch and transmit rabies, especially given the generally positive and benevolent attitude toward cows in India, which may cause people to overlook this risk. In fact, in a multicentric study presented at the 2013 conference on rabies mentioned above, 39% of respondents believed that the bite of a cow cannot cause rabies; lizards and rabbits, who were on the same list, attracted more (unfounded) suspicion.

Returning to dog-mediated rabies, many deaths in India are due to the fact that 79% of dog bite victims receive no rabies treatment (APCRI 2004, 18). Even among the treated patients who nevertheless eventually died of rabies, the APCRI survey (19) found that 82% had never completed the course of immunization and 99% had received no rabies immunoglobulin (RIG), demonstrating gross negligence on the part of the health-care system. In 2017, the same nationwide survey found that the percentage of category 3 patients who received RIG had increased to 16 (APCRI 2018, 41). Official sources state that the use of RIG is particularly low because of its cost, its unavailability, insufficient awareness among medical staff, and the fear of side effects of equine rabies immunoglobulin among professionals (RIA 2011, 48). In fact, thanks to the higher cost of human rabies immunoglobulin, equine rabies immunoglobulin is allowed as a cheaper alternative in India. Nevertheless, a single monoclonal antibody product against rabies, licensed in the country in 2017, has been demonstrated to be safe and effective in clinical trials (WHO 2018a, 212).

At the same time, alternative remedies such as magic and religious practices and herbal therapies continue to be popular, being sought in 29% and

11% of cases, respectively (APCRI 2004, 19). Other studies, however, report much higher percentages of people relying on traditional healing applications—for example, 57% in Dehradun (Ohri et al. 2016, 848) and 55% in Panchkula (Tiwari et al. 2019, 12). In addition to personal preferences for indigenous medicine and traditional healers, people may also resort to them because, while some government hospitals provide the PEP vaccination at low or no cost, budgets are often insufficient, and this results in dangerous shortages and patients' consequent mistrust. The price of a vaccine dose at the drugstore ranges from 300 to 350 rupees (US$4.20–$5). In 2019 the central government considered banning the export of the 30% of the total fifty million doses produced that India currently sells abroad, because the country is facing an annual internal demand of forty-eight million doses, with the result that there is a 20–80% shortage in almost all states (Dey 2019). Moreover, like other Asian countries, India is also affected by the circulation of counterfeit vaccines produced in China (Patranobis 2018).

As in the human medical system, veterinarians are not always adequately trained to deal with rabies (Rani et al. 2010, 1). Because India is a heavily agricultural nation, competency in animal husbandry is the priority in veterinary education. Since rabies mainly affects dogs and is not among the most common pathologies of livestock, veterinary students are not given much training in the disease. Moreover, in 2015 only 70,767 veterinarians and veterinary paraprofessionals were reported to be working in India (OIE 2018). Ironically, in the same period, Delhi alone had more than 50,000 traditional healers for human patients (*Hindu* 2009).

Despite these obstacles, in the past fifteen years India has tried to move forward in its fight against rabies. In 2009, it passed the Prevention and Control of Infectious and Contagious Diseases in Animals Act. During the Tenth Five-Year Plan (2002–7), a program specifically to control rabies was submitted but not approved. During the next Five-Year Plan (2007–12), strategies to control rabies were developed and tested in five cities (Delhi, Ahmedabad, Bangalore, Pune, and Madurai). Once the disease was acknowledged as a major public health challenge, the National Rabies Control Programme was created by the Ministry of Health and Family Welfare under the Twelfth Five-Year Plan (2012–17) and received almost four billion rupees in funding (US$58 million). While the human health component of this initiative has been implemented throughout the country under the National Centre for Disease Control, the animal health component was initially launched in March 2015 in some districts in Haryana.

This initiative was soon discontinued, however, owing to lack of interministerial agreement on funding. In 2017, the Federation of Indian Animal Protection Organizations (FIAPO) launched the Rabies Free Kerala campaign in collaboration with local governments. In 2018, dog bites (though not, curiously, rabies) were included in the Integrated Disease Surveillance Programme of the Ministry of Health and Family Welfare. In the meantime, thanks to the support received by the government of Goa, the UK-based NGO Mission Rabies began experimenting with oral rabies vaccination to control rabies in this state (Gibson et al. 2019). Nevertheless, India has not yet joined the Rabies Vaccine Bank, launched by OIE in 2012 to facilitate the procurement of high-quality dog vaccines. Similarly, India has not yet begun the One Health Zoonotic Disease Prioritization Process recommended by OIE. Interestingly, of the twenty-five countries that have completed this process, twenty-four have prioritized rabies (Shadomy 2019).

Following Rabies

What I have briefly outlined above is a basic overview of the structural elements that compose rabies. The focus of my field research and of this book is the relational dimension of rabies, which necessarily depends on the affiliations between people and animals. Animals have occupied a marginal place in most social studies of health, disease, and medicine; I attempt here to bring them to the forefront, squarely alongside humans. In pursuit of my interest in human-animal social relations, I openly shadowed rabies, people, and animals on the streets of Delhi and Jaipur to observe the moments of interaction and other points of contact among them and to understand how they relate to one another. While this approach may appear at first glance to be focused on micro-interactions, it actually allowed me to broaden what I initially considered to be the borders of a study of rabies. By following the economic, cultural, religious, political, and ecological associations that form the basis of rabies infection, I was able to explore new pathways and intersections that I had previously been unable to imagine, and I discovered that the roads that lead to rabies in India are more numerous than I had anticipated. While following these roads, the big picture that I was aiming for gradually came into view. Moreover, although my approach to studying rabies has been place-based, it has always remained connected to the broader global context (Tsing 2005). Indian rhesus macaques have been shipped to American laboratories, Siberian huskies are imported to Delhi as pets, and beef and carabeef (buffalo meat) from India are enjoyed in Southeast Asian kitchens. The implications of these types of exchanges will become clearer in the following chapters.

Apart from the geographical location of my fieldwork, the only limit that I tried to impose on the size of this picture is its cultural and religious context, by focusing on Hinduism. Yet this should not be understood as a simplification. Hinduism is the most widespread religion in India; it is practiced by roughly 950 million people in an astonishingly high number of personal, familiar, and community interpretations. Owing to its complex, dynamic, multifaceted nature, Hinduism is also extremely challenging when it comes to human relationships with nature and other animal species. Religion deeply permeates the daily lives of orthodox Hindus in particular, thus influencing their behavior, habits, and mindset. An example that gave me food for thought: male public urination is very common in Delhi and indeed throughout India. Isolated walls along pavements are the preferred location. Neither the angry looks of passersby nor notices threatening fines seem to discourage men from urinating by the roadside. But what humans cannot accomplish, gods can. Not a single drop of urine can be found on walls where tiles depicting Hindu deities have been installed about one meter from the ground. After all, as the rickshaw driver who taught me the basics of rickshaw driving in Jaipur used to say, "Indians are and will always be God-fearing people." In a lane not far from Connaught Place, in the heart of the Indian capital, I found confirmation of this claim. "Who can be so mad as to pee facing Shiva?" a passerby asked me rhetorically.

These anti-urine tiles were also scattered throughout Jangpura and Lajpat Nagar, the Delhi neighborhoods where I lived. Located in the north end of the South East Delhi district, they are popular areas that have grown exponentially over the past hundred years thanks to the relocation of the inhabitants of the Raisina Village, who were moved to make way for governmental buildings along the Rajpath, and the accommodation of the refugees who arrived in Delhi when India and Pakistan were separated in 1947. The slum where young Neelam lived was about one kilometer from my place, just behind the stinky drain that trickles toward the Yamuna River along the north side of Jangpura. Along the railway tracks that divide Jangpura and Lajpat Nagar, wherever some land is spared from residential (over)building, more or less improvised slums dot the landscape. Despite the noise created by the 11,000 people—the registered ones—with whom I shared the square kilometer around my flat, one of my most vivid memories of life there is the braying of the donkeys who were kept by the inhabitants of a nearby slum for the transportation of construction material. In Lajpat Nagar, I also lived with the smells of hundreds of dogs, as my flatmates were veterinarians, and their clothes always smelled of sick animals and the operating room.

Taught something new every day about animal medicine and ethology by my flatmates, I blended these lessons with what I knew of public health, Indian religious studies, and, of course, medical anthropology, as I undertook the research for this book. For the multispecies ethnography I carried out in 2012–13, 2015, and 2019, I learned a great deal from Eben Kirksey and Stefan Helmreich (2010) and from the exceptionally stimulating literature to which their work led me. Technically speaking, combining personal stories of human-animal interaction and infection with more general data allowed me to keep a kind of dual, and thus doubly useful, perspective on rabies: in the world of rabies, every infected bite is identical in that it leads to the same end, yet each bite is also different, for it derives from a unique connection between a human and an animal. Until we reach the saturation point, the more stories we collect, the deeper our understanding of rabies becomes, and the better we can comprehend the lives of the people and animals behind statistical figures, which tend to gloss over life's complexity and turn bodies into numbers (Briggs 2016, 157). As Charles Briggs points out, especially in contexts of health and communication inequalities, *each* contribution to knowledge production is key to building a larger "ecology of evidence."

After conducting archival research at the National Medical Library, the Centre des Sciences Humaines, and the Indian Social Institute, I combined qualitative and quantitative research in my fieldwork. The former included minimally structured, open-ended, free-flowing, face-to-face interviews in English and Hindi with a wide and varied range of people: health authorities (among them doctors, veterinarians, primatologists, and public health authorities), dog feeders, monkey trainers, cattle farmers, garbage collectors, cattle shelter directors, Hindu devotees, Hindu priests, staff at cremation sites, animal welfare activists, and pet-shop owners. With respect to participant observation—the primary tool in ethnographic research—I made use of it as soon as I stepped out of my room, focusing my attention on the everyday life, entanglements, and intimacy (Govindrajan 2018) of people and animals. The Ottawa Charter for Health Promotion of 1986 states, "Health is created and lived by people within the settings of their everyday life; where they learn, work, play and love" (WHO 1986), and I took this statement to heart (though I would add "and animals" after "people"). I combined observation with photographic surveying, employed as an unobtrusive research tool. By "unobtrusive research" I mean, following Webb et al. ([1966] 2000), a method of collecting data that does not involve direct elicitation of research subjects but instead uses unusual sources—in my case, this included garbage and food offerings for street animals. Taking pictures occasionally also yielded precious moments of learning about animal behavior—for example, an interaction one day with a young macaque in Connaught Place. At the time, I knew that avoiding eye contact is good monkey manners, but I had yet to witness the agitation caused by the big, zooming eye of the camera. By stepping forward and baring his canine teeth, this macaque taught me a valuable lesson, both as a person and as an ethnographer, that I would not soon forget.

The quantitative methodology consisted of semi-structured interviews and questionnaires. The interviews comprised multiple conversations with the 145 street and slum children I met. I decided to work consistently with these children, not only because they are common victims of rabies in India but also because their voices are not often listened to by anthropologists (Hirschfeld 2002). I met them either in the slums where they lived or, in the case of the street children, in the shelters where they were temporarily housed. Their average age was twelve, males outnumbered females, they were mainly Hindu, and only half of them had ever attended school. Although I am familiar with Hindi (the language mainly spoken in northern India), I sought the assistance of two people for the interviews because these children, most of them migrants from all over India, might have been uncomfortable with my standard Hindi. The translators were fluent in English, Hindi, and their native languages—Punjabi and Sadri. In most of the slums we visited, we were introduced to the local communities by a woman named Kamna, who had been working for a long time as a teacher of the children who could not attend proper school or needed extra coaching to prepare them for the rigid admission exams to private schools.

In the field of human-animal studies, questionnaires are used extensively to collect data about people's beliefs and attitudes toward animals (Anderson 2007). I used ad hoc questionnaires in English—the lingua franca of the Indian university system—to reach 185 mainly middle-class university students living in Delhi and studying in the universities of the city. I have included them in this research not only because they will soon be in charge of Indian politics and economy but also because they belong to a booming and influential class that appears to be reshaping India's culture, ethics, and mindset. The mean age of the students I met was twenty-four; males slightly outnumbered females and they were predominantly Hindu (though most did not consider religion important in their lives); 60% of them were not vegetarians. Many of them declared an interest in animal welfare, but only a tiny fraction were actually engaged in animal activism. Most of our conversations and questionnaire compilation took place over a drink or snack in the square outside the Vishwavidyalaya metro station, which serves the University of Delhi, under an advertising billboard reading, "The biggest gathering of youths of the capital."

My research also greatly benefited from my diverse and extensive experience in three veterinary hospitals and shelters for street animals in both cities where I lived. I agree with Donna Haraway that in order to talk about animals responsibly and usefully we must get "dirty and knowledgeable" (2008, 80). As it is impossible to get dirty without using the body in a direct, close, even intimate way, I always inaugurated my experience in the veterinary hospitals and shelters by performing the grimiest tasks: removing guano from the pigeon cages, cleaning up kittens' diarrhea, bathing mangy dogs, and helping during autopsies. Later, I also bottle-fed dying cattle, assisted in treating worm-infested wounds, counted surgically removed ovaries and testicles, and befriended dogs traumatized by abuse or paralyzed by road accidents. These one-on-one interactions with animals were essential to this kind of research (Sanders and Arluke 1993, 378). I got the chance to interact not only with species with which I was already acquainted, such as dogs, cats, cattle, donkeys, and horses, but also with eagles, monkeys, peacocks, camels, egrets, and parrots, all animals who were collected from the streets of Delhi and Jaipur.

To stay informed about human cases of rabies and human-animal conflict, since 2012 I have systematically searched for all news stories on these topics in the leading English newspapers of India, such as the *Times of India*, the *Hindu*, the *Hindustan Times*, the *Indian Express*, the *New Indian Express*, and the *Pioneer*. Newspaper articles, although they cannot necessarily be taken as unbiased, objective accounts, are nevertheless a valuable source of the perspectives and voices in the debate over human-animal issues within a large setting (Podberscek 1994, 232). In fact, as Amy J. Dickman (2010, 462) rightly notes with regard to the complexities of human-animal conflicts, people base their perceptions and attitudes not only on personal experiences but also on wider societal experiences. Moreover, news articles have allowed me to feel connected with my fieldwork site when I could not physically be there. Even if regional newspapers in vernacular languages have a wider audience, English-language news sources address the urban, educated middle class in which I am interested because of its direct involvement in the hornet's nest of animal-related issues in India.

In my fieldwork, I covered considerable distances within the immense city of Delhi and the overcrowded city of Jaipur. I followed cows on foot for twelve hours at a stretch, registering and analyzing their interactions with people. I rode for hours in the animal hospital ambulances that patrol the streets looking for sick animals and stray dogs to spay, neuter, and vaccinate against rabies. I scoured Old Delhi's labyrinth of narrow lanes looking for dogs to vaccinate with a rabies team from the North Delhi Municipal Corporation. In short, I took to heart the precept of Kirksey and Helmreich (2010, 555) that in order to study animals in their natural environment, multispecies ethnography must be multisited (Marcus 1995). Walking around Delhi was particularly challenging, not only because of the poor conditions of roadsides and the vast size of this city, but also because walking there invariably put me out of place (Douglas 1966, 36), a concept that will reappear throughout this book in relation to the many species I encountered. "In Delhi, only the poor and dogs walk," I was told by the shoemaker who worked on the pavement opposite my flat in Lajpat Nagar, whenever he spotted me coming home on foot. Moreover, except for the areas around schools, markets, and places of worship—all related to easily recognizable female activities—Indian streets are mainly seen as male space. Going out and doing *ghumna-phirna* (loafing around just for pleasure or without a precise aim, as laypeople may perceive ethnographic walking) is a pastime that men generally consider despicable for solitary women like me.

While moving around Delhi and Jaipur looking for contacts between humans, animals, and the rabies virus, it was all too easy to acknowledge that these cities are perfect examples of zoöpolises (Wolch 1998, 119). As a Greek boy who now lives in Vietnam once told me in Delhi, "Compared to where I live, India is another world; it's a world where animals still exist." A zoöpolis is a nonanthropocentric city that is open to nature— or, as Steven Hinchliffe claims, a space where nature does not stop (1999, 138)—in which nonhuman animals are effective members of the multispecies community that accommodates them, and are adapted (or trying to adapt themselves) to the "natural-cultural" (Fuentes 2010) environment in which they live. Following the definition of "hybrid geographies" proposed by Sarah Whatmore, a zoöpolis can be understood as the result of "the heterogeneous [more than human] entanglements of social life" (2002, 3). As Agustín Fuentes (2009, 14) explains, the spaces of these cities are integrative, shared, and shaped by the synergy of humans and animals, who together build and negotiate their co-produced niche, or co-ecology. Not only is this niche a physical space, but it is multidimensional, created at the intersection of ecological, social, cultural, religious, economic, and political factors. Niches, or "zones of sympatry" (Fuentes and Baynes-Rock 2017, 6), are generally imagined as enclaves within a larger space, as areas of limited geographical expansion. Based on my exploration of Delhi and Jaipur, which I do not claim was exhaustive, these two densely inhabited cities appeared to me as zones of sympatry in their entirety. I struggle to recall a portion of their urban landscape that could be described as a zone of allopatry (i.e., lack of geographical overlap), where no dog, macaque, or cattle was around. These three animal species, together with humans, were ubiquitous co-inhabitants of their cities, ever present co-residents of their overlapping spaces.

As imagined by urban geographers, a zoöpolis demolishes the "ontological exceptionalism of humans" (Houston et al. 2017, 1) by refusing persistent dualistic notions, translated into boundary lines, such as domesticated/wild, familiar/out of place, natural/cultural. Consequently, it takes for granted that "gaps" between these abstract categories are actually the norm in typical (that is, fluid and unstable) landscapes (Nading 2014b, 19). For example, as Melanie Rock and Chris Degeling (2016, 70) observe, in a zoöpolis, free-roaming dogs perfectly exemplify how nonhumans easily bridge the divisions between otherness, liminality, and kinship that people create for their own convenience and think they can impose on their passive co-existing species. Even more fitting and telling is the example provided by the cattle who live in Delhi and Jaipur: they may be owned yet neglected, unowned yet well cared for, worshipped yet exploited, slaughtered yet protected by law.

Another artificial construction is the public/private dichotomy, which for the purpose of this book needs to be clarified briefly. Apart from animal hospitals and shelters, I carried out most of my fieldwork in what legal language would define as public spaces, mainly on the street. Yet it immediately became obvious to me that I was navigating ideas of public and private very different from those I grew up with in northern Italy. I felt embarrassed whenever my eyes involuntarily fell upon scenes of people urinating and defecating not only in public spaces but in public view. I felt equally embarrassed whenever, invited to visit people I had just met, I was received for a chat, a chai (Indian tea), or even an entire meal sitting on their beds, occasionally with a half-naked, half-asleep relative in the bed next to us. By contrast, entering a kitchen was usually more complicated, and every time I did so, it was evident that I was crossing the threshold of domestic intimacy. With regard to human-animal-rabies relations, it will become clear as this story unfolds how porous the boundaries between public and private spaces are.

Outline of the Book

Although I aim in this book to present a multispecies narrative, its division into single-species chapters, though they are not meant to describe discrete worlds, has been necessary for the sake of clarity. Chapter 1 presents the human component of the relationship with other animals, focusing on the living conditions of street and slum children and the ideology evident in the lifestyle and language of middle-class youth. It also introduces more fully the towns where I carried out my research, and, in the case of Delhi, it describes the discriminating attitude of people who, idealizing globalist, capitalist modernity, insist on a utopian division between species and spaces. Finally, it concisely outlines the basic concepts of Hinduism relevant to the subject of this book, and related issues such as vegetarianism and animal activism. Chapter 2 describes the role of food as the central knot in the network of interspecies connections considered in this study. In fact, it is largely around food that people's and animals' lives intersect in Delhi and Jaipur. This chapter does not look at animals as sources of food for humans but, more intriguingly, at how people voluntarily and involuntarily feed their neighbor animals. I pay particular attention to the plenitude of garbage on Indian streets, the widespread Hindu practice of offering food to street animals, and the unprecedented abundance of cattle carcasses, which contributes to the proliferation of dogs and the consequent problems of bites and rabies. Relevant but often overlooked factors such as open defecation, human/animal scavenging, the presence of unburned human bodies floating in rivers (per Hindu death customs), and the improper disposal of animal carcasses are also discussed, as they are crucial to understanding the complexity of rabies.

Chapter 3 outlines the role of dogs in Hinduism, with special reference to Bheru, a god associated with these animals. It also describes the extremely ambivalent attitude toward dogs in India, focusing on the contrasting lives of overpampered purebred pet dogs and the despised Indian street dogs whom most people consider responsible for bites and rabies. Moving among dog lovers, animal rights activists, and dog haters, it presents the strategies currently being implemented to control the population of street dogs and rabies. Chapter 4 first presents the main motives behind the arrival of macaques in Indian cities (deforestation, illegal monkey training for entertainment purposes, the use of macaques in Indian and international laboratories, etc.) and the "menace narratives" and episodes of mass hysteria that have resulted. It then addresses the widespread cult of Hanuman, a simian god who indirectly guarantees food, shelter, and legal protection to his flesh-and-blood representatives. The chapter closes with a look at the measures used to manage the continuous, and occasionally "biting," tug of war between humans and primates within this unique context. Chapter 5 deals with Indian cows, animals who have been protagonists of one of the most heated and prolonged debates in the history of anthropology. This discussion has revolved around their supposed sacredness, sometimes attributed to economic factors, sometimes to religious ones. I do not engage with this rigid and somewhat abstract dichotomy, instead looking at the real life of street cows, which is closely connected to complex issues such as urban poverty, environmental deterioration, and growing health risks—for cows, as they choke to death on plastic garbage, and for their coexisting species, as they die of rabies. The chapter explores the reasons why cows end up roaming around and the attempts to remove them from the streets and from the risk of catching and transmitting rabies.

Chapter 6 addresses rabies more directly, through the data I gathered by talking with street and slum children and middle-class university students. It describes how rabies is perceived, what is known about it, how people view rabid dogs, how animal bites are treated, and the main reasons for the vulnerability of rabies' most common victims—male children. The chapter analyzes the unique belief that dog bite causes a terrifying puppy pregnancy in humans and the role of this belief in the fight against rabies. It also provides a comprehensive look at the typical interactions between the four species examined in this study that contribute to the transmission of rabies.

CHAPTER 1

HUMANS

With more than 1.3 billion people, India is the second-most populous country in the world. It is also, demographically speaking, a very young nation, with an average age of twenty-seven years. Since the economic liberalization of 1991, India has become one of the world's fastest-growing economies, although it continues to face severe challenges such as malnutrition, inadequate health care, pollution, and sharp social inequality. In fact, it ranks 130th—in a list of 188—in the United Nations Human Development Index (UN 2015, 210). India spends just 1.04% of its GDP on the health of its citizens, or less than three rupees (US$0.04) per person per day (Dey 2018). According to 2016 World Bank data, 268 million Indians lived on less than US$1.90 per day in 2011. According to the 2011 census (the latest available), the literacy rate in India is 74%, with notable disparities between Kerala, the most literate state, and Bihar, the least literate. Such remarkable differences among the states are largely due to the fact that India is a federal republic, consisting of twenty-nine states and seven union territories.

One of the seven union territories is the National Capital Territory of Delhi (commonly called Delhi, or Dilli in Hindi), which is the most spread-out Indian city (1,484 square kilometers) and has a population of about nineteen million, a figure that increases to almost twenty-six million if we consider its entire metropolitan area. Compared to other Indian cities and towns, Delhi attracted the highest number of immigrants for decades after independence in 1947, mostly from Pakistan and from the poverty-stricken countryside of northern India. In 2007, it was estimated that about 1,300 immigrants arrived in Delhi every day (Sengupta 2007, 107). Consequently, the overall population density of Delhi increased from 9,340 people per square kilometer in 2001 to 11,320 in 2011, or the highest density of all the states and union territories (GNCTD 2014, i). Eight of the eleven districts of Delhi are governed by the Municipal Corporation of Delhi (MCD), which in 2012 was trifurcated into the North MCD, South MCD, and East MCD. Until 2012, the MCD was among the largest municipal bodies in the world. The remaining districts fall under the jurisdiction of two other municipalities, the New Delhi Municipal Council (NDMC) and the Delhi Cantonment Board. Within the National Capital Territory of Delhi, New Delhi is the capital of India; it is also one of the eleven districts that make up Delhi. It is administrated by the NDMC.

Southwest of Delhi lies Rajasthan, the largest Indian state in terms of area. Its capital is Jaipur, which as of the 2011 census had a population of 3.1 million people, making it the tenth-most populous city in the country. Known as the Pink City by the millions of tourists who visit it every year, Jaipur offers a spectacle that other Indian cities, where modernity has overtaken tradition, can no longer offer. In the usual multispecies entanglement of Indian bazaars in the heart of the city, sellers, buyers, rickshaw drivers, beggars, and tourists share space with skinny dogs, macaques who live in the nearby Galtaji temple, hungry cattle, donkeys overloaded with bricks for construction sites, goats with colorful "skirts" around their udders to prevent their kids from drinking their milk, camels who pull carts, and elephants whose stables were, until recently, next to the main road of the old town, Surajpol Bazar Road.

The Indian Capital: Ugly or World-Class?

The first time I set foot in Delhi, as a tourist in 2007, I felt happy only when I left it three days later. To my eyes, this city looked inhospitable, inhumanely huge, exhausting, and impossible to understand. Five years later, my relationship with it changed considerably, though I cannot dispute the claim of Delhi-based reporter Sam Miller that "nothing in Delhi is, I decided, quite as it seems" (2008, 185). Nor can I disagree with Ajay Gandhi and Lotte Hoek, who write that Indian cities "defy the anthropological tendency to make every subject a comprehensive repository of culture. In these places, residents easily concede their inability to fully explain or anticipate the social" (2012, 4). Even the chief minister of Delhi at the time, Sheila Dikshit, described Delhi as "a vast, impossible city" (Luce 2011, 215), mainly because of its sprawl, overcrowding, constant and often unrestrained expansion, and rapid changeability. This ferment reached its apex in October 2010, when Delhi hosted the 19th Commonwealth Games (CWG). Since then, a notable number of scholars, mainly Indians, have seen in this controversial event the clearest and most worrisome application of the latest social and environmental policies implemented by the government of Delhi.

When Delhi was chosen to host the games, this was seen as an unparalleled chance to show the world the pride of a country that longs for international recognition and esteem, and of a capital that wants to be seen as a "world-class city" (Bhan 2009, 140). "Delhi: From Walled City to World City" was in fact the slogan of the "Chalo Dilli" (Let's go, Delhi) campaign hosted by the *Times of India* to advertise the renewal of the city for the CWG. On the official CWG website, the mascot Shera explained the mission of the event with similar enthusiasm. Among the ambitious objectives listed there were "Projecting India as an economic power," "Projecting Delhi as a global destination," "Showing India's cultures and traditions," and also "Leaving behind an old-fashioned legacy." The *CWG Guide to Delhi*, drafted by the Delhi Tourism and Transportation Development Corporation, ended with these words: "The 2010 CWG light hope in Delhi's heart. If the rumours about 'an Asiatic century' are going to come true, the future is undoubtedly here." Sheila Dikshit expressed the hope that the games would make Delhi a place "which *everybody* loves and feels happy in" (*Times of India* 2013e, emphasis added).

A massive campaign to "beautify" Delhi was implemented in the run-up to the games (Kalra 2010, 66), but it might have been more fitting to describe the process as "de-uglification." In fact, Delhi did not simply clean up its public spaces, improve its services, and showcase its many highlights; it also attempted to hastily remove, or at least hide, its flaws. The first targets were the thousands of Delhiites who make up the exploited workforce of the city, working as rickshaw pullers, ragpickers, street vendors, street cleaners, unskilled workers, servants, taxi drivers, and even as laborers for the CWG. The ranks of this vulnerable group are swelled further by the immigrants who constantly pour into Delhi, so much so that job vacancies are an illusion, and stable accommodations remain a dream for most of these people. In fact, 22% of the people who live on the streets of Delhi, on its pavements and under its overpasses, have been living there for more than a decade (I. Singh 2006, 219). Similarly, in the period from 1991 to 2001, the number of slum-dwelling residents of Delhi grew at a pace double that of the rest of the city (Agarwal and Taneja 2005, 233). In 2016, several years after the beautification and demolition drive that preceded the CWG, the Delhi Urban Shelter Improvement Board claimed that the city still had about 330,000 slums (Haidar 2016).

Before and during the CWG, in the areas of Delhi that were being used for the event or were within the sight of international visitors, fifty-three slums were demolished (Srivastava 2009, 341), affecting approximately 450,000 people (roughly the population of Miami), several overnight shelters for street dwellers were closed, and beggars found in so-called no-tolerance zones were sent to special beggars' homes (Nair 2009). In other words, the city that the CWG presented to the world was *not* for everybody, as the chief minister had hoped. After all, "We cannot present to the world a capital of the second-biggest global economy dotted with slums, and dotted with pockets [of poverty] we don't want to see," said the director of the games (Majumdar and Mehta 2010, 28). In order to hide "slums and other unsavoury sights," the media reported, the Delhi government bought large bamboo screens from the governments of Assam and Mizoram, which were installed along main roads (*Hindustan Times* 2009). The most direct consequence of this treatment of Delhi's poor is that between 2001 and 2011, the population of the city declined by 25% in the New Delhi district and 10% in the Central district, which is the flood-lit heart of Delhi, and increased by 31% in the South West district, 28% in the North West, 27% in the North East, 21% in the South, 19% in the West, 17% in the East, and 13% in the North (Pandit 2012). It was easy to relocate the poor to these fringe areas of the city, where the lights of the CWG did not reach.

Another aim of the Delhi makeover was to make the city green and clean through an "ecological transformation" (Srivastava and Bartaria 2010, 38). Thus placards inviting Delhiites to "plant a tree, at least one" became omnipresent on roadsides and roundabouts, the color chosen for traffic signs was green, the logo of the NDMC was a tree, and the "Greening Delhi Action Plan (2005–2006)" announced proudly that greenery covered 11%

of the city. However, while visitors—myself included—were indeed quite pleased to find Delhi (or at least some areas of it) relatively greener than other Indian towns and metropoles, several of the Delhiites with whom I discussed this issue admitted sadly that, compared to the past, the situation had actually gotten worse year after year. In fact, Dikshit's promise in 2011 that 30% of Delhi's territory would be covered by greenery remained largely unfulfilled (Singh 2012). Not only that, but after an impressive increase in the amount of Delhi's tree cover, from 6% in 1999 to 20% in 2009, it has steadily decreased for years, mainly owing to road-widening projects (Singh 2013). The Delhi Forest Department says on its website that tree cover managed to reach slightly above 20% again only in 2015.

In the first weeks of July 2010, in order to prevent the spread of dengue, a severe mosquito-borne disease that has been a growing concern in Delhi for more than a decade, the MCD took advantage of the games to cleanse and disinfect roads, railway stations, bus stops, markets, and temples. The CWG organizing committee also included in its regulations a prohibition on spitting, urinating, and defecating outside "the places and facilities arranged for this need." Similarly, the regulations of the brand-new underground forbade, and still forbid, the introduction of cow dung and human ashes into metro stations and coaches.

Cleanliness and disinfection were among the reasons for the massive demolition of the Yamuna Pushta slum area in the years preceding the CWG. In fact, as part of a broader drive to achieve the "purification of space" (Sibley 1988), slum clearance has been undertaken to ensure "a clean and green riverfront" (Jamwal and Tebbal 2004); this includes the removal "of squatters and encroachers" and the "reclaim[ing of] public spaces for the use of *proper* citizens" (Chatterjee 2004, 131, emphasis added). Slum dwellers were seen as encroachers and polluters and were blamed for the exorbitant levels of pollution of the Yamuna because of their close proximity to the river and the poor sanitary conditions of the slums. Nevertheless, Nidhi Jamwal and Farouk Tebbal of the UN-Habitat Programme (2004) observed that "the Pushta clearance is a horrendous distortion of reality. ... The government is carrying out a war-like operation against its own citizens for pursuits that will further aggravate Delhi's problems." According to Amita Baviskar (2011a), paradoxical measures such as slum clearance and eviction can be explained by the concept of "bourgeois environmentalism," that is, the (ab)use of environmental discourses by a privileged minority to arbitrarily regulate the use of urban spaces and dictate standards of order, hygiene, cleanliness, and safety. The economic, social, and political power of these elites, who often have privileged access to the media and the courts, is reflected in the frequent description of the poor who live on public space in Delhi as a "nuisance" (Baviskar 2011a, 392). But the most glaring evidence of this condescending type of environmentalism is probably the large number of gated communities in Delhi, which are used by the privileged as a tool of estrangement and separation from the nuisance of the poor, of which slums are seen as the most disturbing symbol (Waldrop 2004).

Under section 3 of the Slum Areas Improvement and Clearance Act of 1956, slums have been defined as residential areas where dwellings are unfit for human habitation for reasons of dilapidation; overcrowding; faulty arrangements of buildings; narrowness of streets; lack of ventilation, light, or sanitation facilities; or any combination of these factors that are detrimental to safety, health, and morals. As Asher D. Ghertner (2008) and Gautam Bhan (2009) point out, behind the tendency to translate "poor" as "slum dwellers" there is the propensity to look at these people as part of the urban social structure only when they stop being seen as individuals who contribute to the functioning of the city and become part of the blurred load of encroachers and polluters for whom the rest of the citizens have little tolerance. The residents of gated communities—middle- and upper middle-class areas much in vogue in Delhi's peripheral neighborhoods—resort to every solution to avoid seeing these people and the slums they are invariably seen as "stuck to." These attempts to make the poor invisible include high walls that hide slums, patrolled gates that screen unwanted incomers, flowered gardens that scent the polluted air, air-conditioned apartments that keep sticky humidity outside, swimming pools that wash away outside dirt, video-surveillance systems that promise safety, and garbage-collection services that provide a sense of cleanliness. The billboard I saw for months in the Lajpat Nagar metro station advertised the New Rajneegandha Greens as nothing less than "a joint venture with nature," and thus as nothing further from the image that people usually have of slums. In Jeremy Seabrook's view, the people who live inside the utopian parallel world of gated communities "cease to be citizens of their own country and become nomads belonging to, and owing allegiance to, a superterrestrial topography of money; they become patriots of wealth, nationalists of an elusive and golden nowhere" (1996, 211).

As far as Delhi is concerned, this last statement is not quite true; these superterrestrial enclaves do not completely abstract residents from their surroundings. Delhi neighborhoods use resident welfare associations (RWAs) to represent their interests when it comes to broader urban policies and local governance. These civic bodies are not official organs of government, although the Delhi government increasingly involves them, particularly those based in planned neighborhoods, in making decisions. Interestingly—in that 76% of Delhiites, referred to as "unscrupulous elements" in the legal discourse of the city (Ghertner 2008, 64), live in unauthorized colonies (Ahmad and Choi 2011, 78)—members of the recognized RWAs constitute only a small elite of "proper" citizens. Despite their numeric weakness, recognized RWAs enjoy considerable power in issues that often go beyond the limits of their own neighborhoods, intertwining their worldview with the lives of those who live nearby. As Seabrook notes, RWA members, especially those in gated communities, want to remain proud citizens of their country, but from their privileged, geographically isolated control tower. In fact, as Ghertner observes in the context of some thorny legal cases over Delhi urban planning, "The primary avenue by which slums are demolished today begins when a Resident Welfare Association files a writ petition praying for the removal of a neighbouring slum" (2008, 57). For example, the Ashok Vihar RWA filed a petition complaining about the residents of the adjoining slum, who were bathing and defecating in the open area near the border of their neighborhood, which, the petition stated, "has made the lives of the RWA residents 'miserable' and has 'transgressed their right to very living'" (Ghertner 2008, 60).

Street and Slum Children

The average age in India remains low thanks to more than twenty-seven million births per year, according to the 2011 census. While 70% of Indians still live in rural areas, a growing number are constantly moving into towns and cities. Between 2001 and 2015, the number of children in urban areas increased by 10%, while in rural areas it decreased by 7% (Singh 2015). Most of the migrants in northern India, who often end up in Delhi, come from Bihar, Uttar Pradesh, Rajasthan, Jharkhand, and Madhya Pradesh. For instance, one study showed that 44% of Jaipur's street children come from the Rajasthan countryside and 39% from Bihar (Arora 2013).

Among the street and slum children I met in Delhi, the main reasons for migration were poverty, hunger, parents' unemployment, health issues (e.g., mental retardation and other handicaps), relatives' unwillingness to take care of them in case of their parents' death or imprisonment, domestic violence (often linked to alcohol and drug addiction), family breakups, peer pressure to run away, drought, strained relationship with stepparents, forced child labor, sexual abuse, poor education facilities in villages, fathers' pursuit of work in cities, fights with relatives over inheritance issues, sale of children into prostitution and forced labor, and the wish to experience urban life and independence. It is also not unusual for children to get separated from their families during long train journeys, political rallies, and religious gatherings, or to be kidnapped by criminals.

According to the United Nations Children's Fund (UNICEF), street children fall into three categories: "street-living children," who have run away from their families and live alone on the streets; "street-working children," who spend most of their time on the streets fending for themselves but return to their family on a regular basis; and "children from street families," who live on the streets with their families. Children in the first category are usually called "children of the street"; for them, the street (meant in the broadest sense of the term) is their substitute for a family and their only living environment. The children in the other categories are "children *on* the street," in that they have families. Taking a census of street children, and particularly of "children of the street," is anything but easy. Most of them lack identification documents (this is true of 83% of the people living on Indian streets, according to I. Singh 2006, 219), are instructed by their employers to give their age as nineteen in order to avoid legal prosecution, are constantly on the move in search of better shelters or jobs, fear the police, and are afraid of being found by their relatives or sent back to their villages. Moreover, as reported in *Surviving the Streets*, a much-awaited census of street children carried out in Delhi in 2010 (to coincide with the CWG) by the Institute for Human Development, cleanup drives make it extremely difficult to contact and register street children because they and their families are periodically sent away from their usual residing place. Ironically, again owing to the governmental policies implemented for the CWG, the researchers who conducted this census faced the opposite issue: "Since our field work took place at the time when civil work for the Commonwealth Games was in the final stages of completion, many laborers had been brought from villages in neighboring states with their families, including children. These children were on the street" (IHD 2011, 34).

Surviving the Streets calculated that about 51,000 street children live in Delhi, most of them between the age of seven and fourteen (IHD 2011, 26): 36% were children of street families (who often ended up living on the street when their slums were demolished without any rehabilitation plan—Sheikh and Banda 2014), 29% were street-working children, and 28% were children of the street (IHD 2011, 26–27). One-tenth of the children surveyed claimed that they lived completely alone, not even with fellow street children, and thus were totally cut off from their families (8). Finally, 40% of the street children slept in slums, 4% in shelters provided by NGOs or the government, and the rest in public places (pavements, bus and train stations, places of worship, markets, parks, abandoned buildings, construction sites, garbage dumps, or beneath overpasses) (35).

The weaker the bond with their families, the less support these children receive in the way of education and health care, two issues that are directly linked to the incidence of animal bites and rabies, and in Delhi the lack of both is particularly severe. Only 71% of the total children in Delhi attend school (Pietkiewicz-Pareek 2012, 983). Half of the street children surveyed for *Surviving the Streets* were illiterate, 23% had received informal education by NGOs, 13% had attended nursery school, 4% had gone to primary school, and only 2% had reached middle school (IHD 2011, 30). Most of these children displayed little or no interest in school and, as the authors of the study observed, "the attitude of the school authorities may have had something to do with this too." In fact, "Teachers were reported to be unsympathetic to the children's inability to buy books and other study material, and appeared to pay little attention to them in class" (30).

When they lack supervising parents and teachers, street children are not trained to take care of their health or to ask for help in case of need. When they do not feel well, they first resort to self-medication, using remedies known from home or easily available in the marketplaces; only at a later stage of illness or injury do they seek proper medical advice. In most cases, they take care of their health only when their pain becomes unbearable, they realize the disease is not getting better by itself, they are unable to work, or someone else persuades them to seek treatment (McFadyen 2005, 128, 135). The authors of *Surviving the Streets* point out that the children they met defined illness not as having a cold or fever but as being bedridden. Alarmingly, the children "did not report any skin-related problem [e.g., dermatitis, wounds, animal bites] as a health issue or a condition of sickness, because it was very common among them" (IHD 2011, 53). The minimal attention street children pay to their health is evident also in their expenditure pattern (48). Of the 2,240 rupees (US$32) they earn a month on average, the amount spent on medical care (1.8%) is higher only than the amount given to the police (0.5%), and well below the money allotted for food (47%), parents (33%), clothes (7%), drugs (3%), supervisors (2.5%), entertainment (2.5%), and shelter (2%).

When in need, these children usually turn to private clinics or informal health providers such as medical camps, family-planning centers, or NGOs (40). Fewer than 4% of them go to public hospitals, because of the time and expense involved, along with the overcrowding and mismanagement they perceive at such hospitals and their lack of confidence in hospital doctors. In fact, Lori McFadyen (2005, 140) describes the medical negligence of unaccompanied children, while the Society for Nutrition, Education, and Health Action for Women and Children (2008, 13) reports that street children fear that their organs will be stolen for illegal organ transplants. In more general terms, these kids are understandably reluctant to open themselves to ill treatment, scorn, and prejudice from service providers owing to their substandard status in society (Aptekar 1994, 214). A study carried out in an unauthorized slum in Sangam Vihar (South Delhi) revealed that 39% of children surveyed had turned to unregistered physicians and 27% to home-based remedies, while only 18% took advantage of services from government hospitals (Gupta 2012, 640). Informal private practitioners were generally considered more approachable, familiar, economical, safe, and trustworthy. Interestingly, this was the case even with children who lived with their families.

According to the Global Slavery Index, India has the highest number of people (eighteen million) living in conditions of slavery (Walk Free Foundation 2016, 108). India also has the largest number of child laborers aged five to fourteen (about thirteen million), and, predictably, a portion of them are engaged in hazardous occupations. Roughly 20% of Delhi's street children work as ragpickers, as this is one of the easiest jobs to get (IHD 2011, 31). Scrounging rubbish dumps and gutters makes ragpickers susceptible to wounding themselves with needles, nails, broken glass, and other sharp objects. Lack of hygiene in their living environment increases the chance that these wounds will get infected, go untreated, and get worse. Almost all the young ragpickers I met in Delhi streets and slums had their hands and feet covered by so many scars that they could not remember when or how their wounds had occurred. In fact, young ragpickers hardly ever use gloves while working (Hunt 1996, 116). Additionally, they are exposed to toxic materials, bacteriological infections, worm infestation, and toxic fumes from burning dumps. Finally, the unbearable working conditions often push young ragpickers into taking drugs or sniffing whitener fluids. Chapter 6 explores another important but rarely acknowledged occupational risk for ragpickers: animal bites and the possibility of contracting rabies. As written on the website of I-India, an NGO that works for street children in Jaipur, "Rag-pickers can be seen alongside pigs and dogs searching through trash heaps on their hands and knees."

Middle-Class Youth

In the past two decades, several studies on the internally highly differentiated social group referred to as the "Indian middle class" have set out to understand its size and to provide a profile of its history, composition, values, consumer trends, and cultural practices. Despite their heterogeneity, most of these studies have reached a common conclusion: it is difficult, perhaps impossible, to provide a unanimous, unambiguous, coherent definition of this slippery social category, especially if class is not seen solely as a matter of income. This difficulty is also due to the fact that, as Andre Béteille observes, the Indian middle class is "certainly the most polymorphous in the world" (2011, 79). Without losing sight of these facts, and making every effort to avoid seeing India's middle class in static, well-delineated, or absolute terms, it has proved fruitful to look at this class as an interesting cultural "container" with reference to the subject of this book. I see a parallel case in Philip Lutgendorf's (1997) work on the Hindu religion and the Indian middle class. Lutgendorf initially had his doubts about the usefulness of the concept of the middle class in that context, but his research on Hanuman worship among middle-class Indians has proved to be of exceptional value. When I use the term "middle class" in this book, I am mainly referring to the middle-class people living in Delhi. Needless to say, I cannot claim to speak for each and every one of its members.

The 1990s were a pivotal decade in shaping the identity of what we nowadays call the "new" Indian middle class, and an important turning point for the "old" middle class, which until then had consisted mostly of civil servants and professionals whose offspring, already at an advantage over most of their countrymen, greatly benefited from the economic liberalization of 1991 (Fernandes 2011, 58). The international openness of Rajiv Gandhi, prime minister from 1984 to 1989, and the Indians who supported him opened the way to the enjoyment of the benefits offered by the new global economy. The Indian middle class started to purge itself of the social stigma associated with the pursuit of wealth during Mahatma Gandhi's time and looked with interest at the stimulus proposed by Western countries. Before 1991, says a Delhi-based writer and history teacher, "autarky . . . was the state of grace to which we collectively aspired. Scarcity was ideologically sexy because it was the price we paid for self-sufficiency" (Kesavan 2016). Later, when the wounds of colonization started to heal, India soon began to experience what Dipankar Gupta calls "westoxification," meaning infatuation with "a superficial consumerist display of commodities and fads produced in the West" (2000, 21). He coined this term to describe the post-liberalization sociocultural change that became possible thanks to higher income, widespread access to the internet, and a general increase in exposure to foreign lifestyles and models. Simultaneously, the members of this privileged class started to transform their attitude of inclusion toward their poorer fellow citizens into a mindset of sharp exclusion (Waldrop 2004, 97) or, as the political scientist Rajni Kothari (1993) put it, "growing amnesia." Béteille (2011, 82) described this change as a shift from a harmonic system to a totally disharmonic one, and Paolo Favero noticed it particularly in Delhi, which he defined as "a symbol of post-1991 India" (2005, 10). Leela Fernandes (2011, 59) claims that the main features of the Indian middle class are the modalities it uses to create social inequality and to reinforce hegemony (e.g., through the aforementioned RWAs). For the members of the lower middle class, slums represent the boundary against which they struggle to define their identity and stress their superior position.

From a different perspective, John Parker (2009) defines this class mainly through economic criteria: its members manage to float above poverty and can easily afford their "bread and butter" (an expression widely used in India, meaning basic needs) and their lodging and thus can spend about a third of their income on nonessential needs like leisure, elective medical treatments, higher-priced clothes, and higher education. The great importance that middle-class people give to education is evident in the results of a 2014 survey by the Lok Foundation in Delhi and the Center for the Advanced Study of India at the University of Pennsylvania, investigating the correlation between Indian aspirations and anxieties and class status. As Devesh

Kapur and Milan Vaishnav (2014) observe, "Middle-class belonging also increases with educational attainment: the more educated one is, the more likely she is to claim to be middle class. However, 47% of individuals with less than one tenth of the standard education—those we do not typically associate with middle-class status—still claim such an affiliation."

Within this class, higher education is seen as instrumental for self-fulfillment and social recognition, which in turn are considered fundamental achievements in life (Fernandes 2004, 2418). For this reason, middle-class families put a lot of effort into building strong, spendable, and profitable cultural capital in their offspring. As an example of the tools needed to attain this goal, Fernandes (2000, 95–97) mentions the many courses offered by private institutes in Mumbai, where middle-class youths get an education in manners, style, and taste that is considered essential for those who wish to enter, stay, and prosper in the middle class. Similarly, Delhi's bookshops often prominently display English books on self-management and business, with titles like *How to Be Successful in Life*. Middle-class success is measured in diplomas and degrees in disciplines like information technology, business administration, economics, engineering, law, and medicine. The importance attached to these achievements is so great that, in my experience, the question "What is your qualification?" is much more common than the simple "What do you do?" When they talk about their academic education, people in India not only mention their field of study but specify the level they have achieved within the myriad of university and other courses offered in Indian cities and towns. These attainments are usually written in full detail on visiting cards and, quite often, on the doorplates of private homes.

Satish Deshpande (2003, 136) claims that the "middle-class" label is more useful at a symbolic level than at a factual one, and Sanjay Srivastava (2009, 364) considers it amorphous from an outside perspective but potentially interesting if we look at it from the perspective of its members. I decided to take Srivastava's advice and collect some attempts at self-definition from my middle-class acquaintances in Delhi. One of my flatmates in Jangpura, a young woman from Kolkata, told me that while there are many gradations within the Indian middle class, what distinguishes these people both from the poor who live in slums and on the street and from the broad category of the "filthy rich, the VIP [very important people], and the VVIP [very, very important people]" is that they live in a multiroom flat in a modern neighborhood, have a car, wear nice clothes, speak good English, and have some money to spend for sheer pleasure. While talking with Himanshu, a young Punjabi who lives in the heart of Old Delhi, about the purchase of his first car, he admitted that buying a big car was foolish because of Delhi's traffic congestion and lack of adequate parking, but could not get past his feeling that "small cars are disgusting" and thus that "having a big car is a must in Delhi in these days." Pradeep, a man in his forties who lives in Greater Kailash 1 (South East Delhi), provided a definition of his class that went beyond material belongings and called into question the values, attitudes, and behavior of its members. Pradeep loved living in his middle-class colony because of the relatively abundant space and the quality of housing, but he also described his neighbors as very hostile, intolerant, selfish, and uncooperative. "If you ring a bell in South Delhi to ask for help," he observed, "you can be sure that the person who opens the door is already angry with you, without even knowing your needs. . . . You see, in South Delhi there are mainly middle-class people and their middle-class ego is the problem there."

From an opposite perspective, the diplomat and former member of Parliament Pavan K. Varma devoted two of his best sellers to the portrayal of urban Indians (2004) and urban middle-class Indians (2007), focusing on what they "really" are and not on what they think they are, as the back cover of *Being Indian* explains. The overall aim of his work is to demolish the abundant misconceptions about India and its people, seen both in foreigners' stereotypes of them and in Indians' own myths about themselves. Varma sets out to analyze the paradoxes and contradictions that characterize their attitudes toward many aspects of their life. He writes, for example, that "most Indians are 'other worldly' [spiritual] only in their indifference to anything in the external milieu that is not of direct benefit to their immediate and personal world" (2004, 7). "Altruism," he observes, "the ability of an individual to act in the public good without a self-serving ulterior motive, is deeply suspect" (37). In Varma's 2007 book, *The Great Indian Middle Class*, he addresses middle-class myopia with respect to the poor, who "have been around for so long that they have become a part of the accepted landscape." This myopia, he says, "has its advantages[:] the less one noticed, the less reason one had to be concerned about social obligations; and the less one saw, the less one needed to be distracted from the heady pursuit of one's own material salvation" (137).

During my stay in Delhi, this view of the selfishness and blind individualism of middle-class Indian people was a source of great confusion to me. In fact, I have always been amazed by the quantity and quality of unsolicited help that I received while traveling and living in India. This conviction of mine started to waver when I began to talk about it with university students and middle-class acquaintances in Delhi. The vast majority of them were visibly puzzled when I told them how much willingness to help and genuine concern I had encountered in their fellow citizens. The most diplomatic among them acknowledged this only with respect to rural India, clearly seen as a symbol of righteousness and good nature. My more skeptical acquaintances laughed at me, claiming that my idea of India had nothing to do with reality. After countless conversations on this issue, I still have only a tentative answer to this conundrum. When it comes to the poor people I met in rural villages and urban streets and slums, I believe that their generous and helpful manner toward me sprang mainly from their open and welcoming dispositions, and maybe also from a hope of karmic reward. With respect to the middle-class people I met in Delhi, I suspect that Soumya, an anthropology student at the University of Delhi, may be on to something. She believed that two factors were at work in the open, helpful attitudes I perceived: one was that these people were in effect pretending to be polite and helpful because this is how well-educated, open-minded, modern Western people are expected to be. The other was that, insofar as middle-class Delhiites responded to me with genuine openness and generosity, it was only because I was a foreigner with a useless degree in anthropology and thus presented them with no threat of competition in their quest for social status and success.

Describing civic insensitivity and indifference to the common good among the middle-class denizens of the large industrial city of Ludhiana, Pankaj Mishra writes that "it wasn't for lack of money that such appalling civic conditions were allowed to prevail. If anything, the blame lay with the sudden plentitude of money: far from fostering any notions of civic responsibility, it had encouraged in its beneficiaries only a kind of aggressive individualism" (1995, 9). In Delhi, one can see this attitude in the growing power of RWAs, the mushrooming of gated colonies, the ubiquitous desire for Delhi to be a world-class city, and the antidemocratic measures of cleansing, removal, segregation, gentrification, and other forms of "beautification." At the Indian Institute for Human Settlements, faculty member Gautam Bhan claims that "certain built environments associated with the poor, their modes of employment, indeed their very presence in the city, must literally stay out of sight as new flyovers and expressways allow the nonpoor to move from one enclosed bubble to another without having to encounter the city they drive through" (quoted in Majumdar and Mehta 2010, 81). As Hiranmay Karlekar puts it, referring to the self-enclosed bubbles they try to create for themselves, "Most middle-class persons are not Indians because they are for themselves, their family members and no one else" (2011c). "Otherwise," he continues, "there would not have been compulsive consumption on a gargantuan scale when a vast majority live below the poverty line."

In Delhi, not only do slums and social housing have to stay out of sight, but often they are not even taken into account in urban planning. In fact, the unplanned expansion of the city, the chronic lack of space for immigrants, and the overcrowding of slums is largely blamed on the shortcomings of the Delhi Development Authority (the agency that owns and manages city land in partnership with private builders) in failing to allot the mandatory 25% of residential land to what are called in Delhi the "economically weaker sections" and "lower-income groups" (Ghertner 2008, 61). In 2016, a committee set up to address the problem of inappropriate land management in Delhi described the Development Authority as a "developer" focused on commercial gain rather than "a facilitator and a regulator" (Gupta 2016). In fact, according to the *World Cities Report* drafted by the UN-Habitat Programme in October 2012, the livability of Delhi is hardly damaged by the fact that its urban planning revolves around the real estate market, which predictably gives priority to the interests of well-to-do Delhiites (Jamwal and Tebbal 2004). The result of this process is "bourgeoisification," or "the expansion of the social space occupied by the middle class and its increasing size and salience in terms of the power and influence it wields in economic, political, and social dimensions" (Lobo and Shah 2015, 5).

When it comes to politics, the impossibility of describing the middle class as a homogenous group becomes particularly evident. Karlekar (2011b) ascribes this to the withdrawal of middle-class people from political life, mainly because they are too busy attending to their own problems to have much time left over for the country's. While many of them, Karlekar continues, are socially responsible and politically correct, most of them simply "rely on Public Interest Litigation, to mould society after their values" (2011b) and are complacent with respect to the powerful and exploitive toward the vulnerable. On the other hand, in his 2015 article "Green Politics and the Indian Middle Class," Ashok Lahiri sees increased engagement in environmental issues among the middle class—especially in local "not-in-my-backyard" issues, which Emma Mawdsley confirms

(2004, 81). This interest, however, does not compare to the commitment demonstrated by the "empty-belly" environmentalists who, for example, joined the famous Chipko forest conservation movement of the 1970s, or the Narmada Bachao Andolan, a coalition that opposed large dam projects on the Narmada River in the 1980s and '90s. Lahiri sees the potential for effective middle-class political activism to develop—for example, in green political parties—but for the time being, middle-class attitudes toward environmental protection appear to be largely self-centered and materialistic, suggesting no willingness to sacrifice modernity and development to environmental considerations (2015, 41).

By emphasizing the "ugly face" (Béteille 2001) of the Indian middle class, I do not mean to suggest that this social group has no redeeming values. Indian middle-class people are also creative, intrepid, enterprising, talented, pragmatic, and hardworking. While they are a fundamental driving force behind Indian economy, their kids struggle, beginning in kindergarten, to get into the best schools, urged on by an education system that leaves no room for mercy. Moreover, intoxication with the consumer culture of the West is only one aspect of their identity; another one, particularly in recent years, is sincere pride in being Indian, which has led to increased confidence in India's capabilities, a consistent preference for homemade products (e.g., personal care products, traditional clothes, etc.), and growing interest in local roots and cultural heritage. Interestingly, as Béteille writes, "what appears as the lack of values in the Indian middle class is often the result of a conflict of values rather than their absence" (2011, 84). This inner conflict seems to be confirmed by the results of a Pew Research Center survey (2007), which found that 92% of middle-class Indians wished the state could help their poorer fellow citizens in a more concrete and committed way. This strong preference for government action, and this palpable discrepancy between theory and practice, ideal and reality, will become particularly evident when we come to the issue of managing street animals and rabies.

The Basics of Hinduism

A brief introduction to the key concepts of Hinduism will be of help in understanding the social, cultural, and religious context in which rabies is embedded in India. Hinduism is the dominant religion in India—or, as many Hindus love to say, their way of life. The 2011 census found that 82%

of Delhiites and 78% of residents of Jaipur identify themselves as Hindus; the figure for the country overall is 80%. Despite the saying that there are 330 million deities in Hinduism, most Hindus ultimately believe in only one supreme absolute being, called Brahman. The other deities—the chief ones being the trinity of Brahma, Vishnu, and Shiva, along with the goddess Devi—only represent the many aspects of Brahman. Bheru and Hanuman, the gods dealt with in chapters 4 and 5, respectively, are part of this complex divine multitude.

Within the wide range of traditions and ideas that make Hinduism a colorful and vibrant mosaic, four concepts are prominent: *dharma*, *moksha*, *samsara*, and *karma*. Dharma is the principle of harmony and order that makes life possible; it is an impersonal, universal, natural law that governs the course of things. It is often described as a sociocosmic order, but no fewer than seventeen translations are provided for this concept in the Monier-Williams *Sanskrit-English Dictionary* (Pankaj 2011, 105, 114). Thus dharma can be thought of as a combination of duties, ethics, virtues, rights, practices, morals, and laws that inform the "right way of living" (Rosen 2006, 34–35). *Sanatana* dharma (the eternal dharma) is not only the term that many Hindus use to describe Hinduism, but it is also the dharma that all Hindus follow. However, within this universal framework there is also another, lower level of dharma, the *svadharma*, that is as important and binding as *sanatana* dharma. Depending on caste, gender, and the stage of life a person has reached, each Hindu is supposed to stick to the *svadharma* that corresponds to his temporary condition. Only in this way can one hope to attain *moksha*, which is the liberation from *samsara*, the endless cycle of death and rebirth that every Hindu experiences. The mechanism that powers this endless cycle is *karma*, the individual deeds, thoughts, words, and intentions that positively or negatively influence the future of each person. Living in a proper, right way, in accordance with *sanatana* dharma and *svadharma*, is the best way to eventually experience final and permanent death. As Mahatma Gandhi explains, "Good and bad are relative terms. What is good in some circumstances becomes bad or sin in different circumstances"; thus one's actions are not to be judged in absolute terms but in terms of how they affect one's karma (Gandhi quoted in Battaglia 2002, 174, my translation). As a result, the *Bhagavad Gita*, one of the central texts of Hinduism, says that "it is better to engage in one's own occupation, even though one may perform it imperfectly, than to accept another's occupation and perform it perfectly" (Bhaktivedanta Swami Prabhupada 1986, 732).

Svadharma is intrinsically linked to the caste system, a rigid social hierarchy that distributes people in four descending social groups (*varnas*) and puts others—the outcastes, pariahs, or Dalits—beyond the borders of humanity. The *Rig Veda* (10.90.12) states that the four *varnas* were created from the body of the Purusha—the cosmic man whose sacrifice gave rise to the universe. The Brahmins (priests) came from his mouth, the Kshatriyas (warriors) from his arms, the Vaishyas (farmers, artisans, and traders) from his torso, and the Sudras (servants of the upper castes, such as laundrymen, tanners, shoemakers, butchers, etc.) from his feet. Within each *varna*, the *jati* is the social group one person belongs to by birth and can leave only by falling out of the *varna* system—that is, by becoming an outcaste. Traditionally, *jatis* are usually endogamous, often linked to a specific occupation, and are rigidly closed groups as far as food exchange and commensality are concerned (i.e., who can cook for whom and who can eat with whom).

Nowadays, the constitution of India forbids caste-based discrimination (article 15) and prohibits untouchability (article 17) and thus the use of the term "untouchable," as the Dalits were formerly called. Despite the current legal prohibition, ideas of purity and pollution have for centuries been "elaborated and systematized—one is tempted to say rationalized—to an unusual degree" in India (Béteille 2011, 83). In the post-Vedic era, the purity-impurity concept that had previously applied only at an individual level (e.g., in relation to food choices or personal cleanliness) began to be used as a basis for social ostracism and thus for the hardening of caste discrimination, which reached its apex during British colonization (Riser-Kositsky 2009). As Dina S. Guha says of intercaste food exchanges, "Taboos were erected, so that lower castes or outcastes by virtue of heredity and occupation became pollutants. Their presence, their shadow or touch on cooked foods, or use of water source was held to be contaminated. . . . The mind of the high-caste Hindus actually believed that the laws of *karma* chose to give people birth in the outcaste structures of society. . . . The entire Hindu caste consciousness became permeated with the dichotomy of pure and impure, in the context of food and social contact" (1985, 148–49). Social relations continue to be saturated with the dread of interpersonal pollution, because troubles and unfortunate events are generally seen as coming from the outside, as undermining what is scrupulously protected inside (Raheja 1988, 47). In fact, in her anthropological analysis of the employer-servant relationship in Madurai, Sara Dickey observes that "servants represent the dirt, disease and 'rubbish' of a disorderly outside world that employers commonly associate with the lower class and that pointedly contrast with the ideal cleanliness, order, and hygiene of their own homes" (2000, 462).

It goes without saying that physical, moral, spiritual, or social pollution has nothing to do with actual dirt, which is much less worrisome. The best example of this clash between pollution and dirt, one that is often cited, is the poor condition of the Ganges River. Hindus look at the Ganges not only as a river but as the embodiment, in the divine figure of the Maa Ganga, of a mother's caring love for her children. The *Bhagavata Purana* (5.17.1) celebrates the saving power of the Maa Ganga, saying that it is so strong that she has even mercifully come down to earth to wash away all human sins. The fact that this river is one of the most polluted in the world and represents a severe risk to public health worries thousands of people in India, many of whom have devoted their lives to the cause of cleaning it up, but this does not seem to be a priority for the millions who worship the Maa Ganga every day. In the words of the Hindu scholar Swami Srivatsa Goswami, "Hindus have become champions at raping their own mother" (*Down to Earth* 2000b). Although deeper understanding and concern regarding the condition of this river have grown over time, in 1986 then prime minister Rajiv Gandhi inaugurated the Ganga Action Plan, the first of many government programs for the protection of the Ganges, by saying that "the purity of the Ganga has never been in doubt" (Alley 1998, 171). As Jonathan Parry (1994) explains in his masterly book *Death in Banaras*, many worshippers of the Ganga acknowledge that the river is filthy, but they do not see it as polluted; the problem does not exist, in any case, for the solution is already there, intrinsic in the river's self-purifying power. For orthodox Hindus who believe in the river's power to cleanse and redeem all human depravities, it is difficult to imagine that it is vulnerable to such down-to-earth issues as urban garbage, untreated sewage, decomposing bodies, and chemical waste.

"Are You Veg or Non-Veg?"

I lost count of how often I was asked this question in India. For an Indian, figuring out the food preferences of a fellow citizen is usually child's play. Trained from childhood to identify immediately a person's social position in the caste hierarchy, they are exceptionally good at reading external signs like surname and clothing to guess others' faith, caste, and diet. Understanding food preferences is important in social relations, especially for vegetarian Hindus, who may refuse to sit at the same table with a person eating meat. In fact, many restaurants in India have one room for vegetarians and another for meat-eating customers, and they often announce this on their signs. The same concern can be seen on restaurant menus and on all packaged food. As per the Food Safety and Standards (Packaging and Labelling) Act of 2006 and the Food Safety and Standards (Packaging and Labelling) Regulations of 2011, each food item must be labeled with a small red circle if it contains meat ingredients and a green circle for items that contain only vegetarian ingredients. Eating habits also tend to be among the topics of the long interrogation through which many landlords put their potential lodgers, at least in the two middle-class neighborhoods of South Delhi where I lived.

But despite this legal and social respect for vegetarianism and the widespread belief throughout the world that Indians are vegetarian, only 20% of the population abstains from meat and fish consumption (Natrajan and Jacob 2018, 55). I look at this issue more deeply in chapter 5. For now, suffice it to say that although this 20% figure reflects the largest concentration of vegetarians in the world, it can still seem anomalous and surprising. In fact, eating meat clashes to some extent with the important ethical tenet of *ahimsa*, which is generally translated as "nonviolence" and can be understood as the absence of a desire to kill or harm (Chapple 1993, 10). Causing injuries, in whatever way and to whatever living being, produces the accumulation of *papa* (demerit, sin) and subsequent rebirth in a worse existence, according to karmic law. As the *Bhagavata Purana* (11.5.14) explains, "Such sinful persons [who kill animals without any feeling of remorse or fear of punishment], in their next lives, [will] be eaten by the same creatures they have killed in this one" (Rosen 2006, 183). Despite the force of this warning, it is not the case that vegetarianism in India depends only on a willingness to protect and safeguard animals' lives, as advocates of animal welfare would say, or on a more generic love for animals, as animal lovers would say. It has a lot to do with caste hierarchy as well.

Laws and Animals

Thanks in part to its cultural and religious heritage, India gives outstanding legal attention to animal welfare issues. In fact, it is one of the very few countries in the world to address the subject in its constitution. Although

India's governance is formally secular, the well-known Hindu practice of cow devotion (discussed in detail in chapter 5) is responsible for special attention to this animal in the constitutional section titled "Directive Principles of State Policy" (Chigateri 2011, 142). Article 48 is directed at the animals used in agriculture, cows in particular: "The State shall endeavour to organise agriculture and animal husbandry on modern and scientific lines and shall, in particular, take steps for preserving and improving the breeds, and prohibiting the slaughter, of cows and calves and other milk and draught cattle." Article 51, paragraph (g), on fundamental duties, broadens the scope to include all animal species (and natural resources as well): "It shall be the duty of every citizen of India to protect and improve the natural environment including forests, lakes, rivers and wild life, and to have compassion for living creatures." Articles 25–28 defend religious freedom, allowing Indian citizens to profess, practice, and propagate in their own ways any religion of their choice—provided that it does not collide with issues of public order, morality, or health. These injunctions are directly related to the custom of feeding street animals, an issue that arises again and again in the following chapters.

In addition to these constitutional declarations, in 1960 New Delhi passed the Prevention of Cruelty to Animals Act, a milestone in the area of animal welfare. This is a fairly comprehensive statute that defines cruelty and sets forth detailed rules regarding the many human uses of animals. It is important to note, however, that although article 3 of this act declares that "it shall be the duty of every person having the care or charge of any animal to take all reasonable measures to ensure the wellbeing of such animal and to prevent the infliction upon such animal of unnecessary pain or suffering," exceptions are made when protecting an animal's well-being interferes or conflicts with the constitutional right to freedom of worship.

On March 19, 1992, in compliance with section 4 of the act, the Indian government founded in Chennai the Animal Welfare Board of India (AWBI), which currently has more than 3,000 affiliated animal welfare organizations (AWOs). While many of them were founded and are run by foreigners, the biggest AWO in India is People for Animals, guided since 1992 by Maneka Gandhi, the widow of Sanjay Gandhi (Indira Gandhi's son and a member of the Nehru-Gandhi political dynasty), a high-ranking politician herself and India's most famous animal rights activist. In September 2017, India's first Centre for Animal Law was established at the National

Academy of Legal Studies and Research University Law in Hyderabad. In October 2019, some Mumbai-based animal welfare activists launched the symbolic All India Animals Party to stress the need for animal rights to be included in political manifestos.

The Prevention of Cruelty to Animals Act of 1960 was soon followed by a dozen more specific laws regarding animal protection, among them the Prevention of Cruelty to Animals (Dog Breeding and Marketing) Rules and the Prevention of Cruelty to Animals (Regulation of Livestock Markets) Rules, both passed in 2017. They emphasize the importance not only of animal protection but also of animal welfare in more general terms.

The concern for animal welfare, and the compassion for animals seen more broadly throughout India, is reflected in a sentence handed down by the Tis Hazari Court of Delhi in March 1992, in which the judge wrote:

> This fundamental Duty in the Constitution to have compassion for all living creatures thus determines the legal relation between Indian Citizens and animals on Indian soil, whether small ones or large ones. . . . Their place in the Constitutional Law of the land is thus the fountainhead of total rule of law for the protection of animals and provides not only against their ill treatment, but from it also springs a right to life in harmony with human beings. If this enforceable obligation of State is understood, certain results will follow. Avoidance of this [export of live animals for killing] is preserving the Indian Cultural Heritage. . . . India can only export a message of compassion towards all living creatures of the world, as a beacon to preserve ecology, which is the true and common Dharma of all civilisations. (Shiva 2016, 69)

A veterinarian who works at Jeevashram, a shelter for street animals located in Rajokri (New Delhi), made the same point when I interviewed him. It is worth quoting him at length:

> In Hindu culture, or let's say in the culture of India, there is the idea that kitchen scraps are for animals . . . you know, like feeding street dogs, putting some food on the roof for birds or grains for peacocks, keeping bowls of water [in the garden, for squirrels and birds]. It's something we have in our blood, in our culture.

Now things are changing, we are developing, we are going towards modernization, everybody is running short of money and time, everybody is worried about his bread and butter. . . . But the love for animals is not under discussion, it remains. We were born with this instinct.

CHAPTER 2

FOOD IN THE MIDDLE

Why include a chapter on food in a book about rabies? What does rabies have to do with food? The food that I discuss in this chapter is not even food for people, which is quite unusual when it comes to studies on the relationship between animals and humans. In fact, most anthropological research looks at animals as food for humans. And so do most people: in a world in which the consumption of meat, and other products of animal origin, is increasing day by day, the idea of humans as a *passive* part of the food chain, as food to be eaten by animals, is the opposite of what our anthropocentric view of the world has accustomed us to, and it sounds rather disturbing.

But food is a key link between human and nonhuman inhabitants of Indian cities and towns. While the people of Delhi and Jaipur probably see their lives as totally disconnected from those of the street animals around them, in reality these animals feed mainly on the outcomes of several types of human behavior. The most direct one, and the easiest to sense, is the waste that humans produce in quantities that other species cannot even imagine. As this chapter shows, however, there are many other sources of food that people make more or less consciously available for their neighbor animals. Although rabies is not a food-borne disease, the ecological condition of Indian towns, including street animals' vast accessibility to food, is what sustains the animal population and at the same time makes it difficult to control rabies. If we are to pursue the One Health strategy of eliminating rabies, the environmental component cannot be ignored: while rabies does not make the environment sick, a sick environment helps rabies to thrive. Claude Lévi-Strauss's description of Indian towns is useful for pinning down the ecological context of rabies in which this research takes place: "Filth, chaos, promiscuity, congestion; ruins, huts, mud, dirt; dung, urine, pus, humors, secretions and running sores: all the things against which we expect urban life to give us organized protection, all the things we hate and guard against at such great cost, all these by-products of cohabitation do not see any limitation on it in India. They are more like a natural environment which the Indian town needs in order to prosper" (1992, 134).

Within such an ecological community (by which I mean an assemblage of at least two populations of different species in the same geographical area), a food web results from the complex interconnection of several linear food chains. Besides the well-known herbivorous and carnivorous feeding habits, there is also saprophagy, the eating of nonliving organic material. One type of saprophagy is necrophagy, the consumption of human and nonhuman animal flesh in a more or less advanced state of decomposition. Finally, another feeding habit is coprophagy, the eating of feces. All of these food choices can be seen on the streets of Delhi and Jaipur.

When Vultures Are No More

When I visited Mumbai for the first time, in 2007, I immediately headed to the Hanging Gardens on the advice of my trusty Routard guidebook, which recommended this place for the unique natural spectacle it offers: the circling vultures who come down to the Towers of Silence to eat the corpses buried in the sky by the Parsi community. I remember that I spent almost an hour taking pictures of the birds, trying to observe them as carefully as possible despite the dazzling sunlight. Now, thirteen years later, I know that my ornithological efforts were completely useless. They were not vultures at all, for India had experienced the most rapid and alarming catastrophe in the history of ornithology a decade earlier.

The devastation concerned three species of vulture endemic to south Asia: the Oriental white-backed vulture (*Gyps bengalensis*), the long-billed vulture (*Gyps indicus*), and the slender-billed vulture (*Gyps tenuirostris*). In 2007, what had once been described as the most prominent bird species in the world was put on the Red List of critically endangered species, a list drafted by the International Union for Conservation of Nature. As Vibhu Prakash of the Bombay Natural History Society observed at the screening of Mike Pandey's documentary *The Vanishing Vultures*, a picture taken at the Timarpur garbage dump in Delhi in the 1970s captured thousands of vultures in a single shot. At that time, India had perhaps forty million Oriental white-backed vultures, but thirty years later its population had crashed, falling by more than 99.9%. For the other two vulture species, the collapse reached "only" 97% (Prakash et al. 2007, 132).

Vultures can no longer be seen in any of Delhi's garbage dumps, and in Lodhi Garden, one of the city's most famous parks, a sign sadly reads: "Huge groups of vultures were a common sight on Lodhi Garden Tombs till 1999. Since then, due to reasons not yet clear, rarely sighted." Although vultures are not among the animals I studied, I was very interested in knowing what people thought about their sudden disappearance. The various opinions I randomly collected mirror the bewilderment that Delhiites experienced at the time: "If now there are so many corpses that remain in the open without being consumed by vultures, the reason is that those people committed so many sins that even vultures refuse to touch them! Now these things happen, but they did not happen in the past"; "Some white people must have come and taken the vultures to their country. This proves their utility"; "I think they left our country because of pollution"; "I heard Chinese people took them."

The real reason for their death is diclofenac, a nonsteroidal anti-inflammatory drug (NSAID) widely used in several human and veterinary medicines. Diclofenac was first introduced in India as an analgesic and antipyretic for use in humans. It was then launched and mass-produced for veterinary purposes in the 1990s, mainly for the treatment of inflammation (especially in mastitis—Senacha et al. 2008, 158), fever, pain, and injury in domestic livestock. Soon thereafter, its toxicity to vultures began to decimate the vulture population. Surprisingly, while these birds are exceptionally resistant to lethal bacteria such as anthrax thanks to their strong stomach acid and high body temperature, they are unusually sensitive to diclofenac. In fact, within a few weeks of consuming meat from the carcasses of livestock recently injected with the drug, they develop visceral gout and die of kidney failure. Even small doses of diclofenac are fatal to vultures, so given their habit of feeding in large groups, even a tiny portion of the ungulate carcasses available to vultures is enough to deliver a lethal dose. Moreover, these birds are more vulnerable than other species of scavengers because they are usually the first to arrive at a carcass and they consume most of the flesh, particularly the soft visceral organs that contain high concentrations of the drug.

In 2003, diclofenac was found to be the cause of the shocking decline in the vulture population, and on May 11, 2006, India's drug controller general revoked all licenses granted for the manufacture of diclofenac for veterinary use, a process to be completed within three months. At the same time, it began promoting the production and sale of meloxicam as a vulture-safe alternative. But because diclofenac is cheap and effective, it is hard to replace—and its human formulations are still legal. So even after the ban, diclofenac labeled "for human use only" has continued to be widely sold in pharmacies without a doctor's prescription and purchased by (often unregistered) veterinarians and livestock owners to be used illegally for veterinary purposes. Only in 2015 did the Ministry of Health and Family Welfare ban the manufacture and sale of convenient multidose vials of human formulations of diclofenac (Venkateshwarlu 2015)—too late. In 2019 a new article reported a still alarmingly low number of vultures (Prakash et al. 2019, 55). Meloxicam has now replaced diclofenac, but other NSAIDs (aceclofenac, carprofen, flunixin, ketoprofen, and nimesulide) widely used in livestock have also been found to be toxic to vultures.

What played a critical role in the widespread diffusion of diclofenac was not only its affordability but also the position of cattle in both the Indian economy and Hindu culture and religion. Chapter 5 delves more deeply into these issues, but for now it will suffice to mention a few key points. Cows sustain life in rural India by providing milk and ghee (clarified butter), which are used both for nourishment and in religious rituals, and offspring that represent a guarantee (females through their milk and males through their draft power) of the families' future. Cattle also provide dung that is used as fuel. On a symbolic level, cows are thought to embody many positive qualities, which explains why Hindu farmers in particular do their best to assure them a life without suffering and, in the end, a natural death without pain, as euthanasia is not a legal option in most Indian states. This is why many cattle carcasses show very high residues of diclofenac, which is uselessly administered to dying animals and thus remains active in their bodies after their death, when vultures have easy access to them. Because most Indian states forbid the slaughter of cattle and the sale of their meat, cattle carcasses are not disposed of in a controlled manner. Instead, they are left in the open in rural areas or in carcass dumps throughout urban areas for vultures and other scavengers to feed on. Occasionally, their hide and bones are removed by specialized collectors, who work as intermediaries with the leather and gelatin industries, but their flesh is often left for scavenging animals.

Among the many scavenging animals in India and worldwide, vultures are obligate scavengers—that is, eating carcasses is their normal feeding behavior; they do not opportunistically alternate between predation and scavenging. This method of food procurement is the reason for their well-adapted physical features, such as the long, unfeathered neck, which allows them easily to reach the internal organs of dead animals, and the strong gastric acids that digest decaying meat. These characteristics contribute to making vultures nature's most efficient scavengers. Now that vulture populations have been decimated, secondary scavengers such as crows, egrets, rats, pigs, and, especially, dogs are filling the niche they have vacated, benefiting from an unprecedented lack of competition over carcasses, which is continuously guaranteed by India's elevated number of livestock (512 million) (Ministry of Agriculture 2012, 14). This increased availability of food occurs on the streets, dumping sites, and open fields of both urban and rural India. In fact, according to a study of the value of vultures as scavengers, a vulture is worth 696,000 rupees (US$10,000) in urban India and 585,000 rupees (US$8,500) in rural areas (Shrivastava 2016). Similarly, the problem of the widespread use of diclofenac to treat cattle has been found to be the same in both urban and rural areas (Senacha et al. 2008, 158). Indian towns, let us remember, fit the description of zoöpolises (Wolch 1998, 119).

As far as environmental and health hazards are concerned, the replacement of vultures with dogs is problematic on many levels. First, since dogs are not as efficient as vultures at carcass disposal, rotten and potentially infected carcasses can spread diseases to wildlife, livestock, and humans and can contaminate water and land. Second, dogs breed much faster than vultures do, so an abundance of food can boost their population exponentially. Third, because dogs are the main carriers of rabies in India, their population increase can lead to an escalation in the number of bites and potential rabies cases. Moreover, while vultures, being birds, cannot contract rabies by feeding on the flesh of a rabid animal, dogs can; even if this risk is statistically low, it must be considered. Some scholars (Markandya et al. 2008; Prakash et al. 2003) have already drawn a direct connection between the disappearance of vultures, the increase in the dog population, and the growth in the number of dog bites and rabies deaths. In May 2019, a village in western Uttar Pradesh experienced this connection firsthand, and in the worst way, when a seven-year-old girl was mauled to death by a pack of hungry street dogs while she was walking through the fields to deliver food to her father (Trivedi 2019). Also in 2019, a six-year-old boy was killed on the outskirts of Bhopal by street dogs, who also attacked his mother when she tried to save her son (*Times of India* 2019b). Tragic incidents like these should remind us that no matter how cute and docile our "best friends" can be, dogs are predators. In situations of distress, conflict, competition over resources, and human violence or neglect, their predatory instinct can prevail.

Decaying Bodies

Saprophagous animals like dogs find easy food not only at sites where dead livestock are dumped and vultures are no more. Riverbanks where deceased Hindus are paid their last respects and Muslim cemeteries can be equally profitable for starving dogs. While I was working as a volunteer at the animal rescue NGO Help In Suffering in Jaipur in 2013, a veterinarian approached me one day with a poster in his hands and bitterness in his eyes. The poster had been given to him by a spokesperson for the Muslim community who lived near the animal hospital. Low-quality amateur pictures showed dogs digging up graves in a nearby Muslim cemetery, unearthing the bodies, eating them, and carrying the decaying remains around. In Delhi, a similar violation of burial sites is common on the sandy shores of the Yamuna River, in and around the Wazirabad barrage and the Nigambodh Ghat (a ghat refers to the sacred shore of a river). One morning I was chatting with the priest who oversees a small cremation site in that area, when suddenly he apologized and walked away, grumbling something about the danger represented by dogs. He walked toward two men whom I had seen arriving an hour before, one with a small red bundle in his arms and the other carrying a shovel. Now they were near the shore, engaged in tense discussion. When Manish reached them, he invited them to move some meters away from the waterline and pointed to a spot among small heaps of stones and shabby shrubs where stuffed toys were hanging. When he returned, he explained that he had had to intervene because the men were about to choose a site near the water where the earth is too soft, and dogs would soon have removed the stones placed on the grave and dug up the baby they were burying.

Hindu funeral customs have three procedures for the disposal of corpses. The most common is cremation, but certain categories of people either do not need or are not allowed to go through the fire purification—for example, *sadhus* (ascetics), babies under the age of two, women who die during pregnancy or childbirth, lepers, and people who die of snakebite or infectious diseases such as smallpox. These people are either buried or disposed of through *jal samadhi* (water burial, typically in a river). Fire usually takes no more than five hours to burn an adult body to ashes and small bony slivers that are then thrown into the river. But cremation does not always proceed smoothly. If the quantity of decent-quality wood—at least 400 kilograms (880 pounds) of good logs for an adult body—costs more than a family can afford, corpses remain partially unburned and are thrown into the river, occasionally with a stone tied to them to keep them from surfacing. Destitute families that cannot pay for a proper funeral, which costs 3,000 to 7,000 rupees (US$45 to $100), and make the painful decision not to cremate their beloved using garbage or tires simply float their loved ones down the river in the dark of night.

A priest who manages a temple just a few meters south of the massive Wazirabad barrage on the Yamuna told me that while corpses are thrown into the river all year round, they become particularly visible in the dry season, when the water level drops, and at the peak of the monsoon season, when the power of the Yamuna, swelled by the heavy rains, moves the corpses hidden beneath its surface. His colleague, who works at the cremation site on the opposite shore of the river, came to me holding a box full of pictures showing some of the corpses he and his staff had removed from the river in previous years at the request of municipal authorities. This man, who felt a deep sense of personal responsibility, had photographed the more or less identifiable bodies he and his staff had disposed of, both as a matter of conscience and as proof that they had retrieved and buried the bodies properly. Nowadays, he told me, the rules have changed, and whenever he spots a corpse in the river he must call the police, who attempt to identify the body. He is also particularly scrupulous when corpses are buried in his cremation ground, as he knows that dogs constantly scour the shores of the river in search of food. He has several dogs himself, who live with him at the cremation site and rummage in the ashes as soon as the funeral pyres are extinguished. But he clarified immediately, "The dogs who eat people are not mine. Those are *jangli kuttas* [literally, dogs of the forest, i.e., wild dogs]. They come out at night in packs of twenty or thirty. For my dogs I cook good food, a lot of food, so they aren't hungry and don't eat people. The food I cook for them is non-veg—although I am veg—so they don't need to eat other meat."

According to a survey carried out in Delhi in 2009, 7% of 1,004 respondents admitted that they dispose of dead bodies (especially of children) in the Yamuna. In percentage terms, these data are not particularly impressive, but considering that the population of Delhi is almost nineteen million, the number of decaying bodies available to scavenging animals is not negligible. It is particularly important to note that only 12% of respondents said that they do *not* perform religious rituals in the Yamuna, and even fewer, 0.8%, claimed that they were open to the possibility of burying at least animal carcasses instead of dumping them in the river (PICT 2009a, 53). The Central Pollution Control Board claims that disposal of infant corpses in the river is practiced along the entire length of the Yamuna, and that floating "human dead bodies partially eaten by animals and in a rotten state are generally observed in the lower part of the river" (CPCB 2006, 21).

This wretched state of affairs is not limited to the Yamuna or to Delhi. The Ganges, which flows for 2,500 kilometers through most northern Indian states, providing water to about four hundred million people, suffers from the same situation. The *Water Quality Studies Ganga System Status Report*, published in 1987 by the then Ministry of Water Resources, opens with a picture captioned "dogs and predatory birds feasting on floating corpses in Ganga at Varanasi." In Kanpur, the second-largest industrial town in northern India, the NGO Eco Friends has launched annual cleanup drives since 1993 to cleanse the river of dead bodies, both human and animal. Its website reports that in 1997 the group removed 180 human corpses, over the course of three days, from the ten-kilometer stretch of the Ganges that flows through Kanpur. About ten years later, the number of human and animal corpses fished out of the river had been reduced by two-thirds, but the disposal of corpses in the Ganges has never entirely ceased. On January 14, 2015, more than one hundred unidentified skeletons and uncremated bodies, mostly of young women and children, surfaced in a shallow minor tributary of the Ganges between Kanpur and Lucknow. Television and newspaper reports showed these bloated corpses, in an advanced state of decay, being eaten by dogs and crows. In Agra, the stretch of the Yamuna that flows placidly between the world-famous Taj Mahal and the Agra Fort is dotted by garbage and, occasionally, stinking human corpses and animal carcasses. In Varanasi, where pious Hindus queue up before charitable institutions to be sure to die in the holy city, the situation is even worse. The two main cremation ghats—Manikarnika and Harishchandra—are overworked, with pyres that burn day and night and *doms* (members of the caste traditionally responsible for disposing of corpses) who are predictably interested in speeding up the roughly 30,000 funerals they oversee each year in order to maximize their income.

In Delhi, as in Varanasi, electric crematoriums have been built near traditional cremation sites to solve the problem of half-burned corpses and to provide cheaper funerals to destitute families. Previously, in 1986, the Ganga Action Plan had resorted to another solution: *Nilssonia gangetica*, or flesh-eating turtles. These twenty-kilogram, eighty-centimeter-long soft-shelled animals were once quite common in the Ganges and its tributaries, but about 40,000 turtles were purposely bred on government farms as part of this plan and released into the river. The turtles posed no danger to humans, but they were efficient underwater scavengers. The India Water Portal website says that this breeding program was suspended in 1993 but resumed in 2005, with at least 1,000 turtles introduced into the river every year. According to the *Times of India* (2011), however, this intervention has been undermined by the poaching and marketing of these turtles in West Bengal and Bangladesh. Thus the food chain envisioned by the Ganga Action Plan turned on itself, offering for human consumption the animal that was to have eaten them.

As noted above, rivers and riverbanks have become dumping grounds not only for human corpses but also for animal carcasses. According to Hindu precepts, animals should not be burned, and cows in particular should be given *jal samadhi*, or water burial. From a practical perspective, dumping dead animals in rivers is also the easiest and quickest way to dispose of them. In Delhi this is illegal, and people can phone municipal collectors and ask them to remove the bodies of animals, both large and small, from the places where they have died. In spite of this, it is not uncommon to spot the decaying carcasses of goats, pigs, and dogs in garbage heaps that float on the Yamuna and accumulate along its shores. During the period when I was a regular visitor at the cremation site on the Yamuna near the

Wazirabad barrage, the carcass of an adult horse was stealthily unloaded one night about a hundred meters away from the funeral pyres. For a week I went daily to check on the state of that carcass, and every day I saw at least one dog feeding on it. Animal carcasses are found not only in or along rivers. Animals killed by cars and those who have died from other injuries or diseases are often spotted on the streets of Delhi and Jaipur, occasionally being fed upon by other animals. Near one of the gates of Jawaharlal Nehru Stadium in Delhi, I once saw a skinny puppy being eaten by his even skinnier sibling.

Eating Shit

Within the food web that nourishes street animals, humans become a source of food not only when they die but also during their lives, through the feces that they introduce into the environment. In India, the debate about the harmful effects of human excrement on the environment and public health is usually linked to the compromised state of many water bodies. In many Indian cities and towns, including the capital, New Delhi, the lack or inadequacy of sewer systems is a major problem. India generates 1.7 million tons of fecal waste each day, but 78% of its sewage is untreated and goes directly into open gutters along streets, canals, rivers, and lakes (Rohilla et al. 2016). In Delhi, for example, the city's twenty-one treatment plants can manage only 48% of the 3.8 billion liters of sewage produced every day (Global Interfaith WASH Alliance 2014, 11, 16). Consequently, in the twenty-two-kilometer stretch of the Yamuna River that flows through of the city of Delhi, the river receives 79% of its pollution between Wazirabad barrage and Okhla barrage (Central Pollution Control Board 2006, 19). When the river leaves Delhi south of Okhla barrage, its biochemical oxygen demand value (i.e., the amount of dissolved oxygen needed in water if is to be safe for drinking, bathing, etc.) reached 144 milligrams per liter in February 2006; the permissible value for direct human contact is three milligrams per liter. A similar situation prevails with respect to fecal coliforms, which in Okhla in February 2005 reached the exorbitant count of almost two billion per deciliter, the highest count of all the rivers in the country (PICT 2009b, 30). This level is far too high to be safe even for farming (where the limit is 5,000 per deciliter), let alone bathing (where the limit is 500), never mind drinking (where the limit is 50). The result is that the Yamuna is biologically dead in most of Delhi, as its oxygen level has been stable at 0% for too many years in a row (PICT 2009c, 9). As Sushmita Sengupta (2015) observes, the river ceases to exist at Wazirabad, before entering Delhi. It was precisely at this location, at the Nigambodh Ghat, that I rented a boat to row across the Yamuna and observe its water close up. That night, I wrote in my fieldwork diary, "It looks like a boiling and foamy vegetable soup that has the color of asphalt and stinks of a mixture of something chemical, rotten, and revoltingly sweetish." Sadly, 4% of the Delhiites surveyed by the Peace Institute Charitable Trust agreed that "draining sewage in river Yamuna is a benefit of having a river in Delhi" (PICT 2009a, 30).

Human excrement pollutes the environment not only by ending up in rivers through inefficient sewage systems but also through the practice of open defecation. This means that people do not use a toilet to defecate; to *latrine karna* (literally, "to do latrine"), they take advantage of fields, bushes, forests, roadsides, or other open spaces such as garbage dumps and urban parks. As slums are often located near the railway lines, train tracks are a common site for defecation among the slum dwellers I met in Delhi. This adds to the problem that the Indian railway system, which carries thirty million people daily and relies on open-discharge toilets, was named in 2011 "the world's biggest open toilet" by the then minister of drinking water and sanitation Jairam Ramesh. India accounts for 64% of the 946 million people in the world who practice open defecation because they do not have or do not use private or public toilets (UNICEF 2015, 25). According to the 2011 census, 603 million Indians, or roughly half the population, defecate in the open.

As dogs are coprophagous (they eat the feces of other animals), living alongside humans is greatly advantageous for them. In rural Zimbabwe, for example, human feces make up to 21% of the diet of human-owned but free-roaming dogs, constituting their secondary food source after the porridge provided by their owners (Butler and du Toit 2002, 32). In Indian towns and villages, it is easy to imagine the benefit to dogs of this source of food. If evidence is needed, it is sufficient to keep an eye for a few minutes on a smelly baby diaper dumped on a roadside garbage heap, or simply to talk with slum kids, who will tell you that dogs are a cause of great concern when they defecate on the railway tracks or in the dumping area of the slum, so much so that they usually carry stones to throw at dogs who do not wait for them to leave before pouncing on their feces. Equally telling is the expression "greedier than a dog for the excrement of a young child," used as a biting insult among Muslims.

My ethnographic observations were borne out by an article in the *Times of India* (Mahapatra 2012) reporting on a lawsuit brought by the anti-scavenging NGO Safai Karmachari Andolan that made it to the Supreme Court of India. According to research carried out by this group in 2011, of the roughly 1.3 million dry latrines (i.e., toilets without a flush system) in India, coprophagous animals—mainly dogs and pigs—clean about 497,000, while the remaining 794,000 are emptied by human scavengers, derogatively called *bhangis*. In Delhi the situation is inverted, as animals remove the feces from more than half of the toilets surveyed in the study. Given that one gram of feces, especially children's feces, according to UNICEF, contains ten million viruses and one million bacteria, it is not hard to see why open defecation poses an alarming health threat. In fact, in 2000 the UN set as one of its Millennium Development Goals the eradication of this practice by 2025. In the meantime, dogs are contributing substantially to limiting its ill effects on the environment and public health.

Side by side with dogs, *bhangis* also perform a valuable service to Indian society when it comes to feces disposal (Human Rights Watch 2014; Pathak 1991). Including them in a chapter on the food sources for street animals may seem odd, but it is pivotal to understanding the sociocultural context in which open defecation is practiced. Placed at the very bottom of human society, *bhangis* are not only outcastes, but they also belong to the lowest of the Dalit castes, those traditionally occupied by people who are compelled to do dirty, polluting, degrading jobs that put them in touch with corpses, carcasses, and bodily fluids and excreta. Feces are seen as the worst and most polluting of the twelve secretions produced by the human body. One of the traditional tasks of *bhangis* consists of manually emptying and cleaning the dry latrines of households of higher castes, generally using only a broom, a tin plate, and a basket, and transporting the feces out of built-up areas or to wherever they can be dumped. Until recently, these people had to hang small bells around their necks that informed others of their presence, in order to allow upper castes to keep themselves at a distance. This is no longer required, but they continue to carry their neighbors' feces and discarded sanitary napkins in baskets on their heads.

As the Indian constitution has outlawed the concept of untouchability and the use of the term "untouchable," nowadays the legal term for *bhangi* is *safai karamchari*, or manual scavenger, with no caste connotation. In 1993 the Indian government passed the Employment of Manual Scavengers and

Construction of Dry Latrines (Prohibition) Act (strengthened in 2013 by the Prohibition of Employment as Manual Scavengers and Their Rehabilitation Act), which forbade both this revolting job and made dry latrine owners liable for prosecution. Nevertheless, about ten million dry latrines are still being manually emptied across the country (Sathasivam 2014), and the practice of manual scavenging continues unabated, even if the exact number of people compelled to perform it is hotly debated, with government estimates significantly lower than those put forth by nonprofit groups like Safai Karmachari Andolan. More important, since 1993, not a single person has been convicted of hiring a manual scavenger, which carries a mandatory sentence of a year in jail and a fine of 2,000 rupees (US$30) (*Hindustan Times* 2015b). As a result, hundreds of people who continue to be illegally employed in this work throughout India die every year from asphyxiation (caused by entering septic tanks half-naked and without protective gear), infections and skin diseases, and alcoholism caused by depression, desperation, and social humiliation. Filmmaker Divya Bharathi's documentary *Kakkoos* (Toilets in Tamil), freely available on YouTube, depicts their heart-rending suffering. The practice is not restricted to remote rural villages. In fact, manual scavenging has long been a reality even in Delhi, where in May 2009 the "capital's shame" was reported directly and in detail to the Supreme Court of India (Mahapatra 2009).

Several initiatives have been implemented in the past decade to end open defecation in India. In 2012, a campaign called "Toilets Are Beautiful" was introduced in northern India to awaken public opinion to this taboo topic. In 2014, Prime Minister Narendra Modi launched the Swachh Bharat Abhiyan (Clean India Mission), which aimed to make India free of open defecation by October 2019 by constructing toilets wherever needed across rural India. The effort required to meet this goal was, numerically speaking, gigantic. To look only at Delhi, at least half of Delhiites live in unauthorized human settlements, and 80% of the unregistered slums in the city have no public toilets (PICT 2009b, 13). Of the 3,192 public urinals in Delhi, only 132 are for women (Sheikh 2008, 23). In the Ashok Vihar slum, one latrine is shared by 2,083 people (Baviskar 2004, 89). In rural areas, 60% of households have no access to private or public facilities (Ministry of Drinking Water and Sanitation 2014), in part because public toilets are often used as storerooms for fodder, or exist only on paper (Jitendra, Bera, and Gupta 2014, 34). But statistics alone cannot convey the complexity of this issue. And the reasons for open defecation are not only practical and material, not only a matter of a scarcity of toilets, or of chronic poverty. In fact, televisions and mobile phones are far more abundant than toilets in Indian households (UNICEF 2012, 8). Religious, social, and cultural factors play an equally decisive role, particularly among Hindus. Michael Geruso and Dean Spears note that despite being poorer, Muslims in India are less likely than Hindus to defecate in the open (2015, 1). Similarly, Diane Coffey et al. observe that in Bangladesh, a Muslim country poorer than India, only 5% of people defecate in the open (2017, 59). Pakistan, another Muslim country, fully met the Millennium Development Goals target for sanitation in 2015 (UNICEF 2015, 68).

Several explanations for the persistence of this problem in India have been advanced. First, if they are to be used and appreciated, toilets must be maintained and kept clean. A recent World Bank survey in Uttar Pradesh found that 40% of people with toilets in their homes did not use them because they were considered dirty (Pandey 2018). During my stay in India, I always lived with Indian people, and I witnessed a sort of panic over the task of toilet cleaning quite regularly. As I always lived with middle-class people, they could easily afford at least one housekeeper, for tasks that ranged from cooking to housecleaning and laundry but never included cleaning the toilet, as our helpers were not Dalits and refused to do this job. No one, neither the housekeepers nor my housemates, ever thought of cleaning the toilet except by emptying a bucket of water into it, so the bathroom was always the most neglected room in the house in terms of cleaning. I noticed the same practice in most of the spick-and-span, scrupulously pure houses I visited. Thus I often took this housework upon myself in the shared flats where I lived, which unfailingly caused ill-concealed looks of disdain from my flatmates. Disdain became loathing the day I cleaned our cats' litterbox: my flatmate insisted that this was the task of the housekeeper, who had agreed to do this job rather than clean our toilet. This sort of cultural coprophobia (the abnormal fear of contact with feces) also prevents people from sharing toilets, especially in the case of public facilities, where one does not know who has used them or their position in the caste hierarchy and thus their level of purity. A survey carried out in 2013–14 in rural northern India found that only 7% of the surveyed households with a working latrine reported that people from outside the household (including close relatives living next door) also used it (Coffey et al. 2014).

Relieving oneself in the open is such a long-standing, ingrained behavior that eradicating it requires nothing less than a total change of mindset. When I visited the NGO Sulabh International's Museum of Toilets in South West Delhi, the engineer who showed me the public toilet prototypes they have developed over the years told me frankly that the most difficult job is coming up with a toilet that satisfies men's desire to look around while urinating. He was particularly proud of a spiral-shaped, roofless latrine, made with a curving wall that increases in height until it blocks the user from the sight of passersby but allows him the pleasure of looking out and breathing in fresh air that does not stink of a dirty toilet. This engineer's concern with the cultural acceptability of toilets is well founded: according to a UNICEF study carried out in Tamil Nadu, 5% of respondents claimed that using a toilet was "not in our culture," and another 4% were dissuaded from using one by household elders (UNICEF 2012, 5). Other reasons given for preferring open defecation include saving water, protecting women from the embarrassing sight of men, and the brief respite from annoying wives and mothers (Ramani 2016).

In another study, Diane Coffey et al. (2017, 59) conclude that beliefs, values, and norms concerning purity, pollution, and caste greatly contribute to India's uniquely high rate of open defecation. In particular, they found that the vast majority of people refuse to use the underground soak pits promoted by WHO and subsidized by the Indian government, which are cheap and do not require water. The reason is that they require manual emptying, a job considered too humiliating and ritually polluting for anyone but Dalits. Smaller pits—those mainly built under Swachh Bharat Abhiyan, as their lower cost can be subsidized by this plan, which offers a reimbursement of 12,000 rupees (US$170) per toilet—are particularly disregarded, as they require frequent emptying. Dean Spears and Amit Thorat (2016, 1) conclude that there is a strong correlation between beliefs about untouchability and the practice of open defecation in India, which cannot be explained by economic or educational factors. Several other studies have also highlighted the systemic complexity of setting up an ethically sensitive, scientifically grounded, sustainable, credible sanitation revolution on this scale. The main issue remains the elimination of manual scavenging and the underlying idea that some people come into the world specifically to clean toilets and to die from asphyxiation in sewer lines (Gatade 2015; Prasad and Ray 2018).

On September 26, 2019, two cousins, Roshani Balmiki, age twelve, and Avinash Balmiki, age ten, were beaten to death by two brothers, Hakam and

Rameshwar Yadav, while defecating on a road in Bhavkhedi, their village in Madhya Pradesh. They died on the spot. The children, as their surname suggests, were Dalits, as "Balmiki" is synonymous with "Bhangi." Avinash's mud house, on the outskirts of the village, did not have a working toilet. His grandfather had a toilet built under Swachh Bharat Abhiyan, but its underground sludge pit had flooded during the heavy monsoon rains that hit India in 2019 and was temporarily unusable. The Yadav brothers, as their family name indicates, are upper-caste people and the main landowners in the village. In Bhavkhedi, dry latrines have long since been replaced by toilets that are connected to a sludge pit, but some members of the Yadav family still employ the Balmiki family to clean them for twenty rupees (US$0.30) per household (*Economic Times* 2019b; Lalwani 2019). One week after this incident, the prime minister celebrated the 150th anniversary of Mahatma Gandhi's birth by declaring India free of open defecation thanks to the construction of 110 million toilets in record time. Records indicate that all households in the village of Bhavkhedi have had a toilet since April 4, 2018. Police investigated the murder case to ascertain whether the motive was "superstition" linked to the practice of open defecation or "untouch-ability" (Tomar and Gupta 2019).

This kind of incident is rare, luckily, but children experience several other negative consequences due to open defecation on a daily basis. Girls are at continuous risk of sexual molestation, and both sexes suffer from the lack of adequate hygiene. As I observed in urban slums, young children are generally allowed to defecate whenever and wherever they feel the need. Consequently, they habitually do it alone or are assisted only by a peer. They generally clean their private parts with their hands, their clothes, earth, or plastic scraps. This increases pathways for the transmission of diseases such as cholera, hepatitis A, and, especially, diarrhea. Moreover, because railway tracks are a common defecation site for street and slum dwellers, the children I met experienced constant anxiety about the risk of being hit or run over by a train. Significantly, open defecation also exposes people to dog bites and thus to the risk of contracting rabies. In June 2019, the *New Indian Express* reported the case of a woman who was killed by a pack of dogs while on her way to relieve herself in a field in Odisha. This important causal relationship, explored more deeply in chapter 6, has never been given adequate attention in the studies on dog bites and rabies exposure in India.

Not only defecation but the overall issue of sanitation is considered a socially unacceptable topic in India, particularly among the upper castes.

Bindeshwar Pathak, the founder of Sulabh International, an NGO devoted to environmental sanitation, proper waste management, and other social reforms, was ostracized for his work in these areas and has spent his life fighting this attitude of aversion. He has received several international prizes and awards for his work, and the UN has recognized the toilet technology developed by Sulabh International as a global best practice that could improve the lives of three billion people across the globe. Nevertheless, when he joined the Bhangi-Mukti (Scavengers' Liberation) Cell of the Bihar Gandhi Centenary Celebrations Committee in 1968 from his village in rural Bihar, and when he lived with scavenger families for his PhD research in sociology, people could not believe that a Brahmin was talking about excrement and sitting next to *bhangis* in a temple. As Viswanathan Raghunathan and M. A. Eswaran observe, "We [Indians] think shame lies not in millions upon millions of us defecating out in the open, but with them who clean up after us. In our strange logic, dirtiers are somehow superior to cleaners!" (2012, 19). What Mike Davis says of the urban poor applies equally well to manual scavengers: "Shit still sickeningly mantles the lives of the urban poor as (to quote Marcus again [see Marcus 1974, 185]) 'a virtual objectification of their social condition, their place in society'" (2006, 138). Or, as Apula Singh and Viral Shah (2016) put it, "Our excessive reliance on 'others' to manage 'our' waste has let the situation go out of hand."

Living on Garbage, Dying of Garbage

Quantitatively speaking, garbage is the most important food source for street animals in urban India. Thus garbage production is a pivotal anthropogenic factor (one resulting from the influence of human beings on the world they share with nonhuman others) in the relationship between people and animals. This is particularly evident in the cities, where high human density and lack of space make proper management of solid waste an increasingly challenging task. As India's urban population is growing 3.5% annually, the waste generated in cities and towns is expected to increase by 5% every year (*Down to Earth* 2016). In the past twenty-five years it has more than doubled, reaching the sixty-two million tons of domestic garbage produced in 2014. Given that the production of waste corresponds to family income, urban areas are a bigger concern than rural ones. In fact, per capita waste production is 0.3 kilograms in a slum, compared to

1.5 kilograms in a middle-class colony, and for every 1,000 rupees (US$15) increase in income, solid waste increases by one kilogram per month (Vishwanathan and Tränkler 2003, 40). Delhi ranks first not only in the quantity of solid waste produced but also in the percentage of plastic components it contains, while Jaipur comes in thirtieth (Centre for Science and Environment 2016).

In urban India, the composition of municipal solid waste is undergoing a major shift as the use of plastics and paper grows in proportion to the rise of the middle class and consumerist culture. However, given that most of the Indian population still lives in rural areas and that traditional Indian cuisine is largely based on fresh products, 50% of Indian waste is organic, mostly composed of vegetable and fruit scraps. In addition to private kitchens, other sources of food waste are restaurants and street stalls—which generally dispose of animal offal and bones by simply throwing them at nearby street dogs—and wedding feasts. There are roughly 100,000 weddings and other social events every day in India, where the food offered in buffets aims not only to stuff the guests but, especially, to display the affluence of the host families by providing a spectacular, memorable, and enviable wedding party. One result is that at least a fifth of the prepared food is discarded (Indian Institute of Public Administration 2011, 13). To address this waste, in 2011 the Ministry of Consumer Affairs, Food, and Public Distribution proposed a controversial measure: setting a limit on the number of guests and dishes served at weddings. Needless to say, in a country that revolves around social relationships, this proposal was immediately shot down (George 2011).

The Municipal Solid Waste Rules passed in 2000 by the then Ministry of Environment and Forests required local bodies to collect waste, separate it into categories, and safely transport, process, and dispose of it properly. Delhi, along with many other cities and towns, found it hard to comply with these rules, with the result that only 80% of municipal solid waste nationwide was collected, and only 28% of it was properly treated and recycled (Sambyal 2016a). The Solid Waste Management Rules issued in 2016 aimed to be more effective. However, as the ministry reported on its website in October of that year, the three landfill sites used by Delhi's municipal authority—Bhalswa, Okhla, and Ghazipur (adjacent to the city's main slaughterhouse and near the fish and meat market)—do not meet legal and scientific standards. In fact, Ghazipur landfill was declared saturated in 2002, yet as in the other two, unsegregated garbage has continued to pile up (Adak 2019b). Apart from the natural process of decay and the occasional open burning in bins (sometimes done by municipal workers, sometimes by residents as a means of rubbish removal, and sometimes by street dwellers for warmth at night), only scavenging animals and ragpickers help to keep the situation under control, if barely.

Several factors contribute to the relentless piling up of rubbish. For one thing, finding a proper litter bin in public places can be a challenge. Data from the MCD in 2012 put the number of dustbins in Delhi at 342 (Kumar 2013, 11), or one dustbin for every 32,000 people. One day, while walking in Connaught Place, the heart of New Delhi, I got firsthand confirmation of this poor state of affairs. Strangers in this area have zero chance of walking alone or in peace, for they are invariably accosted by touts, peddlers, and other solicitors who offer to satisfy their every conceivable need—for a price. Given their experience with hundreds of tourists each day, they have a ready answer to whatever protest or objection their marks may attempt. I knew this all too well, but one day when I had just finished eating a fried snack, I discovered to my great satisfaction that there is one thing that will totally throw these hustlers off balance: the request for a litter bin. In the astonishment of the young man who had been badgering me I read not only the disappointment of his hopeful expectation but also dismay at never having been confronted with this evidently unthinkable question before. I later learned, from an amusing anecdote told by Viswanathan Raghunathan (2006, 154), that the use of rubbish bins is not unthinkable but—possibly even worse—unacceptable. When a city franchisee of a national pizza chain offered to place garbage bins along the street outside the restaurant, the municipal officer refused the gift, saying that this would make the street filthy, as people would deliberately throw the garbage around the bins rather than into them. Without such bins, the garbage would be spread over a larger area, making that particular street no dirtier than others.

Another factor that contributes to garbage buildup is that Indian families are not yet used to segregating waste by type, and government efforts to promote the habit have so far been disorganized and ineffective. Rajkumar Joshi and Sirajuddin Ahmed (2016, 6) report, for example, that an attempt in 2009 by the Delhi government to introduce dustbins of different colors was a more or less complete failure. And the practice of domestic composting has not been around long enough to show results on a large scale (Kumar et al. 2009, 885). This is why organic waste easily finds its way first to the mountains of garbage that line Indian streets and surround market areas, and then to the stomachs of scavenging animals who constantly rummage through them. In addition, before municipal collectors move garbage to landfills, there is no organized or formal system to prevent people from dumping it in neighborhood *dalaos* (covered structures for garbage disposal rarely closed to the outside and easily accessible in any case to street animals) or wherever they please. In some residential areas, handcart-equipped door-to-door collectors roam the streets shouting "Kabari," an invitation to residents to hand over their domestic waste. After sorting out what they can resell to recycling centers, however, these collectors empty their carts in the same *dalaos*.

In short, garbage production and disposal are deeply entangled with cultural practices. Indian housewives work tirelessly to keep their houses clean and tidy, in part because Lakshmi, the Hindu goddess of wealth, is known to visit only shiny houses (Leslie 1989, 59). Consequently, there is no reason to run the risk of polluting the house with its own dirt by keeping a bin inside it. As long as it is outside the house, its indiscriminate dumping is a matter of no concern. At most, housewives may worry if their neighbors start grumbling about the nature of the garbage that has been dumped too close to their homes. For this reason, social norms in southern India prohibit putting domestic waste in closed containers, such as bags; instead, it is left open to the vigilant eye of a society obsessed with pollution (Lüthi 2010, 73). In an attempt to sum up the Hindu attitude toward personal, domestic, and environmental filth, it does not seem wrong to speak of an exasperation with the NIMBY (not in my back yard) concept. Dirt does not necessarily need to be removed because it is detrimental to health and hygiene, but pollution must be driven away as far as possible—it does not matter where—because it is too contaminating.

In describing lack of social empathy in the Hindu context, Nirad Chaudhuri wrote in 1951 that "the streets were regularly watered, swept and even scrubbed. But while the street-cleaning ended by about six o'clock in the morning and three in the afternoon, the kitchen-maids would begin to deposit the off-scouring exactly at quarter past six and quarter past three. Nothing seemed capable of making either party modify its hours" (269). I noticed this same indifference toward collaboration and social sympathy every morning during my stay in the flat in Jangpura, when the kitchen lady started peeling potatoes, always dropping the peels on the floor after the cleaning lady, crawling on her bony knees, had just finished washing it. For months I expected her to react with irritation, but she never did.

What prevents Indian streets from exploding like ecological bombs is mainly the "community of silent and invisible environmentalists," a phrase often used to describe ragpickers by organizations that work for the improvement of their working conditions, the uplift of their social status, and the formal recognition of their service. In Delhi, there are about 300,000 ragpickers—men, women, and children who invade Indian cities at night like a brigade of eco-warriors, and who effectively manage almost 1,100 tons of recyclable waste per day (Sambyal 2016b). Scavenging animals are irreplaceable members of this environmentally friendly multispecies community. They play a critical role, and it perfectly complements that of ragpickers, because they sort out the organic waste in garbage heaps that would pose great public health risks if it were left to rot on the streets. Since recyclers, and thus the ragpickers who sell to them, are not interested in this type of waste, it represents a sort of vacuum, filled thrice daily by the kitchen scraps people discharge into the street. Scavenging animals dispose of this organic waste more or less completely, so much so that pictures of cows ransacking garbage heaps have already become ubiquitous in portrayals of India, as well as in many official documents and reports about waste management released by Indian governmental bodies and research institutes.

About 60–75% of the recyclable waste produced in India consists of plastic (Sambyal 2016b), and it is mainly thanks to ragpickers that the country can make use of this lucrative resource through recycling. While citizens do not seem to properly appreciate the ragpickers' contribution, cattle derive great benefit from their salvaging of plastic from waste dumps, for less plastic is left behind for the cattle to ingest. Even so, more than disease, malnutrition, and road accidents, plastic and other inorganic materials (clothes, sand, shards of glass and ceramics, needles, blades, wires, sanitary napkins, and even small electronic devices) are the primary cause of death for Delhi street cattle (GNCTD 2001, 26). Unlike dogs, who use their canine teeth to lacerate their food, and macaques, who use their fingers and nails to meticulously screen it, cattle are not selective eaters and perfunctorily chew and swallow whatever catches their interest, especially when they are very hungry. Rumination represents an evolutionary adjustment among herbivores, who must constantly be on the alert for predators and thus need a feeding behavior that allows them to store considerable quantities of food after rough chewing and fast swallowing. Karishma, a veterinarian I met at Animal India Trust, told me that she had once removed a mobile phone from the stomach of a cow during a rumenotomy (in which the rumen, one of the four compartments of the cow's digestive system, is incised via the left abdominal wall to remove foreign bodies). As cattle are unable to digest such substances, or to excrete them in feces, they form a stiff pack inside the stomach that continues to grow in size as the animal ingests more foreign matter. Many of the cows on the streets of urban India seem well fed, or they may look pregnant, but according to the veterinarian at the Shri Krishna Goshala (Bawana, North Delhi), at least 85% of them in fact experience an excruciating death under the weight of the plastic they have consumed. In September 2016, the *Times of India* published an article about a cow who was found to have 100 kilograms (220 pounds) of plastic in her stomach (Kaushik 2016). The Karuna Society for Animals and Nature, in Andhra Pradesh, had already documented the ordeal of these so-called plastic cows in 2012. Indian cows have been the unfortunate "canary in the coal mine" for one of the major problems of our time: the ubiquity of plastic in the environment and animal bodies, both human and nonhuman.

In 2015, India's Plastic Waste Management Rules went into effect nationwide, increasing the thickness of plastic bags so that their cost would discourage people from using them (Sambyal 2014). In early 2017, increasing environmental concern pushed the National Green Tribunal to ban the manufacture, import, sale, and use of bags, cutlery, cups, and other forms of single-use plastic in the National Capital Territory of Delhi. In Rajasthan, a complete ban on plastic bags was imposed in 2010. In both states, however, the enforcement of these laws has been far from perfect. In the meantime, animal welfare activists continue to urge citizens to dispose of domestic waste in an animal-friendly way, placing edible food in newspapers or on the ground and inorganic trash in hermetic containers and sites dedicated to that purpose. These suggestions have failed to gain much traction with citizens who often consider scavenging street animals an unhygienic nuisance. Paradoxically, the garbage that people produce in growing quantities does not seem to disturb them in the same way. No wonder Minister Jairam Ramesh said, "Our cities are the dirtiest in the world. If there is a Nobel Prize for dirt and filth, India will win it hands down." Ironically, people blame scavenging animals and ragpickers for this state of affairs (S. Singh 2006, 99), when in fact these scavengers contribute substantially to creating the "Clean Delhi, Green

Delhi" that the Delhi government wanted to achieve for the 2010 Commonwealth Games and beyond.

Offering Food

While animal carcasses, human corpses, feces, and garbage are indirect sources of food for street animals, people also intentionally provide them with actual food, as I discuss in more detail in the chapters that follow.

Though dated, Dina Guha's article "Food in the Vedic Tradition" (1985) remains a valuable source for understanding the role of food in Hinduism and its evolution over time. As in many other religious, social, and historical contexts, food in Vedism was utterly essential not only to personal but also to social existence. In Vedic times (1500–600 B.C.E.), the sanctity of food "pervaded man's social dimensions: it create[d] friendship, brotherhood, and the need to be shared with everyone. . . . The social aspects were intensified, as man was not born to be alone or for his own immediate or extended family, nor for his community. The divine substance [food] was for all men" (Guha 1985, 142–43). Within the growing complexity of an agricultural society, the food that until then had "had no hierarchical qualities or attributes" gradually became part of a new socioeconomic order that "produced a separation, and a hierarchy to nature, man, and the social order" (145–46). In the *Chandogya Upanishad*, food for the first time was ordered and labeled according to its supposedly intrinsic qualities. It was divided into three categories: illuminative, thus pure, *sattvic* foods (dairy products, water, legumes, honey, fruits, vegetables, and cereals) were thought to impart vitality, energy, and longevity and to foster spirituality and mental clarity. *Rajasic* foods (fish, eggs, certain meats, sweets, chocolate, tea, coffee, and wine) were believed to cause sorrow and mental restlessness, and sometimes even disease, by dangerously exciting the passions. Stale and reheated, or *tamasic*, foods were thought to cause lethargy and mental dullness; the worst examples of this "putrid food of darkness" (146) were pork and beef, onion, garlic, highly spiced and seasoned food, and, above all, leftovers. All cooked food, irrespective of category, was then divided into *kaccha* and *pakka*. *Kaccha* food was boiled or roasted, while *pakka* food, more elaborate and hence much purer, was fried in lots of ghee, the clarified butter obtained from one of the best *sattvic* ingredients, cow's milk.

These Vedic categories survive in the Hindu beliefs and classifications of the present day. Leftovers, especially if kept overnight, are considered *tamasic*, as they lose their vital essence and may contain microorganisms. As the *Bhavishya Purana* explains, leftovers are *tamasic* (hence impure) not only as *kaladushta* (cooked food spoiled over time) but also as *samsaraga-dushta* (food polluted by impure substances such as saliva). This explains the widespread habit of hawking and spitting in public. The need to get rid of this polluting substance, called *shthivana*, which literally means "eject-able" (Walker 1968, 341), enjoys complete social approval.

Saliva also reinforces the proper order in interpersonal relationships. Eating leftovers polluted by someone else's saliva is acceptable only for subordinated people, such as wives (to husbands), offspring (to parents), or students (to teachers), and especially members of low castes (to high castes). For example, manual scavengers are expected to beg for food from upper-caste households and to collect and clear up the leftovers after wedding feasts (Rashtriya Garima Abhiyan 2011, 10–11). In November 2017, the state legislative assembly in Karnataka passed the Karnataka Prevention and Eradication of Inhuman Evil Practices and Black Magic Bill, also known as the anti-superstition bill. Among other things, it banned the *made snana* (literally, "leftovers bath"), a religious practice that takes place in a few temples in the state where lower-caste people roll on the leftovers of the upper castes after their communal meal on the temple floor. Incidentally, the bill also banned the refusal of medical treatment for victims of snake, scorpion, or dog bite.

Another pair linked by the consumption of leftovers is the one made by a devotee and his deity. In Hindu temples, this ritual reaches its climax when, after waiting in an endless queue, worshippers get to pay their respects to the image of the god and pass to the officiating priest the food (*prasad*) they have brought to honor and serve the deity. The priest hastily offers the food in the direction of the mouth of the god, who tastes and hence transmutes it, and then gives it back to the devotee, who leaves content, the leftovers infused with divine grace and benevolence. While eating another person's leftovers is usually humiliating, when it comes to the leftovers of a divine meal this act becomes one of intentional "respect pollution" (Harper 1964, 181) that is meant to bestow considerable religious merit. In fact, as Lawrence A. Babb observes, "In the presentation of food to the deity, there is a sense in which the deity is being paid for past or future favors" (1970, 296). This important practice of offering food, and gifts in general (Mauss 1967), is discussed in more detail in the following chapters.

As *prasad* embodies the magnanimity of the deity and the devotee's submissiveness, it is an outrageous sin to throw it away, refuse it, or handle it improperly (e.g., by placing it on a polluting surface such as the ground). The symbolic value of *prasad* can be contrasted to food offered as *daan*, which is food bestowed on the poor or needy—including animals—as part of charitable service (*seva*). Unlike *prasad*, which is limited in quantity, *daan* can be given in liberal quantities. The best place in which to observe these different uses of *daan* and *prasad* is at any temple on the day devoted to its god. Since on that day food is offered in lavish quantities, beggars follow the religious map and calendar of the city to go where they will find the most magnanimous divinities and devotees. Devotees dole out their *prasad* on the doorstep of the temple, where the poorest wait patiently. It is important to note that it is only because *prasad* "is in no sense ordinary food" (Babb 1970, 298) that upper-caste devotees lower themselves to offer food to people so much lower in the caste hierarchy. However, as *prasad* finishes early, the most generous devotees usually buy some food in the stalls that sell devotional objects and ritual food to temple-goers and have it distributed by the sellers. Others pay to have food distributed to the poor, a service that some temples provide: after paying the requisite sum, philanthropists can either distribute the food personally or have it done by the temple staff. Enormous quantities of food are thus distributed, sometimes, as in the case of the Hanuman Mandir of Connaught Place in New Delhi on Tuesdays (see chapter 4), far exceeding actual need. Although beggars do their best to stow the food properly (by sorting it into plastic bags according to its nature and how long it can be kept before spoiling), at a certain point food invariably starts to be left on the ground, where it rots.

Food that is offered to animals can also be given as both *prasad* and *daan*. What distinguishes *prasad* given to animals is that it is distributed next to temples or sacred images of the deities, is given in small amounts, and mainly consists of ritual food (e.g., sweets and bananas). Food given as *daan* is generally much more abundant and varied, and it is left in places generally frequented by animals, by roadsides, on sidewalks, perched on walls, or in bowls chained to trees or cemented on the ground. When these food offerings consist of vegetable peels and other kitchen scraps, they can easily be mistaken for garbage, with one important difference: whereas garbage is thrown on the ground with no particular care, leftovers meant as food offerings are not put in touch with the dirty, hence polluting, ground but are placed in a container or on a newspaper or similar surface. Moreover, the food that is offered to animals, particularly to cows (see chapter 5), is often not a leftover but is something cooked on purpose for them.

CHAPTER 3

DOGS

In the Indian clinics that provide first aid to street animals, it is not uncommon to see dogs with their necks cut open, maggots eating the rotting flesh. Embedded deep in the tissue, iron wires are occasionally found, deliberately tied tightly enough to inflict pain on the animal. More frequently, sincere feelings of attachment and care for the dog prompt people to put a collar—generally a simple plastic cord or piece of fabric—around the neck of a puppy born on a nearby street or to a street dog who is considered the family dog. The collar is meant to convey that the puppy is cared for, or at least as evidence of a more or less solid bond with some human. Sometimes this collar ends up hurting the puppy when he outgrows it, the human who put it there having lost interest in caring for the dog, or the dog having wandered away. Eventually, the collar ends up almost beheading the dog. This is what happened to a resilient young street dog whom I met at Help In Suffering, the animal rescue organization in Jaipur, and whom I nicknamed, out of admiration, "Ghigliottina" (guillotine). As physically and psychologically strong as he was, he looked like most street dogs when first brought to the hospital. The only anomaly was the stink emanating from the area around his head. It was soon discovered that embedded in his neck was a plastic thread—a collar in origin—that had been slowly guillotining him for months.

The reason for this sad and paradoxical consequence is the fluidity of human-dog rapport in India. WHO and OIE have acknowledged the complexity of this relationship by establishing a matrix of four categories based on the level of dependence of dogs on humans and the restriction of dogs by humans. Dogs who are owned and restricted by families are totally dependent on their owners, and their movements are restricted and rigidly supervised. Owners provide shelter, food, and water, and they also usually also keep reproduction under control. The second group consists of dogs who are owned but only partially restricted by families; these dogs are heavily dependent on their owners, but their movements are only partially controlled. These dogs can be found roaming the streets, where they can freely reproduce. Their lifespan is long and their success at rearing litters of puppies is high because the essential resources of food, shelter, and protection are provided by their humans (Bögel and Meslin 1990, 282). Nevertheless, these dogs also frequently supplement their diet with street garbage. In rural India, this group includes farm dogs and herding dogs. Because of their close proximity to humans and their exposure to other dogs, this category of dogs is of particular concern when it comes to the spread of rabies. Surplus offspring of partially restricted dogs generally end up entering either the neighborhood (or community) dog population, or becoming feral. Unsupervised neighborhood dogs, the third group, are partially dependent on humans, to whom they have some level of attachment, but their movements are unrestricted (although some of them can be quite accessible to their caretakers). Since these dogs are not supervised, the uncontrolled population growth of this group adds significantly to the increase of the overall dog population. And finally, feral dogs, the fourth category, are independent, or at most they depend only on human waste, and are totally free in their movements. They are usually found in rural areas, since the Indian urban environment rarely allows dogs to live far from humans.

The term "pet"—an increasing number of scholars prefer "companion animal" (Rock and Degeling 2013, 487)—is mainly used with reference to the first category, only occasionally including the second as well. Yet it is evident that in three of the four categories, dogs have a referral household or an attachment to at least one person in a community. It would be misleading, though, to think of these dogs as possessions: most of the people who feed and take care of dogs on the streets build a relation of kinship with them in which the dogs are regarded as something like family members (Warden 2015). Yet this does not necessarily mean that they are properly taken care of, as we shall see.

"Stray" dogs, technically called "free-ranging" or "free-roaming" dogs, are dogs "observed without human supervision on public property or on private property with immediate unrestrained access to public property" (Beck 1973, 3). Dogs can either be born stray or pet dogs can become stray when they get lost or their owners abandon them. All feral dogs are by definition stray, but—significantly—not all stray dogs are feral. In 2001, when the Animal Birth Control (Dogs) Rules were issued, India changed its official language with regard to these dogs. Since then, stray dogs have been considered "street dogs," and dog population control and rabies-control measures are shaped according to the concept that this term conveys. In an article comparing the concept of animal welfare in the United Kingdom and in India, Krithika Srinivasan (2012, 110) observes that the term "stray dog" used in the British context means a dog who is unowned or unsupervised, illegitimate, and out of place (in effect roaming without license on public property), whereas in India the legally meaningful expression "street dog" acknowledges the right of that dog to live on the street. In the United Kingdom, dogs are either pets or strays, and strays are considered a problem to be addressed. In India, street dogs cannot be legally defined as homeless, for the street is acknowledged as their home. But this does not necessarily make things easier, either for the dogs themselves or for the people around them—or for rabies control.

In everyday language in India, the expression "stray" or "street" dog is often used (incorrectly) to refer not to the ontological or legal status of dogs but to their breed. Since most street dogs in India are mongrels (and in some cases "INDogs," described below), these terms are regarded as synonymous and are used interchangeably—despite the fact that abandoned purebred dogs can become street dogs, and mongrels and INDogs can be adopted as family pets. Mongrels are dogs of mixed and often indeterminate breed whose lineage is unknown and whose commercial value is essentially nil. Some of the mongrels who live on the streets of India may have INDog genes in their DNA, but, like stray dogs throughout the world, many of them are just the result of irresponsible pet owners who allow their pet dogs to mate with street mongrels.

Outcast Dogs

INDogs are the indigenous and most common Indian landrace, a term that refers to a domesticated, locally adapted, traditional variety of a species of animal (or plant) that has developed over time through adaptation to its natural and cultural environment. Despite being genetically uniform, specimens of a landrace are more diverse than those of a formal breed. In fact, INDogs are not recognized as a standardized breed by international kennel clubs, but their main physical features are easily recognizable across India. They are a medium-size, slender, short-haired dog with a long and narrow muzzle, usually brown but ranging occasionally from black to reddish, sometimes with white markings. INDogs have almond-shaped dark brown eyes and a long, curved tail, usually held high over the back.

In India, INDogs, like most all street dogs, are usually called "pariah dogs." The term "pariah" probably originally designated a Dalit community of Tamil Nadu, the Paraiyar, heralds who moved from village to village communicating their messages through ceremonial drums called *parai*. Coined by Western travelers and first recorded in English in 1613, the term "pariah" came to mean an outcast, a socially marginalized or ostracized person, and, with reference to India only, a member of the lower castes. Nowadays, outside India, the word "pariah," when used with respect to dogs, is both found in the common language and used by zoologists to describe not a specific breed but native dogs who have served for centuries as scavengers alongside humans in the ecological niche that people have created, characterized by waste from human settlements such as garbage, corpses, and feces.

While outside India the term "pariah" has no particularly negative connotations (again, we are talking only about its use with respect to dogs; the term is of course commonly used to describe ostracized or outcast humans, in which case it has deeply negative connotations), in India it is offensive, for "its metaphorical use is understood still today as a colonialist insult that resumes at its own discretion the Brahmanical vision of untouchability" (Varikas 2010, 31). Nevertheless, while outcastes are now officially known as "Dalit," "pariah" is still used in everyday language in India to refer to dogs in a derogatory way. In a fancy mall in Delhi, I once overheard a short conversation at a stand set up for the adoption of street dogs that illustrates the point. A little girl pointed at an INDog puppy and exclaimed enthusiastically, "That doggy is so cute, Mum!" Her mother replied sternly that he was not a doggy but a pariah dog. Puzzled, the girl asked what that meant and her mother answered that it meant the dog was dirty and lived on the street. I agree with Govindasamy Agoramoorthy (2007) that "the word 'pariah' should not be used in any context—sociological and biological— since it resonates a past humiliating social prejudice." Therefore, I use the term only when necessary to my argument.

At a popular level, INDogs and, more generally, pariah *kuttas* (from *kutta*, the Hindi word for dog) are usually considered just a part of the landscape, in their specific role as street cleaners. "If all the dogs go on pilgrimage to Benares [now Varanasi], who will be left to lick the dishes clean?" (Kipling 1904, 263) used to be a popular saying that perfectly exemplified the idea of dogs as nothing more than scavengers. Within the Indian context, the close link between dogs and waste, dirt, and other impure substances inevitably associates them with the Chandalas, scavengers of human excreta and corpse handlers (called "guardians of the dead" in the *Mahabharata* 13.48.21) and one of the lowest social groups in the Hindu hierarchy. The upper castes see their eating habits as indiscriminate and impure, and they are associated with the color black, the relevance of which is elaborated below.

Sanskrit literature has identified Chandalas with dogs for two millennia. In ancient texts, a synonym for Chandala was *shvapaca*, which means "dog-cookers," "dog-milkers," or "dog-people" (White 1991, 71). According to the *Manava Dharmashastra* (10.51–520), "Chandalas and Shvapacas, however, must live outside the village. . . . Their property consists of dogs and donkeys, their garments are the clothes of the dead; they eat in broken vessels, their ornaments are of iron; and they constantly roam about." The *Manava Dharmashastra* (3.239) forbids Chandalas and dogs to look at a Brahmin while he is eating: the former are thought to spoil with their touch, the latter even with their gaze. It also prescribes that no Brahmin should ever eat food "touched by a dog" (4.208) or by "those who raise dogs" (4.216). Chandalas are also traditionally assigned the task of catching and killing rabid dogs, by hitting them on the head. As Wendy Doniger O'Flaherty observes, "The dog [is] to the cow in the world of beasts what the outcaste is to the Brahmin in the world of men." "To the Indian," she continues, "the dog is the most unclean of all animals, a polluted scavenger, the very image of evil; domestication has not served to bathe away his sins in the eyes of the Hindus" (1976, 173). This opposition between cows and dogs is also evident in the practice of offering the first roti (traditional bread) of the day to cows as a blessing of prosperity and the last to dogs, to placate the ghost world with which dogs are associated. To sum up, "dog and cow, outcaste and Brahmin, excrement and food, are polar opposites" (White 1991, 92).

In India, as John Kipling observed more than a century ago, the dog "has always been on the downhill slope of popular contempt, and it will be long before he can hope to rise. . . . Perhaps it is not too fantastical to say that when compared with the English dog the poor Indian outcast is a pagan" (1904, 266). In fact, although INDogs are ubiquitous, alongside mongrels, in the public spaces of urban India, most people disparage and dismiss this unique and valuable landrace. Several other dog breeds are much sought after, but they are not of Indian origin. Until recently, Indians who wanted puppies of foreign breeds had to import them from abroad. But now that Western-style pet keeping has caught on in Indian cities, the Indian government banned the import of dogs for commercial purposes in 2016 to avoid the proliferation of canine species unsuitable for India's tropical climate. Nowadays, the most popular foreign breeds are bred directly in the country. According to many of the veterinarians and pet shop owners whom I interviewed in Delhi, it is no exaggeration to speak of a well-established dog industry in the city. Anuradha, an elderly woman I met in the Okhla slum, told me that the number of dogs in Delhi has grown exponentially in the past twenty years. "Especially among the ones who live in the big houses [of the rich]," she added, "there is now competition [dekha-dekhi, or envious watchfulness] over keeping dogs inside the house." Anuradha's perception is confirmed by the market intelligence firm Euromonitor International (IIPTF 2013). The Indian pet-care market is growing at a staggering pace, faster than that of any other country. Valued at more than US$1.2 billion, its annual growth rate is above 35% (Hindu 2016).

Breed Matters

INDogs and mongrels are not part of this business: that would be simply unthinkable. Very few people want them, so nobody sells them. Besides, they are ubiquitous, on every street, in every dog shelter. The lucrative industry in dogs specializes in exotic breeds. Large dogs tend to be top sellers, particularly in Delhi, where social prestige is broadcast by huge SUVs, which stand out in traffic jams like elephants among ants, or by owning a farmhouse on the outskirts of town in which to spend weekends in idleness. Ownership of a massive dog completes this delusion of grandeur. German shepherds and Doberman pinschers were a common choice in the 1990s, while more recently Labrador retrievers—nicknamed Labras—and golden retrievers are in great demand, particularly by families with children. At present, the status of the Labrador retriever is unique, as it appears to have become the icon of Delhi's pet dog industry. At the opposite end of the spectrum, small dogs like toy poodles and Lhasa Apsos are also popular and are carried around in tote bags. Proudly keeping his German shepherd on a strong black leather leash, a man whom I met in a pet shop observed that the buyers of these "doggies" are mainly "girls, of course." Not bothering to conceal his disdain, he explained that girls enjoy "going to malls to buy fancy pink dog skirts and treating them like dolls."

Several pet shop owners cited the influence of national and international fashion trends, TV commercials, and Bollywood stars in people's choice of dogs. For example, since the cell phone company Vodafone-Hutch chose a pug as its mascot in 2003, this breed has become the most sought-after pet dog in the country. "They come here and say, 'we want a Hutchwala kutta,'" the owner of a pet shop in Jangpura told me. "Hutchwala kutta" (Hutch's dog) has actually become a kind of unofficial name for pugs in Delhi. For this reason, he admitted, it has become difficult to keep up with the demand for pugs in the city. Yet this situation also has an upside; the popularity of pugs pushed their selling price from 14,000 rupees (US$200) to 60,000 rupees (US$870) apiece. A picture of Cheeka, the pug in the Hutch "You & I" commercial (who follows his young master around with the same loyalty that the service provider promises its customers), became the most downloaded mobile phone screensaver in India in 2005 (Jaypal 2006). In January 2013, when I attended the International Pet Trade Fair in Noida, flat-faced, wrinkly-skinned pugs were the most common four-legged visitors, followed closely by Pomeranians, Labrador retrievers, and golden retrievers.

This obsession with breeds also comes into play when dog owners face the problem of finding a mate for their beloved (yet sexually frustrated and karma-impaired) pet—an issue only for male dogs, who must search far and wide for a bitch in heat. All of the pet shop owners I spoke with told me that male dogs are strongly preferred to females. Data from 1997 show that the sex ratio between unlicensed male and female dogs was not too lopsided (5.79 million males and 4.83 million females), while among licensed dogs, there were almost twice as many males as females (9.69 to 5.16 million) (Debroy 2008, 184). "There is nothing to be surprised about, Deborah! This is India, and here males are always preferred. People want male children and male dogs. The idea is the same: less trouble, less money to spend," observed an animal welfare activist who was clearly fed up with this situation. He added that owners of female dogs must often endure what he described as psychologically unbearable stress about their dogs' chastity, not only because of the practical consequence of unwanted litters of mongrels but also on a symbolic level. "You must know how worried parents are about the virginity of their daughters," this activist continued. "If something goes wrong, you know what I mean, it can become a matter of social stigma. The same also occurs with female dogs. People are really scared that they cannot protect them from male dogs." Bibek Debroy (2008, 110), for example, reports cases in Kerala where upper castes objected to lower castes' keeping male dogs because cross-caste mating could corrupt their female dogs.

Pet shop windows in upscale locales like Khan Market in New Delhi are plastered with dozens of lonely-heart advertisements written by dog owners desperately seeking suitable "brides" for their male pets. Their search is complicated both by the discouraging male-to-female ratio and the desire for a dog belonging to the same breed as the long-suffering "husband." If they fail to find a suitable mate, many veterinarians and animal shelter staff told me, it is not uncommon for the owners of male dogs to let them out on the street to vent their sexual frustration with street bitches. The resulting problem of an unwanted litter of half-breeds is foisted onto the bitches and the community, while the owner continues to search for a purebred female candidate. Since 2008, Delhiites have also had the opportunity to attend, in Ansal Plaza in South Delhi, the biggest mass "marriages" for dogs that have ever taken place in India. Dog owners searching for mates register their pets and send pictures and descriptions of the kind of mates they seek. Organizers then select fitting matches, which they propose to the owners. These events even feature speed-dating in the hope of finding love at first sight. For those who prefer not to have their dogs meet in the flesh, Dogshaadi and Tindog are two "dating" alternatives. Since 2010, Dogshaadi (from *shaadi*, "wedding") has made a name for itself as a website helping people connect their dogs—excluding INDogs, of course. Based on the human hook-up site Tinder, Tindog is a mobile application that allows pet owners to set up profiles of their dogs and look for mates for them, along with human friends for themselves.

The figures presented by Euromonitor International (IIPTF 2013) include all the primary care and additional attention that Indian owners want to provide their dogs, once the matchmaking issue is resolved. The long list of high-end dog luxuries includes a vegetarian version of the main international dog food brands; gluten-free pizza; chocolate-looking cakes; cozy beds; accessories (fur coats, sunglasses, and bathrobes); hygiene products (paw balms that protect footpads from hot surfaces, breath fresheners, and tonics to apply to fur to prevent dogs from licking it); branded garments (counterfeit Gucci being the most famous); clothes for the monsoon season (waterproof cloaks and boots); grooming services (aromatherapy baths, herbal massages, hair coloring, "pawdicures," and *dogZillions*—Brazilian wax to remove hair from the genital area); dog sitting; dog walking; photographic services; birthday party services; psychotherapy; social events (e.g., Pet Fed at Dilli Hat, in New Delhi); pool parties; *doga* (yoga for dogs); the puppy's first bath; dog-friendly restaurants with dog buffets; dog-friendly luxury resorts; air-conditioned kennels; cremation and burial services; and angel-communication healing sessions that allegedly restore contact with deceased or lost pets. At Red Paws, a renowned dog spa in Hauz Khas Village, the trendiest and most Westernized area of South Delhi, grooming services can range from 1,250 rupees (US$18) for a Chihuahua to 3,750 rupees (US$55) for a giant schnauzer.

As the reader may already have gathered, dog sterilization and vaccination are not a priority for the average Indian pet owner for a variety of reasons, ranging from the relative newness of pet keeping as it is understood in Western society to low awareness of dog health and behavior. This topic, which is key to rabies, is addressed in detail below.

Too Many, Too Rabid

What distinguishes pariah *avara kuttas* (unowned wandering dogs) from purebred pet doggies is also the perception of their numbers and the possibility that they carry rabies. Section 399 of the Delhi Municipal Act of 1957 stipulates that pet registration is compulsory in Delhi. It is relatively easy to register a pet and almost free of charge, costing only fifteen rupees (US$0.20) a year. Registered dogs receive a tag that is meant to be hung on the dog's collar, but in all my time in India I saw only one of these tags, hanging from the neck of a lactating bitch who lived on the streets around the Hanuman Mandir of Baba Kharak Singh Marg in New Delhi. None of the hundreds of dogs I saw at the International Pet Trade Fair wore it. In fact, only a small percentage of dog owners actually register their dogs. According to the owner of a pet shop in Defence Colony (South East Delhi), many pet owners think that registering their dogs means buying them a nice Swarovski studded collar. Recent research carried out in a relatively well-off small city in Haryana found that dog owners (68% of whom owned pedigree dogs) preferred to register their dogs with the Kennel Club of India but not with their local municipality, which suggests that registration is considered important mainly for commercial purposes and dog show eligibility (Tiwari et al. 2019, 13). WHO (1988, 8) recommends using the expression "street dogs" only for dogs who do not comply with local regulations, which, evidently, includes most of the pampered yet unregistered pet dogs in Delhi.

One result is that many family-owned dogs are not counted in the official statistics recorded by local municipal authorities. For example, according to a report in the *Hindu* in August 2015, fewer than three hundred pet dogs had been registered in the first half of that year at the North, East, and South MCDs combined (Nath 2015c). These numbers clearly clash with the marketing trends outlined above, which reveal a situation in which the number of pet dogs is increasing by an estimated five hundred per month in Delhi alone, according to Shashank Shekhar (2016). Yet the mushrooming population of pet dogs is not perceived as worrisome, let alone menacing. Street dogs, by contrast, tend to be seen as a threatening invasion, so numerous that they are considered uncountable and out of control. There are no accurate statistics on the population of street dogs nationwide, since only in a handful of locations have comprehensive dog censuses been carried out. According to the 2012 livestock census (Ministry of Agriculture 2012, 14, 89–91, 117), there were 11,673,000 (pet?) dogs and 17,138,349 stray dogs in India, although no definition of "stray dog" is provided, making comparison and further discussion difficult at best. The very precise number of free-roaming dogs is curious, especially when contrasted with that of pet dogs: were the former more cooperative in being counted than the owners of the latter? If we look for other data, estimates range from twenty-four million (Jackman and Rowan 2007, 66) to thirty-eight million (Rupprecht, Kuzmin, and Meslin 2017, 13) to sixty million (Gompper 2013a, 20). Theresa Bradley and Ritchie King (2012), citing market research by Euromonitor International, claim that in the period from 2007 to 2012 India's dog population grew by 58%, faster than any other country's.

Looking only at Delhi, the NGO Wildlife SOS estimated that in 2009 the city had 262,740 street dogs, plus or minus 18,343. In 2012, the livestock census put the number of stray dogs in Delhi—again, without providing a definition of "stray"—at 60,472 (Ministry of Agriculture 2012, 117). An article in the *Hindu* in July 2013 reported that while Delhi had fewer than 300,000 street dogs, "a couple of years" before there had been more than one million (Perappadan 2013), a figure that seems excessive. In June 2014 the then leader of the opposition, Mukesh Goel, told the *Hindu* that while he claimed the number of street dogs was around 300,000, the North MCD maintained that it was half this number (Nath 2014c). Finally, in August 2016, a survey by the Humane Society International on behalf of the South MCD put the number of street dogs in South Delhi at 189,285 (*Indian Express* 2016b). In Jaipur, research published in 2011 estimated the number of free-roaming dogs to be 36,580 (Hiby et al. 2011, 2). In the future, Gurugram could become the first Indian city to know its pet dog population, thanks to the strict rules on pet ownership practices—which also include rabies-control measures—that it imposed in 2018 (Pant 2018).

Where statistics are lacking or inaccurate, rough evaluations abound, adding confusion, and sometimes panic, to an already critical situation. This is exacerbated by newspaper articles that employ catchy headlines conveying anxiety and frenzy—for example, "Street Dog Menace: NHRC Sends Notices to Centre, Delhi Govt." (*Outlook* 2014), "29 Stray Dogs Caught from East Delhi Hospitals" (*Hindu* 2014), and "Stray Dogs Are Terror Threat to Delhi Airport, Says DIAL" (Sharma 2016b). However, it is headlines like "New Delhi: Siblings Killed, Left for Animals to Eat" (*Hindustan Times* 2013) that provoke the most repulsion and hatred toward street dogs. Unfortunate events of this kind, where poverty, starving dogs, and human neglect collide, are reported regularly by newspapers all over India: in Jaipur, "Stray Dogs Mutilate Infant's Body" (*Times of India* 2012c); in Lucknow, "Stray Dogs Mutilate Stillborn's Body Outside KGMU" (*Times of India* 2017c); in Barnala, "Stray Dogs Kill 4-Year-Old Boy, Consume Vital Organs" (*Times of India* 2012b); in Bhopal, "Stray Dogs Drag Body of Newborn in People's Hospital" (*Times of India* 2012a); in Bangalore, "Dog Carries Man's Head, Shocks Bangalore University Campus" (*Times of India* 2013a) and "Stray

Dogs Ravage Abandoned Just-Born Girl's Body" (*Times of India* 2013d), and so on. While Hiranmay Karlekar (2008; 2011a) and Anuradha Ramanujan (2015) claim that it is not uncommon for articles of this kind—often poor in details and context but rich in sensationalism—to be based on unsubstantiated allegations, these events understandably disturb people and incite public rage, though events of this kind are isolated and uncommon, and the dismay they arouse tends to abate quickly.

The fear of being bitten by a street dog is much more enduring. Headlines like "Dog Bites on the Rise in North Delhi" (Jamatia 2013), "1 Dog Bite Every 6 Minutes: Capital Faces Canine Crisis" (Sharma 2016a), and "More Than 225 Dog Bite Cases in Delhi Every Day, Civic Bodies Struggle to Count Canines" (Sharma 2017) clearly depict a tense relationship between people and street dogs. In Delhi, as throughout India, people perceive dog bites as such a menace that in Mumbai, street dogs have even been compared to terrorists: "Dog Bites Killed More Than 2 Terror Attacks," headlined the *Times of India* on March 10, 2016 (Mahapatra 2016). Although there are exceptions (addressed below), Delhiites usually consider street dogs a scourge and a nuisance: they bark day and night, chase cars, topple bicycle riders, cause road accidents, damage property, snarl at children, scatter rubbish around, defecate on doorsteps, and, above all, bite. One of the first things that prospective dog owners in Delhi buy are so-called walking sticks, short plastic sticks similar to riding whips that they use to keep street dogs away when walking their pet dogs.

People fear street dogs not only because of their huge numbers but also because they are considered intrinsically prone to biting and to having and transmitting rabies. A survey in Kerala revealed that 80% of respondents believe that all street dogs are rabid (FIAPO 2017b, 6). It is not my intention to minimize the physical and psychological pain caused by a dog bite— no matter the dog's status—or to deny the importance of seeking medical attention in case of dog bite, but given the many challenges of managing rabies in a resource-limited setting like India, panicking about every dog bite—suspecting rabies in each of them—is counterproductive. On October 13, 2012, the *Times of India* reported that the district hospital in Noida had spent a third of its 2011–12 budget (4.8 million rupees, or US$70,000) on rabies vaccines, yet most of the patients who received the vaccine were driven by phobia and did not actually require it (Ghosal 2012).

As I discuss in detail in chapter 6, there are several complex reasons for this phobia, including an erroneous or inadequate knowledge of rabies and of animal behavior in general. However, fear also feeds on itself, and angst increases exponentially in an atmosphere of alarm and even terror, regardless of the actual risk. When it comes to dog bites, media stories and word of mouth fan the flames, and this does not necessarily result in a better understanding of the actual problem of rabies. An article published in the Kerala section of the *Hindu* in 2014, "Dog Bites on the Rise in District," provides a fitting example (Rajagopal 2014). The article is accompanied by a chart that sums up the main points. Under the heading "BITING SPREE," set in red capital letters, are such items as "increase in dog bites: over a thousand a month," and "anti-rabies vaccine requirement on a high." The article also features a picture of a growling dog of indiscriminate breed, his ears flattened against his head, eyes fixed on his victim, canines bared; drops of blood falling from his teeth have been Photoshopped in. No life-saving information about PEP is provided, and no mention is made of human responsibilities for dogs, such as registration and vaccination. Articles like this arouse the public imagination and foment the demonization of dogs, which are counterproductive responses in the fight against rabies.

Between Love and Hate

In this context of tension and worry, it is not surprising that a wide range of drastic solutions have been proposed to control the dog population and the problem of rabies. Before we look at these proposals, it is important to acknowledge their role in driving a wedge between those who support them and those who disapprove of them. Heated debate over dog population management and rabies control divides the public into "dog lovers" and "dog haters," and the extreme emotion that characterizes both camps tends to undermine the chances of coming up with workable solutions. Each side accuses the other of blindness, fanaticism, and irrationality when it comes to dogs, and in the meantime the rabies virus continues to kill undisturbed.

Those who fear street dogs and consider them a public health threat see dog lovers as naïve in expressing blind trust in these animals, as if humans' having chosen them as their "best friends" would automatically eliminate any risk of interspecies conflict. This kind of caricature of dog lovers is captured in the opening sentence of a newspaper article from January 2013 headlined "Stray Dog Attacks 6-Year-Old Girl in Bangalore": "Her love for strays proved costly." The story goes on to describe Sanjana, a young girl who encountered a stray dog, unknown to her, on the road outside her home. Used to patting and feeding the street dogs in her neighborhood, the girl approached, but the dog attacked her, biting her severely on the face and hand. Sanjana eventually lost four front teeth and her upper lip was partially torn. The article acknowledged that the dog had recently been chased out of his neighborhood, pelted with stones by schoolchildren, and attacked by local dogs. For these reasons, "The dog was not in a mood to take Sanjana's gesture kindly."

Three captioned drawings accompany the text, depicting Sanjana smilingly patting the stray dog on the head, the dog becoming agitated and pouncing on her, and Sanjana running away in tears, "with her hand still in the dog's mouth." The article quotes the joint director of animal husbandry at Bruhat Bengaluru Mahanagara Palika and reports, "BBMP officials said dogs are ferocious from December to February, which is their breeding season. They have suggested that the public be careful on seeing a stray dog." The piece also alludes to five recent instances of dogs' attacking people in a "biting spree," possibly because of rabies (the article does not specify). In closing, it says, "In this dog vs human conflict on Bangalore's streets, it's usually children who are at the highest risk. . . . There is no humane formula for this problem: the argument swings between the live-and-let-live lobby, and the hardline groups who want dogs off the roads" (*Times of India* 2013c).

There is a long and varied history of attempts to control the population of street dogs in India. During British colonial rule, the famous case of the dogs of Mumbai stands out as an example of the pro-killing approach to this issue. To deal with the growing problem of street dogs, in May 1832 the British authorities of Mumbai (then Bombay) expanded and began vigorously enforcing a regulation that had been issued some decades before. Initially limited to the hot season (at the time, it was thought that heat caused dogs to go mad and thus bite and spread rabies), the authorities extended the culling of street dogs "to any time that a nuisance and danger was deemed to exist" (Palsetia 2001, 14). An unprecedented dog hunt thus began on the streets of Mumbai. But what made this event famous were the riots, strikes, and general discontent that it provoked. The measure deeply offended the ethical and religious sensibilities of Mumbai's Parsi community, which has always been very protective of its religious identity. In Zoroastrianism, dogs are held in great esteem and play a central role in funeral rites, as they are imagined as the guardians of the Chinvat (the Bridge of Judgment) and the companions of those who cross that bridge into the afterlife.

The British regulation clashed violently with the local religious and cultural milieu, and the extreme backlash that resulted exposed for the first time the remarkable complexity and delicacy of the issue of dog population and rabies control in India.

A similar dispute over religious beliefs regarding dogs, this time of Hindus, occurred thirty years later in Ahmedabad, a town five hundred kilometers north of Mumbai that was part of the Bombay Presidency under the British Raj. In January 1859, the inhabitants of Ahmedabad petitioned the British governor of Bombay to prohibit the killing of street dogs. The governor agreed, on the grounds that the prohibition would "put a stop to a great uneasiness and mortification to which all the Hindoo inhabitants of this city are subjected." An argument between the governor and the local (British) authorities of Ahmedabad ensued, but eventually the Hindu cultural and religious objection to the slaughter of street dogs prevailed (Ex-Commissioner 1880, 88–89).

Fifty years later, the sensitive subject of dog population and rabies control reemerged, this time in connection with Mahatma Gandhi, the spiritual and political leader of pre-independence India. The trouble started in Gujarat, Gandhi's homeland, when a mill owner had sixty street dogs killed outside his mill. Because his action conflicted with his Hindu faith, the mill owner implored Gandhi for spiritual redemption. To everyone's great surprise, Gandhi expressed his approval of the killing of the dogs. Predictably, he received so many enraged letters and requests for clarification that he took to the pages of his newspaper *Young India* to present his reasoning (Gandhi 1926a, 1926b). With respect to the risk of contracting rabies from dogs, Gandhi explained the difference between violence that causes suffering to an individual and violence that threatens an entire society. Only in the latter case, and in the absence of a more humane method of preventing the spread of rabies, did he support the mass killing of dogs as the only viable solution. In fact, he said, the elimination of starving, sick, injured, ownerless dogs was actually less cruel than passively allowing them to starve, struggle, suffer, reproduce, and eventually die in miserable conditions of neglect. "Connivance or putting up with status quo is no ahimsa [nonviolence]," he wrote. Gandhi made it clear that people who accept the presence of these suffering dogs on their streets are guilty of neglect toward animals. He even went so far as to suggest that those who feed these dogs should be fined for keeping them alive, thus prolonging their misery. To Gandhi, this was a "false feeling of compassion" (Burgat 2004, 225–26).

Defining the concept of responsible ownership long before the term had been coined, Gandhi stated unequivocally that laws allowing municipalities to pursue selective killing (sparing village dogs and watchdogs) were the best solution in cases where more humane measures were unavailable. Ideally, of course, then as now, the best way to prevent the overpopulation, neglect, and suffering of free-roaming dogs is to enforce regulations mandating that pet owners register, sterilize, confine, and leash their dogs; provide and support municipal dog pounds; fund and sponsor animal welfare associations that take care of street dogs; promote dog adoption; and euthanize rabid dogs. Gandhi was ahead of his time in advocating these measures for the control of rabies. But his position that killing street dogs would solve the problem of uncontrolled reproduction and overpopulation, and of rabies transmission, was based on erroneous assumptions that science has since dispelled. The most significant of these assumptions was that mass culling could stabilize the dog population and eliminate rabies.

After India won its independence in 1947, street dogs continued to be killed for decades in horribly inhumane ways. Both local governments and private citizens resorted to clubbing, shooting, strychnine poisoning, starvation, and electrocution. At the National Dog Welfare Conference India in Chennai on January 27–28, 2013, Chinny Krishna, the chair of Blue Cross of India (a well-known animal welfare charity), reported on a Chennai catch-and-kill program that began in 1860. In the 1970s, the Chennai Municipal Corporation was killing so many street dogs that the city's Central Leather Research Institute found it profitable to develop a line of wallets, belts, and other products made of dog skin. By 1995, Krishna reported, the number of dogs killed daily in Chennai had reached 135.

The indiscriminate mass killing became particularly severe in the 1990s, and it continues to occur occasionally throughout the country. In 2015–16, Kerala was often in the headlines for this reason. According to *Outlook* magazine, in the summer of 2015 some village councils in the Ernakulam district proposed reducing Kerala's street dog population by selling stray dogs to South Korea, China, and northeastern India, where dog meat is valued as food. The author of the proposal, K. R. Jayakumar, argued that this would be financially lucrative while at the same time help address "the problem of stray dog attacks on humans" (Outlook 2015c). On July 9, 2015, the chief minister of Kerala ordered local civic bodies to cull more than 250,000 street dogs, declaring that the state, as a member of the Kerala Legislative Assembly put it, had turned from "God's own country"—Kerala's tourist slogan—into "Dog's own country" (Haneef 2015). Three months later, Kerala's leading industrialist and the chairperson of the Stray Dog Free Movement, Kochouseph Chittilappilly, demanded action against street dogs and staged a twenty-four-hour hunger strike to draw attention to the issue (*New Indian Express* 2015a). One year later, members of the Kerala Youth Front Party killed a dozen "dangerous dogs" and paraded their carcasses on the streets of Kottayam to protest against the animal rights activist Maneka Gandhi and the overall political approach to the issue of street dog overpopulation (Babu 2016).

Similar conflicts have occurred, and continue to take place, elsewhere in the country. In February 2012 in Jammu and Kashmir, activists demonstrated against animal rights groups and alleged government apathy regarding the threats posed by street dogs, arguing that "stray dogs cannot be allowed to survive at the expense of humans" (*Outlook* 2012). In November 2017 in Hyderabad, residents alleged that several street dogs were poisoned and removed by the municipal corporation to sanitize the city in advance of Ivanka Trump's visit (Puppala 2017). In January 2019 in Kolkata, two young women bludgeoned sixteen puppies to death. When an onlooker asked them to stop, the women shouted back, asking whether he would protect them if the dogs bit them (Chaudhuri 2019). In March 2019 in a village near Bikaner, more than fifty street dogs were shot dead (*Times of India* 2019a). In September 2019, ninety dogs were found killed with their muzzles and legs tied in a forest area in northern Maharashtra, after they had been captured in a small town on the order of the municipal council (Singh 2019).

In Delhi, following news of a fatal dog attack on a two-month-old baby in June 2014 (Sikdar 2014), a commissioner of the North MCD proposed to address the problem through "passive killing," which means displacing the dogs to areas where they are unable to find food or water or causing them similar indirect harm (Nath 2014a). Passive killing is illegal, however, and so this measure, favored by 49% of Delhiites surveyed (Nath 2014b), was not implemented. One year later, the NGO Society for Public Cause petitioned the High Court of Delhi for the elimination of street dogs who, in its view, not only put human lives at risk owing to the threat of rabies but also defiled the Swachh Bharat Abhiyan (the Clean India Mission launched by the Indian government in 2014 to clean the streets and infrastructures of more than 4,000 cities and towns). With respect to pet dogs, the petition sought compulsory measures such as pet registration and the muzzling of dogs in public places. The authors of this petition claimed that "if animal lovers want to set up kennels they should do so at their own cost and not at public expense" (*Outlook* 2015d).

In May 2016, animal lovers asked the Supreme Court to examine a legal anomaly that was allegedly discriminating against street dogs. The punishment for killing a pet dog can be a jail term of up to five years, as the Indian Penal Code considers it an offense against private property, but the killing of a street dog is covered under the Prevention of Cruelty to Animals Act of 1960, which prescribes a fine of only fifty rupees (US$0.70). Animal welfare activists picketing outside the court carried posters that featured a street dog who asks, "Would you kill a homeless child? Why kill me?" (Choudhary 2016). This legal case reflects the extent to which citizens have become polarized over this issue, and also the juridical void in which street dogs have been placed by the ambiguous nature of dog ownership in India. When no one takes responsibility for paying for their medical care and well-being, whose fault is it when a dog, rabid or not, attacks someone else, whether a human, another street dog, a pet dog, someone's cow, or a wild monkey?

The Key Role of Food and Feeding

Even if many people in India and worldwide regard the mass culling, removal, and relocation of street dogs as good—or at least straightforward—methods of keeping rabies at bay, WHO had already concluded in 1992 that "there is no evidence that the removal of dogs has ever had a significant impact on dog population densities or the spread of rabies. The population turnover of dogs may be so high that even the highest recorded removal rates (about 15% of the dog population) are easily compensated by survival rates" (1992, 31). Evidence from Delhi confirms this: "A concerted effort . . . at dog removal killed a third of the straying dogs with no reduction in dog population" (Reece 2005, 59).

The main reason for this seeming paradox is the widespread availability of food, along with water and shelter, to street dogs. According to the *Guidelines for Dog Population Management* published by WHO and the World Society for the Protection of Animals (now World Animal Protection) (1990, 9), "Each habitat has a specific carrying capacity for each species" that "essentially depends on the availability, quality and distribution of the resources (shelter, food, water) for the species concerned. The density of population for higher vertebrates (including dogs) is almost always near the carrying capacity of the environment." In other words, as long as food, water, and shelter are available in a given area, dogs will take advantage of them—unless a way is found to exterminate all Indian street dogs at once and to prevent any unrestricted and unsupervised movement of pet dogs in public spaces (which would depend on responsible dog owners, still a vanishingly small group in India). In fact, as soon as a biological niche becomes available, dogs rapidly multiply and fill it. Given the free movement of street dogs across neighborhoods and the abstract nature of administrative boundaries (designed to isolate zones that want to remain dog-free despite the alluring presence of food on their streets—a losing proposition), there will always be hungry dogs who struggle to survive and will fight for their lives.

Where does the food available to street dogs come from? In chapter 2, I described the various anthropogenic factors and ecological pathways through which edible items reach the streets of Indian towns, becoming food for the animals who inhabit them. Quantitatively speaking, the major source of food for street dogs in India is garbage (Pal 2001, 70), and the correlation between municipal solid waste and street dog population and dog bites is clear (Chandran and Azeez 2016). People are particularly convinced that dumping of waste by slaughterhouses and meat shops is the leading cause of the increase in dog population—for example in Kerala (FIAPO 2017b, 7). Mutton restaurants (a common name for non-veg restaurants) and Chinese food stalls in particular are blamed for feeding dogs food that not only is plentiful but is also thought to increase their aggression. Other important sources are human excreta, animal bodies, human remains, and deliberate food offerings. Food provisioning varies according to the animal to whom it is directed, but our focus here is on the food offered to street dogs. Since there is an important religious dimension in this gesture, we must examine the unique position of the dog in Hinduism.

Dogs have been seen as both good and bad since Vedic times. Early references to them in the *Rig Veda* are very positive; they are allies of people (2.39.4), guards of the home (7.55.1–4), and full members of the family (7.55.5). The *Rig Veda* also portrays Sarama (the bitch who is the progenitor of all carnivorous animals, according to the *Bhagavata Purana*) as an extremely positive example of the mother figure (10.108.8–11; see also Singh 1997, 143–44). In the *Sabha Parva*, Sarama and dogs in general are described as the personification of *bhakti* (devotion to a favorite deity). Later hymns in the *Rig Veda* (10.14.10–12) tell a very different story about dogs. They are associated with Yama, the god of death, and they begin to be described as black (Bollée 2006, 17). The link with death is mainly represented by the two four-eyed Sarameya (Sarama's sons): Shyama, the dark or black one, and Shabala, the spotted or multicolored one. In hymns 10, 11, and 12 of the *Atharva Veda*, the role of dogs as custodians of the dead is emphasized: "The messengers of Yama, broad-nosed and of exceeding strength, and satiating themselves with life (of mortals), hunt mankind; may they allow us this day a prosperous existence here, that we may look upon the sun (ever after)" (Tulpule 1991, 273). In addition to the connection with death, the *Chandogya Upanishad* explicitly highlights the relationship between dogs and sin, promising a disgraceful "rebirth as a dog or pig to those whose conduct has been evil" (Nelson 2006, 185). The positive association between Sarama and the concept of motherhood found in the *Rig Veda* is limited to this text. In fact, the *Ekagni Kanda* warns the reader to protect all children from the dog spirits that may try to attack them, and these are personified in particular by Sarama's sons, who are said to cause cough and spasms (Singh 1997, 491–93). Sarama's malevolent attitude is particularly evident in the *Vana Parva*, where she is described as a wicked mother or an evil spirit who roams around searching for children and fetuses to devour (Mani 1975, 694).

If we were speaking about a Hindu god rather than an animal, its complex and conflicting attributes could be likened to those of Shiva, a deity who is simultaneously generous, hot-tempered, salvific, and destructive. Thus it is no accident that in contemporary Hinduism dogs are often associated with Shiva: they are seen as both unpredictable attackers and loyal companions and they are accepted at sites of cremation. In fact, "dogs in India . . . are primarily thought of as necrophagous and associated with beings on charnel fields, such as birds (crows, vultures), jackals and outcasts," and are often referred to as *shava kamya*, "the ones who love eating corpses" (Bollée 2006, 33, 11).

In Delhi, Shiva is particularly revered in his fierce manifestation as Bheru, also called Shvashva, "whose mount is a dog" (Bollée 2006, 96). Bheru, who is also known as Bhairon, Bhairava, or Kala Bhairava, is addressed as "the terrible," "the frightful," or, according to a man whom I often used to encounter at the Bheru Mandir of Bhairon Marg in Delhi, "the god of dread and panic." Based on the information I gathered in this temple, in the epithet "Kala Bhairava," the black color (*kala*) recalls not only the idea of death but also the unforgivable sin of cutting off one of the five heads of the god Brahma, by Shiva's order. From that day on, Brahma had only four heads; the fifth one appears in the hands of Kala Bhairava in most of the statues that represent him. The *vahana* (the vehicle or companion animal) of Bheru is generally a black dog, whose collar clearly indicates that he belongs to his master, with whom he has a close relationship. Bheru is often worshipped at cremation sites, such as in the one in North Delhi where I carried out part of my fieldwork. In the Hoysaleshwara Temple in Halebidu, a statue depicts Bheru's dogs devouring the leg of a corpse (Debroy 2008, 125). Bheru's temples are among the few that can be founded by outcastes and that welcome and even revere dogs, as at the Bheru Mandir in Delhi, where dogs are ubiquitous and well fed (White 1991, 102–3).

Although Bheru primarily represents the terrifying and aggressive aspects of Shiva, having been born of his blood (Bunce 2000, 76) or his wrath (Bhattacharyya 2001, 51), his role is nevertheless positive and protective. In fact, Bheru's intercession is helpful in destroying illusion and ignorance; at a more mundane level, he promotes health, wealth, success, and the evasion of a violent, untimely death (Dwivedi 2006, 132). In particular, Bhutanatha Bheru is worshipped for his power to cure hallucinations, insomnia, and spontaneous miscarriages. In his form as "Svarnakarshana" (the one who attracts gold), Bheru is venerated by Hindu merchants who wish to increase their fortunes (Jacobsen 2009, 489).

As dogs are the intermediaries between Bheru and humans, it is not uncommon for people to offer them food in an attempt to secure themselves a long, prosperous, and healthy life. Given their strong symbolic value, black dogs are usually favored. It is believed that if dogs eat the food offered to them, they symbolically relieve all of the giver's pain and sorrow. In other words, in what appears to be a gesture of pure generosity, these animals are actually fed a poisonous morsel. One of the most common reasons for feeding black dogs, according to Delhiites who feed them (particularly in low-income areas), is the hope of a cure for male sterility (or suspected sterility). "Giving milk or rotis to a black dog on Saturday [considered an unlucky day]: this is what a man has to do if he wants to solve his problems," an elderly woman whom I regularly ran into at the Bheru Mandir recommended. When a newly married couple want to conceive a child—or, owing to social pressure, feel they must—it is not uncommon, she told me, to see the man distributing rotis and loaves of bread to street dogs. Astrologers, who prey on hopeful newlyweds, offer the same advice. Although there may be other reasons for such offerings, I witnessed this behavior fairly frequently, particularly in the early morning at bus, taxi, and rickshaw stands, where men waited for the right dog to come along. He had to be black and, even more important, hungry. One man told me that if a black dog is not available, the food offering may still be efficacious, but if the dog, whatever his color, does not eat it enthusiastically, this is cause for concern. Although it was early in the morning, I often saw dogs too full to eat another bite, thus disappointing the would-be father's hopes.

In the scant scholarly literature on dogs in Hinduism, there are a few references to the practice of offering food to street dogs. They are fed during funerals to prevent them from feeding on the soul of the deceased (Bollée 2006, 36), in case of indigestion (Walker 1968, 289), and on Sitala Saptami, the feast day of the goddess Sitala, a folk deity and incarnation of the supreme goddess Durga worshipped in northern India for providing protection from pox, sores, pustules, and other contagious diseases (Bollée 2006, 21). Finally, because of their connection with death, "the dogs of Yama are worshipped with offerings of *pinda* (i.e., rice-balls) so that they might not bark at or molest those who convey the sacrifice to the *pitri* [ancestors] in the other world" (Walker 1968, 289).

People feed street dogs not only in the hope of relief from pain and suffering, but also to get rid of their sins and thus improve their karma. In fact, street dogs are also fed because of their pariah status. Sacred texts give precise instructions on this matter. The *Manava Dharmashastra* (3.92) recommends that householders "should also gently place on the ground offerings for dogs, outcastes, dog-cookers, persons with evil diseases, crows, and worms" (Olivelle 2005, 113). Yet the purpose of such offerings is not to benefit the recipient—whatever the species—but to enhance the karma of those who give it. In fact, this apparent act of generosity is considered a rite, called *vaishvadeva*, recommended by many Sanskrit texts (White 1991, 89).

If we consider this opportunistic aspect of dog feeding in light of the broader issues of dog population control and reducing rabies, it appears paradoxical. People feed street dogs for their own personal advantage (including their health), but in doing so they directly contribute to sustaining the dog population and they exacerbate the problem of rabies, about which they vehemently complain. There are no large-scale data to quantify this complicated situation. No definitive survey has ever been carried out at the city, state, or national level to accurately gauge public opinion on the management of street dogs and rabies control. However, we do have some idea of how many Delhiites feed street dogs. The 2009 Wildlife SOS survey found that 66% of Delhiites claimed that they feed street dogs on a more or less regular basis (Bhasin 2009). In 2013, the veterinarian who runs the Animal India Trust shelter for street dogs estimated the number at around 60%. My survey of university students found that 69% of them feed street animals, though not on a regular basis. Dogs are the most commonly fed animals (63%), followed by cows (42%), birds (19%, mostly pigeons), and cats (18%).

ABC-ARV

In short, the wide availability of food on the streets increases the dog population; Mahatma Gandhi considered feeding street dogs an irresponsible and hypocritical act; many Indians feed them for religious and cultural reasons and out of compassion; at the same time, people complain about the ubiquitous presence of street dogs in public spaces, which are also filled with garbage. To complicate matters even further, the Animal Welfare Board of India and the AWOs that follow its guidelines claim that feeding street dogs is *not* counterproductive in terms of demographic control and the elimination of rabies. On the contrary, in its *Revised Module for Street Dog Population Management, Rabies Eradication, Reducing Man-Dog Conflict* (AWBI 2016), the AWBI states that feeding them is useful and beneficial if it is done within the broader animal birth control (ABC)–anti-rabies vaccination (ARV) program that it promotes. During my fieldwork in 2019, some people also pointed out the role played by the Swachh Bharat Abhiyan (Clean India Mission). They claimed that dog bites and attacks have increased since 2014, as improved garbage management and cleaner streets are leaving dogs hungrier.

Before we examine the details of ABC-ARV, it is important to note that not everybody in India agrees on this strategy. Its opponents include both those who advocate mass culling for the purpose of controlling rabies and those researchers and NGOs that blame ABC-ARV for illogically perpetuating the problem instead of addressing its root causes. The latter argue that dogs are domestic animals, that the "street dog" label is counterproductive, and that there is nothing scientific or compassionate about condemning them to a life of homelessness, hunger, mistreatment, and suffering while pretending that feeding them is good for them, their human neighbors, the human-dog relationship, or rabies control (Uniyal 2019). Moreover, opponents of the ABC-ARV approach maintain that feeding dogs in public places poses risks for other animals, especially wild species, and thus contravenes article 51 of the constitution—the same article that ABC-ARV supporters take inspiration from.

Finally, these critics point out that the Animal Birth Control (Dogs) Rules of 2001 actually contradict in several places the Prevention of Cruelty to Animals Act of 1960 that they build upon. For example, section 2(f) of the 1960 act says that the caretaker of an animal "includes not only the owner but also any other person for the time being in possession or custody of the animal, whether with or without the consent of the owner." As Abi T. Vanak, Aniruddha Belsare, and Meghna Uniyal (2016) observe, this means that once municipal authorities and AWOs pick up free-roaming, ownerless, unclaimed dogs from the streets, they lawfully become the owners of these animals, and according to chapter 3, subsection 11 of the same act, they commit an offense when they "abandon any animal in circumstances which render it likely that it will suffer pain by reason of starvation or thirst." International rabies scholars, most of whom are actively involved with WHO and GARC, likewise do not recommend ABC-ARV if rabies control is its first or only goal. Epidemiologists have not yet determined the exact relationship between rabies control and sterilization efforts, but they do not consider them strongly linked (Morters et al. 2013, 12). Thus rabies experts, and WHO itself, consider vaccination the most direct, efficient, and cost-effective solution to dog-mediated rabies, particularly in resource-limited settings (Cleaveland et al. 2014, 189). Sterilization has collateral advantages: it reduces the number of females in heat and consequently competition over them, thus resulting in fewer bites to both people and other dogs; it reduces dog turnover and thus the number who require vaccination. But at present there is no scientific evidence to support it as an essential component of rabies control (Knobel et al. 2013, 599), and it is expensive, time-consuming, and labor-intensive (Fitzpatrick et al. 2016, 14577). Let us turn now to the specifics of ABC-ARV.

The animal shelter and veterinary clinic Help In Suffering in Jaipur is one of the best places in which to see the ABC-ARV policy at work. In the HIS operating room—surrounded by the pungent smells of antiseptics and burnt flesh and hypnotized by the colonies of ticks trying to escape from the sedated and thus inhospitable bodies of the dogs—I learned most of what I know about it. The animal birth control–anti-rabies vaccination strategy prescribes that dogs must be counted and surveyed within a given area; humanely caught by properly trained dogcatchers (with the exclusion of visibly pregnant or lactating bitches and puppies less than six months old); safely transported by van to the ABC-ARV center; properly housed; either identified by a collar with specific color coding or given a distinctive V-shaped notch in the left ear and an alphanumeric code tattooed inside the same ear; spayed or neutered in a safe, hygienic, and well-equipped operating theater; given adequate postsurgical care during the recovery period (four to six days); inoculated against rabies; and taken back to the exact location of the town from which they were collected. When the right-flank approach is used to spay female dogs, for a period after the surgery they are easily recognizable by their shaved flank.

For each dog who undergoes ABC-ARV, a detailed form must be kept in a register. It consists of a health report and identity card for each animal. In fact, one of the essential principles of ABC-ARV is that there is a strong connection between dogs and their place on the street. If this link is broken, ABC-ARV cannot work, resulting in a loss of time, money, and other resources. I occasionally joined the HIS staff during the release process and was consistently amazed by the meticulousness with which they carried out this task. While in Delhi, I helped the manager of the ABC clinic Animal India Trust update the clinic's registers, and I began to know the city as I never had before. In transcribing the addresses of more than 4,000 releases, I began to see Delhi from the point of view of the dogs. The most frequent points of reference for the staff during the release process were not the ones with which people are usually concerned, such as shops, tourist spots, and civic landmarks. They were the ones that matter to dogs: *dalaos* (areas for garbage disposal), *dhabas* (roadside eateries), markets, subways, and landfills.

If an ABC-ARV project is to succeed, at least 70% of the total dog population must be sterilized in each area within a time frame of six months (AWBI 2009, 5). Six months corresponds to the breeding cycle of most breeds, even though most Indian street dogs reproduce only once a year (Pal 2001, 71). After the first rabies vaccine shot, which is given when the dog is sterilized, dogs should be revaccinated against rabies every year, as the long-term efficacy of rabies vaccines is uncertain and remains a matter of debate. The 70% figure ensures a stable dog population, since any successful mating of the remaining 30% yields a birth rate that does not exceed the natural death rate, thus not producing an increase in the total number of dogs (provided, of course, that the cycle repeats, with at least 70% of new births also being sterilized, and so on). At the same time, the sustained immunization of at least 70% of the dogs in a given area breaks the transmission of rabies even in a country like India, where the disease is endemic. Successful ABC-ARV programs require dog population density and ecological studies both before and after implementation, since rabies-control initiatives need to be adapted to the local dog ecology (Kappeler and Wandeler 1991, 8). To ensure that these studies are accurate, responsible pet registration—of both pet dogs kept inside homes and those who roam freely—is imperative. Pet registration can also be used as a tool that helps sterilize and vaccinate pet dogs and to inform the public about the importance of these measures. Registration also plays a vital role in controlling the spread of rabies, because it links a specific street dog to its respective owner or caretaker, making it easier to localize the animal in case of bites or for the necessary anti-rabies boosters.

If the sterilization goal of 70% is not reached within a certain area, the number of dogs in it will increase until the carrying capacity of that area is fully exploited. This population growth is due to the longer life expectancy of the remaining unsterilized dogs that results from decreased competition over food caused by sterilization. In contrast, if an area is left vacant by mass killing, new dogs, who may not have been sterilized or vaccinated, will fill the vacancies. These dogs inevitably destabilize the unique balance of any given area, by breeding, spreading disease, competing with the local dogs for dominance in the new neighborhood, and behaving aggressively toward unfamiliar human residents. Similarly, if vaccination does not reach the 70% threshold, the rabies virus can circulate freely, with fatal results.

In India, mass culling was admitted to be a complete failure in the early 1990s and was soon replaced by ABC-ARV. Delhi was the first city to implement ABC-ARV, in 1993, soon followed by Jaipur and Chennai, which started their model programs in 1994 and 1996, respectively. In November 1997, the AWBI began supporting the implementation of ABC-ARV by AWOs all over India. One month later, ABC-ARV was adopted as the official dog-control policy of the entire country. On December 24, 2001, the Ministry of Culture issued the Animal Birth Control (Dogs) Rules (or ABC rules), pursuant to the Prevention of Cruelty to Animals Act of 1960. These rules made it a crime for individuals, resident welfare associations

(RWAs), and municipal corporations to kill, relocate, beat, or drive away street dogs, whether sterilized and vaccinated or not. Citizens may only report what they perceive as a nuisance to the municipal authorities, who in turn should operate a dog pound. The rules make an exception for terminally ill dogs, who can be euthanized. Yet dogs suspected of being rabid must be caught and kept in isolation for ten days, until they are either declared uninfected or die an atrocious death. Dogs may not be euthanized just because they are perceived as aggressive or bad-tempered.

Feeding street dogs is believed to play a key role in helping with the implementation of ABC-ARV. Yet in recent years this issue has led to a fierce debate and more acrimony between those who feed, defend, and support street dogs and those who view such actions as irresponsible lunacy. Supporters claim that ABC-ARV promotes more stable human-dog coexistence, and that feeding street dogs reduces their fear of humans and makes it easier to catch them for sterilization and vaccination. They also point out that hungry dogs are more likely to fight, bite, and contract and transmit disease, risks that increase when they must forage for food in garbage. Tired of being verbally and physically harassed by ABC-ARV opponents, several of Delhi's dog feeders submitted a petition to the High Court of Delhi in 2009 seeking permission to feed street dogs undisturbed and protected by law (Rajagopal 2009). In its ruling on that petition, the court took a stand on this issue when it acknowledged that feeding street dogs provides a "great service to humanity." The court ordered police protection for those feeding dogs and asked the AWBI, in cooperation with RWAs and the local police, to identify legitimate dog-feeding sites in various neighborhoods where dog feeders are entitled to take care of street dogs. Since then, dozens of these feeding sites have been created in Delhi, particularly in the south. The Jawaharlal Nehru University campus was one of these sites until March 2017, when the university administration forbade feeding dogs on its premises. The court ruling specified that feeding sites must be located away from busy streets, footpaths, and children's parks, and that feeding must be carried out in a responsible and hygienic manner and must not cause any public disturbance.

In 2012, the AWBI also obtained permission to issue a "colony animal caretaker card," an ID card recognized by the then MCD and the Delhi Police that provides further protection to dog feeders. The law made it a punishable offense to restrict, prohibit, or cause inconvenience to any card-carrying person feeding a street dog. According to a notice "regarding curbing cruelty against animals" issued on February 2, 2012, by the Municipal Corporation of Gurgaon (a suburb of Delhi, now Gurugram) to the presidents of its RWAs, dog feeding is a "social service" and a constitutional duty (according to article 51, which mandates compassion for animals).

While dog-feeding sites are common in many Indian cities, the colony caretaker card is, to my knowledge, unique to Delhi. These measures were intended, on the one hand, to benefit dogs, and, on the other hand, to help defuse tension over the issue of street dogs. As an article on dog-feeding sites in the *Indian Express* put it, "The dog-feeders and dog-haters of Delhi can breathe easy for now" (Sinha 2010). Similarly, the NGO People for Animals informs visitors to its website that the colony caretaker card "comes in useful if people complain to the police or neighbors and animal haters prove to be a nuisance." At the same time, however, there are mixed feelings about this card even among defenders of street dogs. One staunch animal welfare activist told me that he did not like the idea that people who were not really animal lovers, let alone activists, could now present themselves as animal caretakers solely through possession of this card. He accused such people of wanting to flaunt their alleged love for dogs merely because it gives them social prestige within their social circles by officially designating them as philanthropists who spend their time and money on possibly the worst-treated animals in India. He and hard-core activists like him, he said with pride and disdain, do not have time to leave the dogs they take care of to go and apply for this card.

Gaps Between Theory and Practice

In Delhi, the strain over the management of street dogs and rabies is palpable. Each side in the debate regards the other with suspicion, hostility, and mistrust and accuses the other of politicizing and intentionally inflaming this issue. Religious beliefs, cultural norms, and the hardships of poverty also contribute to the disagreement over how to manage street dogs, making it difficult to find a solution that satisfies the majority. The British veterinarian in charge of the ABC-ARV program at Help In Suffering in Jaipur has no doubt that this strained and divisive atmosphere is the chief obstacle to the efficient management of street dog population and rabies in India. "The majority of people would say that street dogs are a bad idea," he observed (see also Beck 1973, viii), but in Jaipur the opposite is actually true. For all the people who want to see dogs on the street, there are as many others who, he said, "would like them to be dead today if possible. The rest of the population who sit in the middle are tolerant. Because Indians are extraordinarily tolerant!" The same situation exists in Delhi and, very likely, throughout India. Predictably, this plurality of viewpoints is particularly pronounced in urban settings, which bring together people with different cultural backgrounds and diverse level of exposure to animals and animal-related issues.

I witnessed this dynamic repeatedly, each time I joined the HIS staff in the ABC-ARV catch-and-release process. In some areas—particularly the lower-income ones—the community objects to the catching phase, as residents do not want the dogs to be taken away. For decades they have watched municipal authorities round up street dogs who are never seen again, so their opposition is understandable. In other neighborhoods, HIS staff face resistance when they release the dogs after neutering and vaccination. Those who object are constrained by their Hindu ethics from demanding that the dogs be killed; instead, they favor their relocation. "Don't release the dogs here—release them somewhere else": HIS staff hear this every day. The problem, of course, is that *somewhere else*, no matter how far away, they will encounter the same complaint. "So," the veterinarian concluded, "they are stuck!" In yet another instance of "not in my back yard," people do not want the dogs to be killed, but they do not want them around, either. "Let's not say 'remove,'" a Hindu man, worried about his karmic balance sheet, suggested. "I prefer saying 'take them to another place.' It sounds better, you know." As with garbage management, which Viswanathan Raghunathan describes as "not a garbage disposal system but a garbage redistribution system" (2006, 77), so with dog population and rabies control: out of sight, out of mind.

In Delhi, the variety of opinions on street dogs is even larger and more fragmented. This is particularly the case within the middle class, which, according to most of the animal welfare activists I spoke with in the city, plays a key role in issues of pet keeping and street dog management. As the manager of a clinic for street dogs in Lajpat Nagar (South East Delhi) told me, middle-class ideas about pet keeping are often irresponsible. There are exceptions, of course, but most middle-class dog owners see their dogs mainly as desirable status symbols. So "why should people take a street dog?" she asked me rhetorically. People spend 40,000 rupees (US$580) for a Saint Bernard or 60,000 rupees (US$870) for a Siberian husky, ignoring the fact that summer temperatures in Delhi can easily reach 113 degrees Fahrenheit (45 degrees Celsius). They want a pug only because "it is so cute," or they take a Labrador retriever to a flat hardly big enough for a Chihuahua. Then, she goes on, "the grandma gets sick and they come and ask me where they can leave it."

I was told a similar story by a woman who lives in an affluent neighborhood of South Delhi with her elderly mother, about two dozen dogs, and more cats than she can keep track of. By nature very emotional and extremely sensitive to animal suffering, her eyes filled with tears even before she began her story. In a nearby house there lived a family that she described as "filthy rich." Sometime before, this family had bought a Labrador retriever who she knew was ill, for the servant who walked him had told her that they were trying to cure him of cancer. One morning she had seen the *kabariwala* (someone who goes door to door collecting household garbage) putting the dog on his rubbish cart. In a broken voice she described how she had run into the street and asked where he was taking the dog. He replied that the lady of the house had hastily told him to take the dog with him, giving him no chance to object. "I couldn't say no," he told the bereft neighbor. She took a deep breath and told me, "It's true, he could not say no; you cannot win with these people. They are so rich and they have so many possibilities, but as soon as the dog is ill, they kick him out."

The day I brought one of our cats to Friendicoes, I witnessed firsthand the unfortunate fate of many Delhi dogs. Friendicoes is an animal welfare organization, located under the overpass that divides Jangpura from Defence Colony, that runs a shelter for street dogs and a veterinary clinic for pets. Such places were not new to me. I had already spent time at HIS in Jaipur and Animal Aid Unlimited in Udaipur, and I was used to seeing street dogs arrive at those shelters in the worst imaginable condition. But the vast majority of the dogs in Jaipur and Udaipur were INDogs or mongrels. What I saw for the first time at Friendicoes were dozens of foreign-breed dogs, mainly pugs and Labrador retrievers but also a Saint Bernard and a Great Dane. In most cases they had ended up there (and in similar shelters) because their owners had abandoned them when the fashion changed or their fascination waned. Or when they realized how demanding and expensive a dog's upkeep is, or when they learned that dogs, too, can get sick (and foreign-breed dogs usually contract illnesses more frequently than local dogs). Or even just when their cute little puppy grew up and was no longer quite so adorable. As early as 1962, K. B. Roy had already written of India, "In our urban society, ownership of a dog has become a symbol of respectability even for people who neither love a dog nor can afford to keep one decently" (141). I have no historical data available, but I assume that this syndrome has not gotten any better. A study carried out in Chandigarh on dog-keeping practices provided alarming results on dog vaccination awareness. A fifth of the dog owners surveyed did not know the vaccination status of their dog, and 66% never provided their dog with the necessary boosters after initial immunization (Singh et al. 2011, 113).

Of course, the abandonment of pet dogs has direct and significant repercussions for the overall issue of dog population control and rabies elimination. Not only are more dogs added to an already large population of street dogs, but these new entries are not always sterilized and they will mate as soon as they learn how to survive on their own. Initially, being unaccustomed to fending for themselves and to the harshness of street life, these dogs are completely hopeless in regard to the search for food, water, and shelter. Since their previous life, often as lone pets, may not have socialized them to other dogs, they may be relationally ignorant and may not know how to find a place for themselves in a territory already occupied by a pack of dogs. Violent fights are thus not uncommon, and in their fear, hunger, and pain, these dogs can direct their aggression toward people by biting them. At present, the proportion of abandoned dogs in the overall street dog population is limited, but given the growing trend of pet ownership in India and the preference for foreign-breed dogs, it is likely to increase, and this factor must be considered in view of the composite project of dog population control and rabies management. More than a third of the university students I interviewed personally knew people who had abandoned their pets. The most common reasons given for abandonment were lack of time, dog health problems, and behavioral issues.

Although no precise data are available, some of the breed dogs found on Indian streets were not abandoned by their owners but are victims of illegal breeding. Given the high demand for certain foreign breeds, unregistered, improvised, and unscrupulous "puppy mills" are flourishing in India. To obtain the adult dogs they need for mating, breeders occasionally steal pet dogs, and once these animals have served their purpose, they kill or abandon them. Breeding markets are mainly located in and around Delhi—for example, in Gurugram, Ghaziabad, Narela, Meerut, Faridabad, and Rohtak (Shekhar 2016). The Prevention of Cruelty to Animals (Dog

Breeding and Marketing) Rules of 2017 now prohibit breeding activities and owning or housing dogs for breeding or sale without updated registration and proper records.

The main strength, but also the greatest weakness, of ABC-ARV is the intricate interplay of its many components, which all must work smoothly if this strategy is to work. In fact, since dog population management, dog bites, and rabies are issues of wide and multidimensional scope, their management invariably calls for a multipronged strategy that does not focus solely on dogs. The interrelations include those between dogs and people, dogs and other animal species (such as the disappearing vultures), street dogs and pet dogs, pet owners and prospective pet owners, dog lovers and dog haters, patients seeking health care and health-care providers, dog feeding and garbage disposal, accountable pet ownership and responsible public spirit. Appreciating the importance of all these factors and their complex interactions is probably the main challenge that India must face if it wants to fight rabies. Lack of accurate information, confusion spread by media, and the deeply emotional nature of these issues further complicate this matter. The ABC-ARV strategy cannot succeed if even one of the processes involved is not carried out properly. And even if the ABC-ARV method works smoothly, results cannot be expected overnight; at least a decade is necessary. ABC-ARV is by nature and by definition a long-term, systematic, and well-organized project that takes several years to pay off—and that is assuming that everything goes according to plan. The strategy must be carried out scrupulously, with no interruptions or even slowdowns. It requires forward-looking planning, maintaining a delicate balance between all the component parts, and a great deal of patience. Finally, ABC-ARV needs a multispecies approach for best results, as the rabies virus is not picky about choosing its hosts.

Given the difficulty of keeping so many moving parts working together in a well-oiled machine, ABC-ARV often breaks down even before reaching the public. In fact, there is widespread failure to comply with the Animal Birth Control (Dogs) Rules of 2001 by the very municipal corporations and animal welfare organizations responsible for transforming ABC-ARV from theory to practice. Within the circle of virtuous AWOs, news often circulates about municipal dog pounds where dogs are not sterilized and vaccinated, as per the law, but are instead starved to death, or are reduced to eating their own puppies (Voice of Street Dogs 2011). Moreover, many of the AWO managers I met in Delhi and Jaipur told me that municipal dogcatchers often work on call—that is, they catch dogs randomly whenever irate, influential citizens ask them to intervene, turning ABC-ARV into a haphazard mess. One cost of these random roundups is that sterilized, vaccinated, healthy, well-fed dogs may be killed, since their trust in people makes them easy to catch. I vividly remember returning to the HIS shelter in Jaipur one day after we had released some dogs neutered, vaccinated, dogs. We got stuck in traffic just behind the dark green van used by the municipal corporation for the same purpose. The HIS dogcatcher driving our van wondered sadly how long it would take the municipal crew to round up the dogs we had just released.

To make matters worse, AWOs themselves do not always operate properly. Accounts sometimes circulate of sterilized bitches found on the street with gaping wounds because of untrained medical staff, poor surgical materials, insufficient medical care, and lucrative same-day release. Incompetence and mismanagement is one culprit (Srinivasan and Nagaraj 2007, 1085), but intentional misconduct is also often a factor, as demonstrated by an internal review of the ABC-ARV program conducted in 2008 (Uniyal and Vanak 2016). In Delhi, Jaipur, and many other Indian cities, local government typically appoints AWOs to carry out ABC-ARV, paying them 800–1,000 rupees (US$11–14) for each dog they sterilize and immunize. At HIS and Animal India Trust, government inspectors used to come regularly to check the registers and the reproductive organs preserved in formaldehyde. Despite these methods of strict (and theoretically foolproof) control, AWOs and municipal dog pounds sometimes alter their registers to show sterilizations that were never performed (Kumar 2016). Rumors about such practices predictably increase tension over rabies and dog population control.

Even apart from the cases of incompetence and malfeasance, ABC-ARV suffers from critical logistical and operational challenges baked into its very conception. Funding from the central government is woefully inadequate, so much so that in 2016 an AWBI report concluded that "successfully conducting a viable animal birth control programme through out [sic] the country is not possible in these circumstances" (AWBI 2016, 155). At the base of this problem is serious institutional conflict over who is financially responsible for implementing ABC-ARV. While the human medicine sector bears the brunt of rabies costs in terms of human rabies deaths and PEP, the costs of ABC-ARV fall on the veterinary sector, which has limited interest in safeguarding the health of dogs because of their low economic value in

India (Cleaveland et al. 2014, 189). Such a bottleneck is often the primary challenge to controlling neglected tropical diseases around the world (Bardosh 2014, 4).

Another tricky issue is that although the AWBI protocol envisions a dog population estimate before ABC-ARV can be implemented, the small minority of AWOs that provide such data have only "unreliable and imaginary" information (Uniyal and Vanak 2016). The same lack of proper data and records plagues the vaccination process, periodic revaccination, and the final intervention evaluation. Other challenges include the difficulty of catching unowned or loosely owned dogs in open areas (mainly in rural India, far from where ABC-ARV is currently being tested), roaming dogs' increasing wariness of catching teams, and the requirement for a large number of skilled dogcatchers per vaccination team. Finally, while the AWBI says that "no street dog can be pronounced rabid unless a scientific test is conducted" (2016, 43), postmortem autopsy and lab testing of brain samples present challenges in terms of time, money, staff, and logistics that put them out of reach of many AWOs. The incineration of the carcasses of rabid dogs and the handling of dog-related complaints prescribed by the AWBI (2016, 137, 139) create an additional drain on short-staffed, underfunded agencies. In short, when we remember that ABC-ARV is supposed to address some sixty million dogs in India, the problem looks formidable, the outlook grim.

There is some good news in localized areas, however. After a tough period of adjustment, ABC-ARV has produced positive results in the areas of Jaipur where HIS has been operating since 1994, reaching and often exceeding the goal of vaccinating and sterilizing 70% of an area's dogs. By 1999, after five years in force, no human deaths from rabies were reported in those areas. By contrast, human losses continued and even increased in the non-ABC-ARV areas of Jaipur. Similarly, the number of reported dog bites declined from seven per thousand in 1997 to less than three in 2015 (Reece and Chawla 2006, 381). Yet, interestingly, the Jaipur Municipal Corporation continues to receive at least two complaints about street dogs each day (*Times of India* 2018). Moreover, despite the laudable efforts of HIS (in collaboration with the Jaipur Municipal Corporation), no dog population management program is currently in effect in Jaipur as a whole, as the Rajasthan state government has failed to allocate funds (AWBI 2016, 206). Rajasthan is not alone in this failure in combatting rabies: a mere 2.4% of the street dogs in all of India were vaccinated by the AWBI, through its

AWOs, in the decade 2008 to 2018 (Kukreti 2018). As if this percentage were not low enough, the possibility of nonresponders and immunologically challenged dogs must also be taken into account when vaccination programs are evaluated. A study conducted in Chandigarh showed that of one hundred street dogs tested, only one had antibodies above protective levels (Singh et al. 2011, 112). Moreover, when the 70% vaccination objective is set, particular attention must be paid to which dog subcategories to include—for example, unsupervised free-roaming dogs have a high rate of population turnover (Vanak 2017). Therefore, there is no blanket strategy for the entire country and its diverse dog population.

The situation in Delhi is even more complicated than the one in Jaipur. After the last survey of street dogs there, in 2009, the MCD was split in three (into North, East, and South Delhi), which made the systematic collection of data on street dogs, bites, and rabies cases even more difficult. In 2015 the South MCD invited bids for carrying out another survey and received no response at all (*New Indian Express* 2015b). Without a reliable estimate of the city's total dog population, figures on how many dogs AWOs manage to sterilize and vaccinate are not particularly useful. Even less useful are misleading proposals such as the one made by the New Delhi Municipal Council in November 2015, which infuriated Delhi's animal welfare activists. It sent residents a mobile phone text message asking, "Should NDMC [New Delhi Municipal Council] relocate stray dogs to sanctuaries? Please send response. . . . Regards, Chairman NDMC" (Nath 2015b). While the aim was to collect citizens' feedback for India's Smart Cities Challenge (in which cities competed for government funding for sustainable urban renewal projects), the text message solicited opinions on a practice that not only has been proved ineffective but is in fact illegal under the Animal Birth Control (Dogs) Rules of 2001.

In 2015, the South MCD opened a new dog sterilization center in Bijwasan, in addition to the nine already located there (some managed directly by the South MCD, some by NGOs), and asked the Delhi Development Authority to provide land for more such centers. There is also a sterilization center in the jurisdiction of the North MCD. No centers have been opened by the East MCD yet, but the *Times of India* (2016) reported that the East MCD had in 2016 approved the establishment of the first pound in the city for terminally ill and rabid dogs, where ABC-ARV will also be carried out. By the way, the North MCD and the East MCD are the areas of Delhi with the highest number of dog bite cases, 37,915 and 24,802, respectively (*Hindustan Times* 2015a). In January 2019, for the first time, the Delhi government announced an integrated plan, which it called the Animal Health and Welfare Policy, to tackle the many animal-related issues that bedevil the city. The development minister at the time also suggested that the Animal Husbandry Unit of the Development Department should be renamed the Animal Health and Welfare Department (GNCTD 2018).

Whose Life Matters More?

In addition to the massive conceptual and practical problems outlined above, the most fundamental obstacle to the success of ABC-ARV—but also of its vaccination component only, should this measure be implemented on its own—lies in how the issue of rabies control is framed. Invariably, the issue comes down to the question "Whose life matters more, that of the dog who bites and transmits rabies or that of the person who is bitten and dies of rabies?" This question, and the choice it poses between dogs and people, arises in informal conversations, media reports, municipal councils, and courts of law. What many people fail to see, however, is that this is a false distinction based on faulty reasoning. Scientific research and successful rabies-control programs (such as those by WHO in South America—Del Rio Vilas et al. 2017) clearly demonstrate that when dogs are vaccinated, the incidence of dog-mediated rabies in humans drops to zero. If rabies is eliminated in dogs, it will also disappear in the human population. Unfortunately, in India this fact is often overlooked, lost in the confusion over ABC-ARV and the vitriolic disagreement between "dog lovers" and "dog haters." The debate over rabies and dog population control measures easily becomes personal, losing the objectivity and scientific rigor it needs in order to bear fruit. In the meantime, the large number of rabies cases in humans, and the high incidence of dog attacks on humans and human violence to dogs, continue unabated. And this situation cannot help but further pit humans and dogs against each other, obscuring their mutual interests in the fight against rabies and reinforcing the erroneous suggestion that human life and dog welfare are incompatible.

Class and socioeconomic inequalities add fuel to the fire. As in other countries, there are deep inequities of wealth, power, and related freedoms in India. Despite being ideologically far apart, the various factions in the debate over rabies and dog management—those who champion

ABC-ARV, those who promote vaccination alone, and those who believe in mass culling—have two things in common. First, they are largely composed of (urban) middle-class and upper middle-class people. Second, they often presume, whether legitimately or illegitimately, to champion and speak for those who have little or no voice. These voiceless people are India's urban poor, who live in slums or on the streets. Statistically speaking, they are also the most common victims of rabies. Critics of ABC-ARV accuse its supporters of being heartless elitists who care more about street dogs than they do about people—even worse, about already vulnerable people. In short, they are criticized for being "armchair activists" who dispense their opinions from a privileged position and will never experience firsthand the real needs and afflictions of the unfortunate people whose welfare they claim to protect. With their misplaced priorities, sentimentality, ideological pretensions, antidemocratic insolence, and social and economic advantages, opponents charge, these dog-loving no-kill armchair activists put human lives at risk. It is this pro-dog, anti-poor lobby, not dogs themselves, that detractors of ABC-ARV consider the greatest menace.

The dogs of Lodhi Garden perfectly illustrate the tension and the distance between the dog welfare activists and ABC-ARV champions, on the one hand, and those who favor a more incisive approach to dog management and rabies control, on the other. Lodhi Garden is a ninety-acre public park in the heart of Delhi, near the city's most upscale neighborhoods and its main political institutions. Known for its botanical and architectural heritage, Lodhi Garden is an idyllic setting for the morning walks of Delhiites, especially for the well-to-do residents of the surrounding area. Signs at the entrances announce that dogs are allowed in the park between 8:00 A.M. and 5:00 P.M., provided they are kept on a leash. People who take their Siberian huskies jogging with them, or allow their Pomeranians to stroll among the rose gardens and ancient tombs, often ignore the leash rule. So does the quite stable population of about thirty dogs who have been permanent residents of the park for several years now, roaming free there 24/7. In October 2012, the High Court of Delhi ordered municipal authorities to remove these dogs from the park. One week later, however, it asked the authorities to postpone rounding up the dogs. The reason for the reversal was a plea from prominent animal-loving Delhiites and animal rights activists, who pointed out that the dogs had been sterilized and vaccinated and thus did not need to be removed; in fact, they reminded the High Court,

ABC-ARV rules allow the removal of a dog only when there is a complaint that he has bitten someone or become a nuisance in some other way. As a result, the dogs remained in the park, enjoying Delhi's winter clothed in warm dog coats and regularly fed by nearby residents or their servants, who provided bowls of food to each dog in this pack.

Predictably, many Delhiites were not happy about this. The comments left on the website of the *Times of India*, which told the story of these dogs (Garg 2012b), speak for themselves:

> "You people live in well-off area and travel in cars and wont allow these dogs to enter inside your streets, at least it roams in our streets." (Tamil Nadu)
> "There are more dog lovers in usa than india but such a casul approach is never made. they should be in the homes of the lovers not in the street eating garbage and biting innocent people." (United States)
> "[Maneka Gandhi] should take all the dogs to her house if she loves them so much!! Each dog can cause rabies ensuring a certain death!!" (Uttar Pradesh)
> "Which is better: to have well fed stray dogs spreading Rabies or our countrymen protected from Rabies?" (Bangalore)

Once again, poor people who live and work on the streets are at the center of the issue. ABC-ARV supporters claim that street and slum dwellers are unrivaled in their love for street dogs and their desire to live with them, while skeptics insist that rabies threatens the poor more than any other class of people. Of course, poor people themselves rarely get to express their own actual views. And even when they do, the two factions tend to get in the middle of things. Take the case of Shivalingaiah, an unskilled laborer and father of an eight-year-old girl who was killed by a group of dogs in Bangalore in 2007. In her analysis of the media hoopla over this tragedy, Anuradha Ramanujan claimed that this man was against the mass killing drive that was subsequently organized by the Bangalore municipality, and that he made this clear to television reporters. Yet "his class position, loss and vulnerability were repeatedly invoked by the media and the anti-'stray' dog lobby" to advance their agenda (2015, 225). ABC-ARV advocates, for their part, repeated their argument that the poor actually derive the main benefits of having street dogs around, as they are protected at night, their homes and belongings are guarded, and they have a companion animal they could not afford otherwise. The AWBI (n.d., 25) claims that 88% of community and neighborhood dog owners and caretakers attempt to hide their dogs from municipal dogcatchers out of fear that they may be killed or taken away permanently.

This issue was one of the thorniest I encountered during my fieldwork. I remember well the first time I entered a slum, prepared by WHO data on rabies to encounter the most vulnerable victims of the disease. But I left this slum with a new insight, after listening for hours to people who had experienced the pain of dog bites, witnessed the tribulations of rabies in friends and relatives, and seen the terror of puppy pregnancies in neighbors. I saw the apprehension firsthand, and I heard many fearful stories, but I sensed no hate or violent intolerance toward dogs in the words and attitudes of the people. Much of the general lenience I witnessed toward dogs is probably due to the interspecies empathy that I first saw in children like Neelam, with whom I began this book, described at more length in chapter 6. In the street, a garbage collector pointed out, the poor and the dogs are in the same boat; both have to struggle for resources—from food to love, safety to happiness. And quite often they struggle side by side, rummaging through the same garbage heap, or sleeping together on winter nights to share some warmth and safety. Mishaps like dog bites may happen, of course, but they are mainly due to the harsh conditions of living on the street. "It's nobody's fault," he concluded serenely. I also met dog bite victims who told me, as calmly as this man had, that they had beaten the offending dog to death without the slightest hesitation. Once the culprit has been punished, or the anger discharged, no resentment and intolerance toward dogs as a species is harbored.

Pramod, a veterinarian from Delhi whom I met on an interminable train journey, did not hesitate when I asked him where dogs in Delhi enjoy the best quality of life: with the filthy richest and the poorest, he said. In affluent colonies like Golf Links, Khan Market, and Pandara Park, street dogs enjoy extremely high standards of living because people spend "unthinkable amounts of time and money for them." He described a dozen dog feeders he knew in just one area, and the number of street dogs they take care of on a daily basis, about thirty each. Then he turned to the dogs of the poor. "Even if they are not educated on how to keep dogs, they really love them. . . . They may not have much to feed them, but they keep them anyway and do their best to make them feel good." My ethnographic observations bear this out. In the slums of Delhi that I visited, people showed me the rats, mice, and parrots who were their pets, but dogs were also always present, treated with respect, and introduced as long-term members of the community. For the most part, people did not seem to treat them as pets, if by this we mean that pet dogs have names. In fact, different people, even within the same family, called a given dog by different names, Ramu, Kalu, and Moti being common favorites. I often sensed that people had come up with these names as we spoke, as naming was not important to them and even less so to the dogs. Many people were much more concerned about the presence of a collar on the dog's neck—not necessarily a proper collar, but just a piece of cloth or plastic bag so that "nobody will take them away."

Then there are the in-betweens, my traveling companion concluded, the middle-class people. "You can divide them in two," he explained. "Half go crazy for dogs and sometimes even exaggerate; half are the worst I know when it comes to dogs." In upper middle-class areas, he claimed, people take unimaginably good care of street dogs. In others, such as the one where he lived, he did not even want his neighbors to know that he is a veterinarian. Otherwise, he said, "as soon as a dog barks at night, they come and knock at my door." Hiranmay Karlekar, a well-off journalist who fought for the Lodhi Garden dogs, shared Pramod's view when I interviewed him in February 2013, his adopted dog jumping on and off the sofa in his living room while we spoke. In Karlekar's opinion, the percentage of people in Delhi who love animals is much higher among the poor than among the middle class. "If in India some humanity is left, for sure it is among the poor," he said without hesitation. In his view, middle-class people are so egoistically interested in increasing their material wealth that they are unable to maintain human relationships, given the time and effort they require. When I asked him whether the same was true of relationships with animals, he vigorously assented. "It's not that they don't worry about animals," he clarified, "they don't worry about *anyone*." When I later read his book *Savage Humans and Stray Dogs*, I realized that he had actually been quite measured and restrained during our meeting.

The same disagreement over the management of street dogs and rabies that exists among private citizens is echoed in the legal discourse on these issues. In spite of the government's Animal Birth Control (Dogs) Rules of 2001, which remain in effect, and the AWBI's *Revised Module for Street Dog Population Management, Rabies Eradication, Reducing Man-Dog Conflict* of 2016, adherence is patchy and voices of dissent are regularly raised. The result is an emotional and legal rollercoaster, with continual changes of direction. In September 2013, the Jammu and Kashmir State Human Rights Commission defined the killing of a baby by a pack of (allegedly rabid) street dogs as a human rights violation (*Greater Kashmir* 2013). In August 2015, the following headline appeared on the website of the National Human Rights Commission (NHRC): "Stray Dog Menace: NHRC Calls for a Civil Society Debate on Human Rights Versus Animal Rights; Also Notice to Centre and Delhi Government to Ascertain Their Views." The NHRC, the article stated, "has taken suo motu cognizance of media reports on the stray dog menace and observed that prima facie, it is of the view that Human Rights should weigh above animal rights in a situation where human lives are at risk due to attack by animals." Meanwhile, the NGOs Nyaya Bhoomi and Society for Public Cause asked the High Court of Delhi to address the issue of street dogs and dog bites and to take a stand on the question of the priority of human or animal life. The court replied that the lives of people and dogs were equally important (*Outlook* 2015b). Yet in September 2016, in response to the AWBI's *Revised Module for Street Dog Population Management*, the Supreme Court of India decided that "compassion should be shown toward stray dogs but at the mean time, these animals cannot be allowed to become a menace to the society. A balance needs to be created for dealing with such situations" (*Indian Express* 2016c). Finally, in 2018, the High Court of Uttarakhand declared that the entire animal kingdom is a legal entity with the legal rights of a "living person." This decision was explained by citing article 21 of the constitution: "While safeguarding the rights of humans, [the article] protects life and the word 'life' means animal world" (Santoshi 2018). In the High Court of Punjab and Haryana, Justice Rajiv Sharma issued a similar 104-page declaration in 2019, which ends: "The entire animal kingdom including avian and aquatic are declared as legal entities having a distinct persona with corresponding rights, duties and liabilities of a living person. All the citizens throughout the State of Haryana are hereby declared persons in loco parentis as the human face for the welfare/protection of animals. 'Live and let live.'" While several of these documents address infectious diseases, rabies—the most lethal of them all—is never mentioned.

CHAPTER 4

MACAQUES

When I think back to the first time I met a macaque, I wonder how I managed to spend so much time with these animals. That encounter was anything but promising. On the morning of November 5, 2009, I was an unprepared tourist on a day trip to the Elephanta Caves on a lovely island in Mumbai Harbor, and the monkey—at the time, this term was sufficient for me—was looking for a way to get some food without too much effort. What happened next was my fault: I did not know that eating near hungry macaques is not advisable. The monkey, a rather large male, walked toward me confidently, staring at the half-eaten corncob in my hand, and when it became clear that he meant to leap for it, I clumsily jumped back and dropped my snack. He grabbed the corncob and sat down to eat it while keeping an eye on me. But my lesson was not over: I was also unaware that being stared at is a clear threat signal to a monkey. My eyes were fixed on him in simple fear, but the monkey stood up in anger, baring his canines in all their shining glory. I stepped back in sheer panic and dropped the little jar of antimalarial tablets I was planning to take during the meal. The jar was open and the tablets flew onto the floor, arousing the curiosity of the monkey, who started to collect them. I remember that I was both fascinated by the meticulousness with which he was tidying up my mess—the same way I would have done it—and concerned that he might ingest the tablets. Luckily, a water seller intervened, chasing the monkey away by wielding a stone. I lost all my tablets—and never did start the antimalarial prophylaxis—but at least the monkey did not swallow them. Instead, he moved to the shade of a nearby tree and continued eating my corn.

During the following two months of my journey across northern India, every time I met a monkey, I put into practice the lessons I had learned. Above all, I learned how to recognize a macaque, more specifically a rhesus macaque, from afar. The rhesus macaque, or *Macaca mulatta*, is covered in grayish to brownish fur except for his reddish-pink face, large pointed ears, long nipples, rump, and the palms of his hands and soles of his feet. During mating season, from October to December, the reddish hue of his skin becomes brighter. His thick, furry tail measures between 20 and 25 centimeters (8 to 10 inches). Adult males measure about 55 centimeters (22 inches) tall and weigh approximately 8 kilograms (about 17 pounds). Females are smaller (45 centimeters, or 17 inches) and lighter (5 kilograms, or 11 pounds). They have five long, tapered fingers and toes. Their round, expressive eyes, which range from dark green to brown in color, stand out for their size, between a protruding forehead and flattened nose. Behind light whiskers and narrow lips, the mouth reaches a remarkable size when wide open and contains thirty-two strong teeth, including four sharp canines. They are diurnal animals, both arboreal and terrestrial, and live in well-organized groups of dozens of animals of all ages and both sexes.

Rhesus macaques and rabies are doubly linked. First, as mammals, macaques can catch and transmit rabies. Yet contrary to the erroneous information that I often heard circulating in India, compared to dogs and cows, the incidence of rabies among monkeys is quite low (APCRI 2004, 31). Moreover, in a review of about thirty articles on rabies cases and animal bites in India published over the past two decades, I found that monkeys generally occupy the third position on the list of animals who bite, after dogs and cats. In the multicentric rabies survey commissioned in 2003 by WHO and performed by the APCRI (2004, 27), the percentage of monkey bites was 2%, much lower than dog bites (91%) and cat bites (5%). If we narrow the focus of these studies to specific geographical areas, the proportion of monkeys among potentially rabid biting animals increases, although it still remains quite low. It is 0.4% in Delhi (Chhabra et al. 2004, 218), Jodhpur (Chauhan and Saini 2013, 1090), and Kolkata (Kumar and Pal 2010, 244); 4% in Pondicherry (Naik, Sahu, and Kumar 2015, 503); 10% in Gwalior

(Dwivedi, Bhatia, and Mishra 2016, 102); 14% in Darbhanga (Kumar et al. 2013, 95); and 16% in Haryana (Jyoti, Vashisht, and Khanna 2010, 216).

Although these data confirm that monkeys do not frequently transmit rabies to humans, it is important to note that in countries like India, where rabies is endemic and is mostly spread by dogs, cases transmitted by wild animals tend to be underreported or ignored (Mani, Anand, and Madhusudana 2016, 559). Moreover, according to Rattan L. Ichhpujani et al. (2008, 30), the number of rabies cases involving monkey bites has risen in recent years, mainly because of the increased proximity between people and macaques in urban areas. In Delhi, the data provided by the officer in charge of rabies control at the then MCD indicated that the number of people given anti-rabies vaccine at MCD clinics after being bitten by a monkey more than doubled between 2002 and 2003, from 671 to 1,603 (Dogra and Phatarphekar 2004). In 2014, 1,540 monkey bites were reported by the civic agencies in the National Capital Territory of Delhi (*Hindustan Times* 2015a). The same is true in West Bengal, where monkey bites are more common in urban than in rural areas (Das et al. 2015, 58). As anticipated, monkey bites are also a concern for international tourists. A case of human rabies in Germany was reported to be related to a monkey bite the victim received three years prior to developing the disease (Summer, Ross, and Kiehl 2004), and a young boy in Australia developed rabies following a monkey bite on his finger on a trip to northern India (CDC 1988).

The second link between macaques and rabies lies in the fact that, owing to their physiological similarity to humans, these monkeys have been used extensively in biomedical research to test the efficacy of a variety of rabies vaccines (Lodmell et al. 1998). Yet although these animals have contributed—against their will—to the advancement of rabies control, macaque-mediated rabies is a potential source of great concern, as they constitute the second-largest group of primates in the world, after humans. The natural habitat of macaques ranges from Afghanistan to Japan (although Gibraltar has a remarkable colony of macaques) and includes areas where rabies is either endemic or notably present. In India, the distance between humans and rhesus macaques is steadily diminishing, which increases the chance of zoonotic infection.

There are several reasons for the increased proximity of humans and macaques in India, discussed in more detail below, but the primary one is the increase in the number of urban macaques. Although simian population surveys are difficult to carry out, and available data thus rely mainly on rough estimates, in Indian towns and villages macaques seem to have almost outnumbered their counterparts in the forests. In order to learn more about urban macaques, especially in the complex case of Delhi, I had several meetings with Iqbal Malik, who also shared with me some of her unpublished notes. In the 1980s, Malik was the first female Indian researcher to study wild monkeys for her doctorate, focusing on two colonies of macaques in Tughlakabad Fort, an area in South East Delhi that was then relatively isolated from the city but later became incorporated into the sprawling suburbs of Delhi. In 2002, she also organized what was—and remains— probably the largest project of macaque relocation ever attempted in the world in Vrindavan, a small town located 150 kilometers south of Delhi. Over the past two decades, the name of this primatologist has invariably been linked to the growing human-monkey conflict in the city.

According to Malik, at least 80% of the macaques currently living in India are commensal with humans. The term "commensal" derives from the Latin word *commensalis*, meaning "sharing a table" (*com-*, "together," plus *mensa*, "meal" or "table"). In biology, commensalism is a relationship between two species that live in close association, in which one species obtains benefits from the other without affecting it either positively or negatively. In the case of urban macaques, the main benefit they obtain from humans is food. Although the term "commensal" might have applied to the first macaques who moved into Indian towns decades ago, "kleptoparasitism" (parasitism by theft—in this case, theft of food) seems a more appropriate description of the monkeys' relationship with humans today. In addition to food, humans also provide macaques with shelter and enhanced locomotion, since these animals make good use of the urban landscape for sleeping and grooming (using walls, air-conditioners, cars, terraces, roofs, etc.) and moving around (via light poles, electric cables, gutters, etc.).

When I questioned Malik about the number of macaques in Delhi, her reply was careful and considered. Given the lack of scientific and up-to-date population surveys, she admitted, only estimates are possible. Malik is probably the best-known primatologist in Delhi, and many people trust her assessment of the situation, so she knows that she must be as precise as possible. Moreover, she is well aware of the media's tendency to sensationalize the subject of human-animal conflict and of the risk that this involves. Malik's best estimate of the number of macaques in Delhi is around 6,000, at least 85% of them relying on humans for food. At first, I was surprised by this—in a city of 19,000,000 humans, 300,000 dogs, and 60,000 cows, 6,000 monkeys are a tiny minority. I was confused; I had seen other figures, much higher than Malik's, in many newspaper articles, most of them Indian, a few from outside the country. It was true that some of these news reports seemed to recycle the same information over and over, though others quoted allegedly up-to-date statements from politicians and local authorities. Newspaper articles (discussed in more detail below) typically estimate 25,000 macaques in Delhi, with the most conservative figure given as 15,000.

Setting aside for a moment the question of Delhi's actual macaque population, it is essential to consider the trend of the monkeys' dependence on the food provisioned (directly or indirectly) by humans, which has steadily increased since the 1980s, when the first systematic surveys were performed. For the sake of convenience, I will use the term "commensalism" here, even if the relationship between humans and urban macaques is clearly becoming conflictual, to the extent that by 1989 the expression "weed macaques" had already been coined to convey the fact that macaques, like weeds, were appearing in places where they were not wanted (Richard, Goldstein, and Dewar 1989). In the early 1980s, Malik explained, about 15% of Indian macaques lived in commensal relationships with people. From research done in the 1990s by Charles H. Southwick and Rafiq M. Siddiqi (1994, 226) in northern India, we learn that 49% of the macaques lived in cities, towns, and villages (including temples and railway stations), where they had extensive contact with humans; 37% on roadsides and canal banks, with limited human interactions; and 14% in more or less complete isolation from humans. By the late 1990s, Malik told me, about 30% of them had become commensal with humans, and this percentage doubled in the first decade of this century. In 1980, Delhi had about 2,000 macaques, about 30% of whom lived in close contact with humans. By 1987 this figure had doubled. Ten years later it had reached 5,000, at least half of them commensal with humans. It was at this point that human-macaque conflicts began—and peaceful commensalism ceased to exist—exacerbated by the reduction of Delhi's green cover and the increase of its human population (the rate of which is twice that of the rest of the country). In the following decade, macaques "started getting out of hand," as Malik put it, and a crisis point was reached by 2005, when human tolerance became seriously strained.

Menace Narratives and Mass Hysteria

My conversations with Professor Malik continued to bewilder me for rea-sons beyond the numerical inconsistencies on Delhi macaques. Her calm and measured tone contrasted starkly with the general sense of alarm and chaos depicted in newspapers and newscasts. I asked her how she was able to keep a lid on her frustration, after all the things she has seen happen to people and macaques in her city. "The last thing that I want to do," she explained, "is make things even more messy. A lot has already been said on this topic, and now confusion is everywhere." She was hinting at media coverage, which has largely contributed to creating and reinforcing an atmo-sphere of anxiety and distress surrounding the issue of urban monkeys. This is especially the case in Delhi, where the human-macaque conflict has probably reached its peak.

"Threat narratives" about macaques began to circulate in Delhi in the first decade of this millennium, when the first reports of monkey bites shocked and alarmed the citizenry. In 2001, public anxiety over macaques shot to unprecedented levels. In April of that year, rumors, newspaper arti-cles, and police announcements on TV began to spread the word that a strange monkeylike creature was attacking, biting, and scratching people at night, particularly in low-income resettlement colonies and *jhuggi jhopris* (informal, unplanned shanty settlements). Day by day, supposed eyewit-nesses began outlining the bizarre identikit of the "Monkey Man": it was between one and two meters tall, was covered in thick black hair, wore black clothes, a motorcycle helmet, and steel claws, had shining red eyes, human legs, a typical apelike face, and red and green lights blinking on its chest. Thanks to its astonishing agility, speed, and physical strength, hidden by the dark of night, it could easily leap from rooftop to rooftop, where many people sleep during the humid summer nights, seeking refuge from the heat. Between May 10 and May 25, 2001, the police received 397 calls about this so-called Monkey Man, a reflection of growing hysteria in Delhi (Verma and Srivastava 2003, 355). By then, this terrifying figure had gone viral in the popular imagination and had inflicted real casualties: alarmed by neighbors who were sure they had seen the simian monster, a pregnant woman fell down the stairs and died. In two other incidents, a frightened mob chased and beat up a passerby who was mistaken for the Monkey Man. Two scholarly articles (Edamaruku 2001; Verma and Srivas-tava 2003) described these incidents as a phenomenon of mass hysteria, in which injuries blamed on the mysterious figure were either deliberately or unknowingly self-inflicted. In an article titled "To Catch a Phantom" in the mass-circulation newspaper the *Hindu*, a psychologist expressed concern that the hysteria was actually creating phobias in children (Joshua 2001).

When fear of the Monkey Man eventually abated, real incidents soon began to occupy the Delhi pages of Indian newspapers. In January 2004, a macaque killed a two-month-old girl in her sleep (*Times of India* 2004). Priyanka, my neighbor in Jangpura, still remembers the gruesome details disclosed by the press: the animal gouged out her eye and threw her to the floor before her mother could intervene. But the incident that created the greatest panic in the city occurred on October 21, 2007. The deputy mayor of Delhi, Sawinder Singh Bajwa, slipped and fell to his death from his terrace while allegedly chasing away a troop of macaques that had entered his house (*Times of India* 2007). There are different versions of this story, some of them denying that the macaques caused Bajwa's fall, but whatever actually happened, the incident drew attention to the issue of urban macaques—and for the first time made the point that not even the rich and powerful are exempt from the potentially harmful impact of these animals on people.

A new wave of alarm passed through Delhi in 2012. In February of that year, a nine-year-old girl died after she was attacked and bitten by a macaque in Sangam Vihar, in South Delhi (*Deccan Herald* 2012). Three months later, a less dramatic event occurred in Ghaziabad, a city to the east of Delhi. I was living in India at the time, and I remember reading the news story in the *Hindustan Times* over breakfast. A fourteen-year-old girl had fallen from the fourth floor of her building after fleeing a group of macaques that the press described as "rampaging" (Khandelwal 2012). Also in Ghaziabad, in May 2015, a disabled boy died after being attacked by a monkey (Das 2015). In February 2016, two macaque attacks apparently caused the death of a three-year-old boy, who fell from the roof of his house while surrounded by a group of monkeys (*Hindustan Times* 2016b), and a seventy-year-old man died in the same horrific way (*Hindustan Times* 2016a). The following year, in Gurugram, a city south of Delhi, a headline screamed, "Monkeys Let Loose Reign of Terror in South City, Target Autistic Girl" (Mir 2017).

These events all have contributed to the construction of what can be called a "menace narrative." In fact, "monkey menace" has become a popular expression in newspaper headlines: thus "The Monkey Menace" (Bhatnagar 2013), "No Full Stops to Monkey Menace" (*Times of India* 2013b), "Monkey

Menace Continues to Haunt Municipal Body" (Nath 2015a), and many more. Such articles describe macaques as roaming the streets and attacking in "brigades" (*Deccan Herald* 2012) or "hordes" (Nath 2015a). Predictably, readers have absorbed this language and embellished it with "keywords" that now seem impossible to avoid when discussing the human-monkey conflict in the city. The Delhiites I spoke with about this issue used words like "invasion," "havoc," and "infestation." They described macaques as "naughty," "mischievous," "mad," "misbehaved," "ill-tempered," "unpredictable," "marauding," "vicious," "nasty," "ferocious," and "belligerent" and used such epithets as *gundas* (gangsters, vandals), "bullies," "criminals," "thieves," "thugs," and *dacoits* (armed bandits), and even "terrorists." Macaques are said to roam around in "bands," "tribes," and "squads."

The Way to the City

Why does Delhi have so many macaques? There are several reasons, closely linked, but the first one Malik gave is the exploitation of these animals in biomedical research. As mentioned above, macaques have been used to develop vaccines, test medicines, and study blood constitution (the Rh factor found in certain blood types owes its name to rhesus macaques). Throughout the twentieth century, hundreds of laboratories around the world, particularly in the United States, imported many thousands of macaques captured in the forests of northern India. This caused not only a dramatic decrease in their population but also, more important, a dangerous demographic imbalance due to the phenomenon of "chaotic fission," in Malik's words. Laboratories demanded adolescent males, and this inevitably disrupted macaque social groups, which are based on a rigid hierarchy, and altered their age and sex ratios. In April 1978, India banned the export of macaques for ethical and legal reasons, after pressure from animal rights activists and the prime minister at the time, Morarji Desai. In the thirty years preceding this ban, however, about 200,000 macaques were shipped abroad to research labs (Southwick and Lindburg 1986, 171), mainly from Uttar Pradesh (Southwick, Beg, and Siddiqi 1961, 538). Although export was banned in 1978, the use of macaques in Indian laboratories was still permitted until 2012, using the same methods of capture. Even if the number of monkey captures decreased significantly, it was too late: macaques had already moved into nearby villages and towns, where dismembered packs could find food more easily and establish new social ties, now with humans as well.

Another factor in the migration of macaques to towns, one still very much in play, is the loss of forest cover to make way for roads, industry, mining, development projects, and, of course, people and livestock. Available data are difficult to interpret. The latest report, released in 2017 by the Forest Survey of India (Ministry of Environment 2017, 25), puts the total amount of forest in India at 708,273 square kilometers, or 21.5% of the total geographical area of the country, indicating an average increase of 0.94% nationwide since 2015. Data provided by the World Resources Institute's Global Forest Watch project (Harris et al. 2018) paint a much less rosy picture, one in which India lost more than 16,000 square kilometers of tree cover between 2001 and 2018. This discrepancy is mainly attributed to differing definitions of forest density and to the fact that the Forest Survey of India covers pretty much all vegetation visible from satellites, thus also including man-made commercial plantations and fruit orchards. India is a member of the UN Framework Convention on Climate Change, has actively participated in all Conference of the Parties meetings, and has consistently reasserted its goal of having 33% of its territory covered by forests. Yet wildlife experts, environmentalists, and concerned citizens regularly protest actions that undermine this goal and take the country in the opposite direction. In October 2019, some 2,140 trees were cut down in the Aarey Forest of Mumbai to make way for a metro building—just one recent example. What Mumbaikars consider the green lungs of their city is, to the Brihanmumbai Municipal Corporation, and even to Minister of the Environment, Forest, and Climate Change Prakash Javadekar, technically not a forest (Kukreti 2019). In the meantime, the National Green Tribunal created in 2010 has seen its power increasingly diluted (Sahu 2019).

Meanwhile, the presence of macaques in towns and cities has become good business for *madaris*, or *kalandars* (monkey trainers), and this complicates the already problematic cohabitation of monkeys and humans. *Madaris* buy, train, and use macaques to entertain people on the street and at fairs and festivals, dressing them up as humans with makeup and clothing and making them dance, sing, and perform for spectators. Using wild animals in this way was declared illegal in 1973 by the government's Performing Animals Rules, but this activity, although reduced, is still practiced in tourist locations and along tourist routes, such as the highway that connects Delhi to Agra. During my stay in Delhi and Jaipur, I never came across this kind of show, but in Delhi's slums I saw about a dozen young macaques kept for this purpose. A close friend told me that with the right connections one can arrange a private show—for example, a birthday party—anywhere in the city for a very reasonable price with only a few hours' notice. Most *madaris* keep only a pair of monkeys, but taken together they contribute to the problem of urban monkeys, not only because these trainers bring young animals to the city and acquaint them with people, but also because they abandon the macaques when they become old, sick, aggressive, or difficult to handle. These monkeys have been trained to beg for money and to steal sunglasses and demand money for their return, and they are fearless, even cocky, about approaching people.

A City on a Simian Scale

The combination of media sensationalism and relentless word of mouth has given rise to a trove of stories about the problems caused by macaques, some true, some exaggerated, some made up out of thin air. I heard many accounts of monkeys playing with laundry hung out to dry, uprooting plants from pots, bathing in rooftop water tanks, breaking car mirrors, tearing down electric cables, turning on water taps, ripping the leather seats of two-wheelers, and jumping on people to steal and play with their glasses, phones, cameras, and other belongings. But the most frequent and disturbing trouble they cause is the theft of food. Macaques pilfer food left to dry in the sun, accost passersby for their food, snatch lunch boxes from schoolchildren, and even raid the fridge. Nearly every such story I heard ended with the monkeys becoming violent and biting when interrupted in this foraging.

The bizarre details of many of these stories, especially the ones involving kitchen invasions, initially made me skeptical. But then I saw it for myself. One Sunday morning, my flatmate had left the door of her bedroom open to let the sunshine in. I was writing emails, and our cat, Macha, was ambling around looking for a place to sleep. Suddenly, she ran into my room from the balcony, her fur on end and eyes wide. I rushed to find out what was going on, and as I entered the kitchen I bumped into two adult macaques who were hastening toward the fridge. I immediately stepped back and closed the door that separated my room from the kitchen, but was able to observe the monkeys through the glass. They were both female.

The larger one walked to the fridge and opened it without hesitation. She showed no apparent surprise or dismay as she quickly scanned the contents of the fridge, or any apparent reaction to the wave of cold air emanating from it. In other words, it seemed that this was not her first time raiding a refrigerator. The pair first removed the most recognizable items—a bag of tomatoes and a bunch of green peas. Then they noticed something covered in tinfoil; they quickly tore it open and found the rotis left from the previous night's dinner. They put the rotis on the floor and shifted their attention to a big plate of boiled rice. The younger monkey grabbed it but could not carry it with only one hand, so it clattered to the floor. The unexpected sound scared them; they stepped back and seemed on the verge of leaving. But then the bigger one turned back; she picked up the rice that had spilled onto the floor and began eating it. I took advantage of their agitation to knock on the glass, hoping that this would chase them away. The larger one decided to go, though she seemed more annoyed than frightened. The smaller one followed her, stopping to collect the heap of rotis they had left on the floor. By the time I managed to overcome my fear and reach the balcony, they had disappeared into the urban jungle of Delhi.

In addition to accounts of home invasion and attack, funny stories of monkey mischief are also popular. I heard countless times that macaques love stealing mobile phones because they like the ringtones. Of course, I always asked how it was possible for a monkey to make such intelligent use of a mobile phone; most people told me that they wait for incoming calls to enjoy the music, though some claimed that they are able to navigate the menu and play the ringtones at will. Macaques are also said to splash around in the swimming pools of five-star hotels, to the annoyance of paying guests. I have never witnessed this myself, but at the end of Surajpol Bazar Road in Jaipur, near the path to the Galta Mandir (also known as monkey temple), there is a tank used as a swimming pool by the colony of monkeys who live in and around the temple. I spent hours watching them climb the nearby pole (carefully avoiding the barbed wire that had been twisted around it in a vain attempt to keep them off) and diving with style, like divers at the Olympic Games. There are also less humorous stories of macaques stealing intravenous units from Delhi hospital rooms and drinking their contents. I cannot confirm their validity, but such stories—and the uncertainty about whether they are all true—feed the collective fear and unease surrounding urban macaques.

Macaque troops have established their territory in many parts of Delhi (particularly in and around parks and forested areas), although they are not always immediately apparent. But even when they are difficult to spot at first, their presence is palpable, and they are not hard to discover if you know what to look for. In fact, while it is undeniable that Delhi blatantly exemplifies the Anthropocene—this age in which humans have deeply altered natural ecologies and landscapes, affecting the environment and nonhuman others as never before—it is also true that other animal species are co-creating it with us, although to a lesser extent (Fuentes and Baynes-Rock 2017). Buses and rickshaws feature advertisements for monkey-proof rooftop water tanks. Some people use scarecrows (scare-monkeys?) to try to keep macaques at bay. My neighbors in Lajpat Nagar kept a big stuffed monkey hanging from the railing of their balcony, hoping to keep macaques away from their potted plants. I had a good laugh at that moribund fake monkey, and I guess that the real macaques did too. A few kilometers north, in the narrow lanes of Old Delhi, people had to barricade themselves inside their houses, their porches and windows covered by metal grilles. To protect themselves while napping on the grass in the park, people usually keep a stick or stone at hand, to scare monkeys away.

Although macaques can be found in about 90% of the neighborhoods of Delhi, they are especially concentrated in three locations. The first is the Hanuman Mandir, one of the most popular Hindu temples in the city, where Hanuman (a monkeylike god, described in more detail below) is worshipped. The entry to this temple is in Baba Kharak Singh Marg, a market just southwest of Connaught Place, New Delhi's main square. Just opposite the temple are the expensive state emporiums, which feature prime Indian handicrafts, strategically located in the heart of the city to attract international tourists. The temple is located between a tall building that is home to the popular Regal Cinema and the biggest hub for fake jeans in Delhi, the Connaught Place Police Station, and a small but pleasant neighborhood park. The shrine is run by the New Delhi Municipal Council. It is surrounded by dozens of shops selling ritual handicrafts, new-age CDs, toys, and wedding bangles, snacks, and sweets. In the subway opposite the temple, dozens of homeless people have found a place to live, particularly on Tuesdays and Saturdays—the days devoted to Hanuman—when benefactors come to the temple to distribute food to the monkeys and, while they are at it, to the poor.

Despite its pleasant location, my first impression of the area, in the summer of 2012, was that it looked like a circle of Dante's *Inferno*: a perpetual smell of urine coming from the flowerbeds; the usual cacophony of car horns; police announcements that continuously remind the public of the danger of terrorist attacks; drunken men; disabled people who removed their artificial limbs to inspire pity in visitors; street children collecting garbage while sniffing correction fluid; dying old people who beg with hopelessness in their eyes; an astrologist who for only twenty-one rupees (US$0.30) would predict your future; an army of feeble cleaners; shoe shiners; a huge man with a disfigured face and a hoarse voice trying to keep order among beggars by banging the floor with his scary stick; ear cleaners; *mehndiwalas* (women who make henna tattoos); dogs below and monkeys above; a carpet of banana peels on the ground.

I gradually grew accustomed to this atmosphere, however, and began to seek the best place from which to observe the interactions between people and the roughly 150 macaques who inhabit the 700-square-meter area of the temple. I eventually settled on the short wall behind the roof opposite the temple's entrance, where people left their shoes before entering the sacred space. There I sat, between a hedge and several square meters of carefully arranged shoes. The shoe supervisor was happy to have me, for he thought I might serve as a sort of magnet for curious visitors, who would then be more likely leave their shoes under his protection. Because there was no food in that particular area, the monkeys were not much interested in it, which allowed me to eat the occasional snack and use my camera in (relative) safety. Since offering food is a meritorious act for orthodox Hindus, and since, as Indians love to say, "the guest is god," before collecting their shoes temple visitors occasionally gifted me the *prasad* (sanctified food) they had planned to bring home and distribute among their family members. Others offered their *prasad* to the rats who lived under the roots of the huge Banyan tree on my right.

Thus between the shoes and the rats I found my place at the Hanuman Mandir. I cannot claim that I became part of the monkeys' social world, as Marcus Baynes-Rock (2015) did with the hyenas of Harar, in Ethiopia. Given the large number of people who gravitated toward this temple every day, the monkeys never seemed interested in specific individuals, in getting to know them better or establishing a relationship. To the monkeys, excepting fruit and sweet sellers and food distributors, people were simply members of an interesting and beneficial crowd. I did my best to blend into the surroundings so as not to attract their attention or interfere with them, letting them decide their level of tolerance toward me. As Matei Candea (2010, 246) observed of the meerkats he studied in South Africa, the macaques of the Hanuman Mandir preferred that people keep a "polite distance" from them. They wanted to set the terms of their relationships with humans, making their own decisions about how much proximity they would tolerate in exchange for food. They wanted to be the ones empowered to decide when to be fed and when to be left in peace. As I learned from my first encounter with the monkey who wanted my corncob in Mumbai, the first rule of interacting with macaques is *do not look them in the eye* unless you want to risk a violent confrontation over supremacy. Observing the monkeys of the Hanuman Mandir without making eye contact was one of the most difficult (and ethnographically paradoxical) challenges of my research experience. But I also learned that this kind of detachment is, after all, one way of relating to others (Nading 2014b, 233).

A few kilometers to the south, macaques abound in and around the Rashtrapati Bhavan complex (India's presidential palace), with its adjoining Secretariat Building, prime minister's office, and chief ministries—this is the second area of the city where they can be found in high numbers. Built atop Raisina Hill, these buildings are surrounded by vast gardens and forested areas where macaques sleep at night. During the day they visit the lawns of Rajpath and India Gate, where office workers (on weekdays) and common Delhiites (on weekends) love to picnic. Needless to say, the monkeys take full advantage of the edible refuse left behind. When feeding time is over, the monkeys usually return to the rooftops of the government buildings, where they rest, groom, sun themselves, and play. Macaque troops can appear and disappear in a flash, and thus can transform places, their purposes, and the ways in which humans and other species use them, in the blink of an eye. They are considered such a nuisance in this area, spoiling the intended grandeur of the center of Indian government and annoying its high-ranking officials, that in 2016 the upper house of Parliament invited citizens' "suggestions on the management of monkeys and dogs in MPs' residential areas in Delhi."

To the west of the Hanuman Mandir and Raisina Hill lies the third large macaque population in Delhi: the huge Central Ridge Reserve Forest (commonly called the Ridge), a piece of forest in the heart of one of the biggest and most overcrowded cities in the world. The Ridge is under the jurisdiction of the Ministry of Environment, Forest, and Climate Change, and acts as the green lungs for the city. Macaques are abundant there and can live relatively undisturbed. At night they retreat into the forest, but from sunrise to sunset they congregate on the walls and fences of the Ridge and drop down to the adjacent pathway to eat the food offered to them by passersby. On this pathway, located between the Ridge and an expressway, no commercial activity is permitted given its proximity to the governmental center of the capital. Consequently, this location is free of the usual overcrowding on typical urban Indian streets, and the monkeys' quality of life here seems to be relatively good.

One day I was sitting on the pavement, taking pictures of two macaques grooming each other in the shade, when a man stopped his car and began unloading bags of tomatoes for the monkeys. After a few minutes, I approached him out of curiosity and got a look at the back seat of his car, which still contained at least fifteen bags of tomatoes. We exchanged pleasantries and I naïvely asked him the reason for his generosity. "You know about Hanuman, don't you?" he replied. He turned back to distributing the tomatoes, talking to the monkeys as if they had known one another for a long time.

The Cult of Hanuman

Hanuman is a monkey-like god who, despite being a secondary deity in the Hindu pantheon, has been enjoying great popularity in recent decades. His mixed genetic inheritance makes him neither fully man nor fully monkey: according to popular legend, he is the son of Vayu, the wind god, and Anjani, an *apsara* (celestial nymph), who was cursed to live in the body of a monkey because of her sexual affair with the god. Hanuman's life changed dramatically when, as a young adult, he met the god Rama, who was searching desperately for his beloved wife, Sita, in the forests of southern India. This encounter, narrated in the fifth book of the *Ramayana* (a Hindu epic written in the first or second century B.C.E.), definitively admitted Hanuman into the vast Hindu pantheon. Sita had been abducted by the demon Ravana and taken to the island of Lanka, but Hanuman promised that he would save her. Leading a makeshift but efficient army of monkeys, he leaped over the ocean and reached Lanka, where he defeated Ravana's guards, freed Sita, and set fire to the fortress. He then returned Sita to Rama. In the sixth book of the *Ramayana*, Hanuman cemented his friendship with Rama when he took upon himself the challenging task of running to the Himalayas to collect the herbs needed to heal Rama's sick and exhausted army. Hanuman reached the mountains with extraordinary speed and even lifted and transported an entire mountain, delivering it to the dying soldiers. With this gesture Hanuman proved himself not only a hero of amazing courage and physical strength but also an exemplar of selflessness, loyalty, and dedication.

Centuries later, Hanuman is still worshipped for the *bhakti* (devotion) and *shakti* (physical and mental strength) he embodies in his relationship with Rama. Many other qualities make him worthy of the highest devotion: his pursuit of perfection, control of ego, lack of arrogance, purity of heart and mind, humility, compassion, and moderation. In fact, although his *asthasiddhi* (the eight powers of Hindu deities—e.g., the ability to fly as fast as the wind, to become as light as a feather or as immobile as a mountain, to become invisible, to expand the body) are extraordinary, he never flaunts them. There is no question that Hanuman is revered for his bravery (he is also known as Mahavira, "the courageous one"—Narula 2005, 22), but this quality is accompanied by a well-balanced, reasonable, and intelligent mind. Hanuman is also an expert in grammar, a music lover, and a master poet. He is admired for his communication, oratorical, diplomatic, and logical skills. As an emblem of wisdom and curiosity, he is the tutelary deity of students, musicians, and grammarians. Thus devotees worship him in order to receive knowledge, improve their self-confidence, become fluent speakers, gain courage in facing difficult trials, and find relief from fear of failure.

Hanuman is revered for his immortality: he is one of the seven *chiranjivi* (long-lived or immortal). Yet despite this superpower, Hanuman is also considered a "self-made god." Unlike many other Hindu deities, he was not born into a high-ranking family of divine origin. In fact, not only was Hanuman's mother cursed to look like a monkey, but his biological father abandoned him when Hanuman was a child, leaving him in the care of his foster father, Keshari, forcing Hanuman to live in the forest among monkeys (Williams 2008, 148). Thus Hanuman's success, stature, and popularity are due solely to his firm willpower and diligence.

For this ability to improve himself and fulfill his dreams, Hanuman is the idol of the Indian urban middle class (Lutgendorf 1997). Like him, the members of this growing and increasingly demanding class may be hampered by their humble origins and lack of inherited advantages to smooth their path in life. Middle-class youths naturally identify with him, suspended as they are between a less than brilliant past and the brighter future they long for. They do not seek Hanuman's godly status, of course, but they fervently aspire to material benefits and personal success. They turn to Hanuman for help and support in fulfilling their dreams, and many consider him a kind of personal coach who can teach them how to live up to their potential and show them the way to success. Hanuman can teach them the qualities they need most for their mission in life: mental strength, perseverance, and self-confidence. Although middle-class prosperity has been on the rise since the 1990s, the fear of falling back into financial insecurity or lack of opportunity remains very much alive, thus the need for hope and reassurance.

Hanuman is a very popular deity among India's new middle class also because of his extraordinarily forgiving attitude and the fact that he does not demand the excessive religious zeal that other deities do. In fact, Hanuman worship is said to be one of the most spontaneous and simple to perform. The pocket edition of the *Hanuman Chalisa*, sold both in Hindi and in English in the stalls outside the Hanuman Mandir, contains both the long, regular version of the ritual for Hanuman and a shorter, reader-friendly one. The relative ease and speed with which Hanuman can be approached are particularly important to middle-class people, who do not have much time for spirituality in their hectic, busy lives. In this new context, devotion to Hanuman has become akin to an item of mass consumption.

Hanuman is especially popular among the bureaucrats and office workers in and around Connaught Place, the hub of New Delhi. These workers are easy to spot; the timing of their visits to the temple is dictated by their office hours. They arrive on motorcycles or in small economy cars; before entering the temple they deposit not only their nice shoes but also their helmets and briefcases; they are quick in their prayers and usually buy some *prasad* to distribute to the animals; and they usually linger just long enough to have a quick snack before facing Delhi's impossible traffic in the hope of getting home in time for dinner. The preference of these office workers for Hanuman Mandir has given the temple a new nickname: *sarkari babu Hanuman*, "the Hanuman of government bureaucrats" (Lutgendorf 1997, 312). In short, the recent surge in Hanuman's popularity is closely linked to the growing size of India's urban middle class. This, along with the features of Hanuman described in the previous paragraphs, is key to

understanding the current situation of macaques in Delhi and their relationship with people.

Feeding Hanuman's Army

Compared to other anthropic regions of the world, Indian cities and towns
provide a relatively favorable environment for macaques. The two primary
reasons for this are the cultural and religious propensity for tolerance and
nonviolence toward animals in India, discussed in chapter 1, and the heart-
felt Hindu devotion to Hanuman. The most direct expression of this attitude
is the feeding of macaques. The best place in Delhi to observe this interaction is on the aforementioned pathway near the Ridge on Sardar Patel
Marg, the permanent home of a numerous troop of macaques who receive
daily visits from an equally numerous troop of human monkey feeders.
Near the corner of Simon Bolivar Marg, there is a thriving business in selling bananas to macaque feeders. When I was there in 2012–13, and again in
2015, this business was run first by Prabhu and then by Amit. Prabhu was a
Hindu in his fifties who had left his family in a village in Uttar Pradesh to
earn a better living in Delhi, while Amit was a thirty-two-year-old Muslim
man, who later opened a fruit shake stall in Old Delhi. I met these two
men when I asked if I could join them while they sold their bananas, in
order to chat about the monkeys, talk to their customers, and observe the
interactions between the macaques and their feeders at close range. They
happily agreed, and I spent several days there, sitting between baskets of
bananas and families of macaques. Prabhu and Amit were as pleased with
this arrangement as I was, for they now had someone to talk to, to break
the monotony, and to relieve them when they had lunch or took a nap
while I stood guard over the fruit. Finally, the bargaining skills in which I
had long trained as a customer turned out to be useful for their business.

Early morning was the most popular feeding time; customers explained,
somewhat proudly, that the macaques had gone without food all night and
needed someone to feed them breakfast. Weather also played a role, since
both people and macaques prefer not to eat—or to do much of anything—
during the hottest part of the day. The morning was also best for people
who chose to bring their own food for the monkeys rather than buy Prabhu
and Amit's bananas; they could simply drop it off on their way to work.

A typical Saturday morning there looked something like this (from my field notes of Saturday, March 30, 2013):

6:28: A man spread a few handfuls of chickpeas on the ground.

6:40: A man bought bananas for 40 rupees (US$0.60), tossing some to the monkeys and handing others directly to them.

6:49: A man bought bananas for 50 rupees (US$0.70) and tossed them around.

7:24: A man spent 100 rupees (US$1.40) on bananas and offered some to each monkey.

7:26 and 7:28: A man spent 40 rupees (US$0.60) and did the same.

7:50: A man stopped his motorcycle, pulled a bag of bananas from under the seat, and threw them to the macaques.

8:06: A man on a motorcycle slowed down and tossed one roti to the monkeys.

8:07: An elderly couple opened the trunk of their car and distributed bananas, apples, cauliflower, beans, and three packets of sliced bread.

8:08: A boy emptied a bag of chickpeas on the ground.

8:09: A middle-aged couple threw a few handfuls of chickpeas from their motorcycle.

8:10: A boy bought bananas for 40 rupees (US$0.60) and offered them to the macaques; his mother and younger sister soon joined him.

8:11: A man bought bananas for 50 rupees (US$0.70) and cautiously distributed them to the monkeys, repeatedly asking Prabhu if they bite.

8:12: A man bought bananas for 20 rupees (US$0.30) and tossed them from a distance.

8:36: A young man distributed three packets of sliced bread, bananas, and apples, joined his hands in a quick prayer, and left.

8:37: A young man pulled over and threw some bananas from his car window.

8:41: A teenage boy handed a banana to the first macaque who approached him.

8:43: A man pulled over and threw five rotis from a short distance.

8:44: A man with his daughter pulled over and both threw eight bananas from the half-open window.

9:08: A policeman in uniform threw a packet of sliced bread at the animals.

9:10: A man walked by and distributed a bag of tomatoes by throwing them at the macaques.

9:16: A man dumped a bag of tomatoes on the ground.

This kind of activity went on continuously, each day bringing a parade of people to feed the macaques. Most of them were young and middle-aged men who came by motorbike or car; some of them even had a driver—the distinguishing feature of high-ranking *sarkari babus* (government bureaucrats). Most people began with the intention of feeding the macaques one by one, handing bananas directly to them. This plan would fall apart by around 9:00 in the morning; by then the monkeys were too full to care about more offerings. At half past nine on that Saturday morning, a customer who had just bought some bananas from Prabhu came back complaining that the monkeys were not hungry enough.

Some people were afraid of the macaques and preferred to throw food from a safe distance, some even from their cars. When children were there, their relatives sometimes encouraged them to feed the monkeys themselves, but it was quite evident that everybody was weary and uncomfortable. A few people asked Prabhu and Amit to distribute the food on their behalf, or simply left money for that purpose. Neither Prabhu nor Amit had ever witnessed a monkey bite anyone during those feeding sessions, though they regularly saw the macaques become uneasy, particularly when people approached their infants or were not quick and clear in their intentions to distribute the food. Only a small minority of people looked truly at ease among the macaques, probably because they had been feeding the animals for years. Thanks to their extensive experience with macaques, two of them remarked, they in fact stopped feeding them when too many others began doing it, and focused on giving them water instead. In fact, apart from Prabhu and Amit, who cleaned and filled the big iron pots chained to the trees every morning, very few people gave a thought to the animals' thirst.

On Tuesdays and Saturdays in particular—the days devoted to Hanuman's worship—all the bananas were sold by lunchtime. However, I would estimate that at least a third of the food offered to the macaques went to waste, though some of it was recycled by the sellers, who sometimes collected the uneaten bananas to sell again the next day. By this time of day the monkeys were so overfed, and probably also so sick of visitors, that they would retreat to the woods, leaving behind an impressively colorful mess of banana leaves, half-eaten tomatoes, untouched rotis, heaps of chickpeas, and inedible waste. In fact, most visitors did not bother to take away the plastic packaging from the sliced bread, tomatoes, and other food offerings, or the newspaper they used as plates for the sweets. Even worse, those who brought homemade rotis often threw it from their cars wrapped in tinfoil: macaques could easily unwrap the rotis, but they tore the foil into confetti-sized pieces that were then scattered around the area. Prabhu and Amit were very diligent in cleaning up the garbage each evening and throwing the banana peels into the woods. Even so, the area was never totally free of garbage.

When Feeding Harms

While it is easy to understand how direct conflict produces negative perceptions of monkeys, well-intentioned actions like feeding them can also be problematic (Lee and Priston 2005, 11). Yet there was no sign posted near the banana stand informing people about the impropriety of feeding macaques. Feeding these monkeys is illegal in many parts of India, but Prabhu and Amit were not aware of this, or so they said. Nor was a policeman who bought bananas for the monkeys; when I told him of this prohibition, he said he had no doubt that there was no such law in Delhi.

Actually, the High Court of Delhi banned the feeding of macaques in the city more than a decade ago, both because of scientific concern for these animals' health and behavior and in the hope of avoiding the same sorts of divisions among the citizenry that we saw in the case of street dogs. Feeding macaques does them more harm than good. Even if the monkeys have become accustomed to urban life, they remain wild animals who are not used—or *were* not used—to the quality and quantity of food they are given. In Sardar Patel Marg they mainly received fruits and vegetables, but they were often also fed rotis spread with ghee, sliced bread containing preservatives, and *jaggery* (cane sugar). Although these foods are not good for macaques, they receive food offerings that are even worse for them. In the Hanuman Mandir, they mainly receive the *prasad* that worshippers buy for Hanuman. Unfortunately, Hanuman's favorite food is *laddu*, round sweets made of chickpea flour, semolina, and sugar and then fried in butter or oil.

Moreover, just outside the Hanuman Mandir, several stalls sell ice cream, candies, chocolate sweets, and cola, all bad for macaques and all consumed by them, as they steal them from the customers' hands or directly from the stall. The owner of the temple's shoe depository told me that people sometimes even give macaques alcoholic drinks to make them drunk for their own amusement. As Iqbal Malik explained to me, urban macaques are thus prone to obesity, diabetes, and dermatological problems. She has long since lost any hope of making people understand that *laddus* must not be given to macaques. The people who feed them this food believe that because *laddus* are *prasad*, sanctified food, they cannot, by definition, be harmful. Even those who understand science, she observed, "in a moment of their life which is particularly difficult, would let themselves be blown away by these religious sentiments." As long as Hanuman loves *laddus*, she concluded, people will feed it to macaques. That Hanuman cannot suffer from diabetes or obesity like the flesh-and-blood monkeys makes no difference to them.

The problem is not just the food itself—harmful in both quality and quantity—but also the way in which macaques consume it. In the forest, monkeys spend a considerable amount of time foraging, which entails a low but continuous use of energy and requires small but frequent feedings. The balance between the calories they gain by consuming food and those they spend in finding food keeps macaques in good health. As we have seen all too clearly, most urban macaques are not only fed excessive quantities of food but rarely have to work for it. They are like pampered children who are fed chips and candies while playing video games on the sofa. The sofa, for these urban monkeys, is about three square kilometers, a mere fifth of the fifteen square kilometers a macaque troop would cover while foraging in the forest, Malik explained to me. Moreover, the decreased amount of time needed for foraging increases macaque reproduction (Loudon, Howells, and Fuentes 2006, 9).

What is worse is that these Delhi macaques are overfed in this way only twice a week, on Tuesday and Saturday, while for the remaining five days they are more or less forgotten. In Sardar Patel Marg there are a few people who deliberately bring food on the other days of the week, aware that the monkeys must eat not just on the two days devoted to Hanuman. As a man who worked at the Hanuman Mandir once told me, on the other days of the week macaques rely mainly on "grass. And mud. And . . . [he gestured with his eyes to three garbage bins where two monkeys were scavenging]."

The people who stuff the macaques every Tuesday and Saturday are clearly less interested in the monkeys' well-being than in their own karmic balance sheet, which they hope to augment by Hanuman's intercession. In the experience of Malik, Prabhu, and Amit, there is a very wide range of situations in which Hanuman's help is sought, and hence in which macaques are fed. They have seen schoolboys worried about their exams, housewives concerned about the health or wealth of their families, university students afraid of their future, and, above all, businessmen stressed about their jobs. Interestingly, Malik said that a small but consistent number of these men were Sikhs; she remembered one in particular who used to come every Tuesday with a truckload of food, convinced that this was good for his business even though his faith had no particular connection to monkeys. Ajay Gandhi sums up the situation: "Delhi's simian menace was not wildness threatening civilization," as people like to imagine; instead, "monkeys wrestled with a negativity that was human in origin" (2012, 53).

In the long run, feeding macaques is detrimental not only to them but to people as well. In the rigid macaque social structure, the circulation of food is pivotal in building a strong hierarchy of dominance and in regulating the behavior expected from each member of the group. High-ranking monkeys eat first and are served by those of lower rank, who are submissive in their attitude toward their superiors. When people feed these animals, they enter this complex web of social relations, but they put themselves in the worst position—the lowest one. Moreover, people who offer food tend to be deferential, even obsequious, in their gestures, mainly because they are scared of the macaques—or of Hanuman. They approach the monkeys slowly, hesitantly, quietly, bearing large quantities of food and often offering it from a position of inferiority (e.g., when monkeys are up on a tree branch, wall, or roof). Some people take their deference to extremes, putting their food offerings on newspaper to prevent the food's coming into contact with the ground, or they peel the bananas before offering them to the macaques. Monkeys are flattered by this attention and, owing to their despotic social nature, happy to have a multitude of eager, subservient people at their service.

But when these food offerings dwindle or dry up, hungry macaques are not afraid to confront humans and invade their homes in search of the food to which they feel entitled. Macaques in urban India have long since lost their fear of humans, and this appears to be irreversible. When the monkey population was not as high and potentially dangerous, people were quite amused by and well disposed toward them, often luring them with food. In this way, a vicious circle inevitably began. In fact, many of the people who told me that they occasionally feed macaques in or near their homes confessed their hope that their offerings would placate the monkeys, preventing them from becoming aggressive or causing trouble. A woman in her forties named Nandita, who has lived in Old Delhi all her life and never had any problem with the macaques in the past, told me, "We can't stop feeding them because they go crazy. . . . They become like children when you don't feed them. They get angry. . . . No, it's not a good idea to stop feeding monkeys." If Nandita is fed up with macaques, her son is literally terrified. When he is home alone, he empties packets of biscuits on the terrace floor to keep the monkeys outside the house. Macaques have become very skilled at intimidating people, and people, in turn, have become increasingly scared of them. As I listened to their stories, I remembered my first encounter with the macaque at the Elephanta Caves, when I surrendered my corncob to mollify him and prevent an attack. I was the loser in that interaction, he the winner; I only succeeded in increasing his confidence in approaching humans.

The data I collected from university students demonstrate that the increase in macaques' boldness is directly proportional to the decrease in safety that people perceive in their interactions with the monkeys. Fully 72% of the students considered their presence in the city problematic and felt that they were much more dangerous than bulls, dogs, or rats. Half of these students had witnessed at least one episode of human violence toward monkeys, and 35% gave human fear as the main reason for it. Other motives were the attempt to keep the monkeys at a distance (26%) and punishment of macaques' misbehavior (20%). Of course, what people see as misbehavior could be normal macaque behavior in managing conflict with humans (Malik and Johnson 1994, 237). In the context of increased interspecies competition for space and other resources, humans are growing frustrated and pursuing more aggressive means of dealing with this conflict, while macaques in turn adapt their behavior, becoming more hostile as well, toward both humans and one another (Camperio-Ciani 1986, 438).

Looking for a Way Out

At the end of the twentieth century, the costs and risks of cohabitation with macaques started to worry Delhi citizens, who began to contemplate alternatives and solutions. One possibility was not considered, however: culling. "Why should we kill them?" my flatmate in Jangpura asked. "Monkeys have the same right to live we have. Moreover, . . . harming a monkey brings bad luck. I don't believe in these things, but who knows? It is better not to take the chance." We were discussing the damage that some macaques had done to the water tank on our roof. Jangpura, along with Nizamuddin East and Sangam Vihar, are the areas worst affected by macaques in the South MCD district (Suraksha 2016). My flatmate considered herself an atheist, and she stressed that the widespread opposition to monkey culling is not religiously driven—"It is not a Hindu thing," she claimed—but is linked to Indian culture in general. Kavita, my neighbor in Lajpat Nagar, sees opposition to culling as a simple matter of ethics and common sense, requiring no discussion. "No, no, monkeys can't be killed, as people can't be killed. We Indians are a lot, and so? Should we kill ourselves?" she asked. When I asked for her solution, then, she did not hesitate. "Indira Gandhi . . . got men sterilized," she said with a wicked smile. "If it worked with people, it will also work with monkeys." Kavita was farsighted. In 2019, the Delhi government opted to use injectable contraceptives on its macaques (Adak 2019a).

Earlier, however, in 2001, Delhi adopted its first measure to try and control macaques, hiring langur monkeys (*Presbytis entellus* or *Hanuman langur*) to scare them away. Langurs are bigger than macaques (males can weigh up to seventeen kilograms and grow to be sixty-nine centimeters, or two feet, tall), with coal-black faces and hands. Their black hands and faces are supposed to frighten macaques, which is the key to the plan. The idea was to pay their handlers, the *langurwalas*, to patrol a given area with a langur on a long leash, encouraging the langur to frighten the macaques away. In reality, most *langurwalas* simply tie the langur to a tree on a long leash while they rest nearby, keeping a lazy eye on things. This langur-based solution has not been implemented on a large scale in Delhi, not only because its cost, though modest, is out of reach for many Delhiites but because it is completely illegal. Langurs are a wild species listed under schedule II of the Wildlife Protection Act of 1972, and they are not to be killed, owned, traded, or hired by anyone but appropriate wildlife authorities and those licensed by them. Offenders risk up to three years in prison or a fine. Ironically, both the local and national government bodies in Delhi have made the greatest use of langurs and their trainers, much to the delight of the popular media. The government pursued this approach to monkey control during the 2010 Commonwealth Games in Delhi, employing about forty langurs to patrol the athletes' village and the sport premises in the hope of preventing macaques from spoiling Delhi's moment in the international spotlight (Evans 2010). Similarly, when U.S. president Barack Obama visited Delhi in October 2010, *langurwalas* and their monkeys were used to keep macaques out of his sight (Barry 2015).

Two years later, on October 15, 2012, the Wildlife Crime Control Bureau issued a directive on the "illegal hiring of langur for the security of official buildings," instructing government ministries to cease using langurs for this purpose immediately. On July 31, 2014, the then minister of urban development, M. Venkaiah Naidu, announced that to address the problem of macaques in the Parliament House, the NDMC had hired forty young people to imitate the sounds of langurs to scare macaques away. While this measure had limited success, the business of renting out langurs is still flourishing on the black market; langurs continue to be used in the gated communities, luxury hotels, and government offices of the city, particularly in South Delhi (Shekhar 2017).

Yet the Wildlife Crime Control Bureau directive did have some impact on some Delhiites. In 2013, in the small public park behind the Hanuman Mandir, not far from Connaught Place police station and the NDMC offices in Palika Kendra, Pavan and Arjun lived and worked for some months. Pavan was a twenty-two-month-old male langur named after Pavanputra, one of Hanuman's epithets. Arjun, a quiet man in his thirties who had moved to the city from his village in Uttar Pradesh two years before, was Pavan's handler. Arjun lived in a tiny house in a corner of the park; Pavan's cage, covered by a burlap sack, stood nearby. Arjun preferred to describe himself as a gardener, but when I asked him about his work with Pavan he admitted that he was there "to throw the monkeys out." He never used the term *langurwala* or the expression *bandar pakadnewala* (monkey catcher). Indeed, he emphasized that he had never harmed or even touched any macaque. Arjun took good care of Pavan, scratching his belly continuously during our first conversation, but he also claimed that Pavan did not belong to him and denied that he had bought him. He claimed that the resident welfare association of that area had paid about 8,000 rupees (US$115) for Pavan and had sent Arjun to the Krishi Bhawan, the building in which the Ministry of Agriculture is located, to collect him. Arjun paid for Pavan's support out of the salary he received from the RWA. The park where they worked was owned by the NDMC but, Arjun explained, the plants and flowers belonged to the RWA, and his task was to prevent the macaques from destroying them.

When I saw Arjun and Pavan again some weeks later, I asked Arjun if he knew of other langurs used to control macaques in the city. He told me that it had become increasingly difficult to find langurs because Maneka Gandhi had shut down the Krishi Bhawan. (Of course, the building itself had not been closed, but the supply of langurs had been curbed.) According to Arjun, Maneka had sent the manager of the langur business to jail and set all the langurs free. He expressed great relief that all those monkeys were finally free, but he was worried about the consequences for him and Pavan. He was not terribly concerned that the local police might take Pavan from him, but he knew that anyone could file a complaint (saying, for example, that Pavan was being mistreated), and that "Maneka Gandhi's office" would then come and take him away. Arjun was also afraid that Pavan might be stolen, given the high demand and scarce supply of langurs in Delhi; in fact, this had happened to Bittu, Pavan's predecessor in the garden. Arjun's colleagues, long-time gardeners in this park, remembered the night Bittu was kidnapped. Two men had shown up at the park one night and had struck up a conversation with the gardeners, "as you are doing now," one of them remarked. But whereas I had brought sweets and bananas, the two men had brought good whiskey. They had gotten Bittu's caretakers so drunk that they had fallen asleep. When they woke up, Bittu was gone.

Bittu, Pavan, and all the other langurs in Delhi have been deprived of their freedom—and for no good reason. There is no scientific evidence that macaques are scared of langurs to the extent that people think. On the contrary, research going back forty years has shown that it is not uncommon for macaques and langurs to live in close proximity in the wild, even to the extent that langurs will breastfeed young macaques (Das and Sharma 1980, 124). In her fieldwork on the macaques of Tughlakabad Fort, Malik witnessed macaques mourning the death of a langur who had joined their troop. In a South Delhi slum, I once met a man who owned a langur and brought home a macaque; when he left them together, the macaque had no fear of the langur, who stepped back submissively, despite being much older and bigger. But one does not need to be an expert on ethology to see that the idea of using langurs to frighten away macaques is ludicrous. For one thing, langurs are restricted by their leashes, so macaques—even if they were afraid—can simply steer around them. For another, macaque troops are territorial and learn very quickly to recognize the other species with which they share territory. So even if they are afraid of langurs at first, they soon learn to ignore the presence of the poor tethered creatures who watch them enviously.

The second approach to reducing the macaque problem in Delhi has focused on food. According to Malik and the team of primatologists behind the Prevention and Control of Conflict with Non-Human Primates in Public Spaces Rules proposed in 2005, the key to solving the problem is to stop feeding macaques and eliminate their access to food in human garbage and temples. The scavenging behavior of macaques, along with their taking full advantage of human food provisioning, clearly demonstrates their adaptability and evolution alongside humans (Richard, Goldstein, and Dewar 1989). It also proves their ability to compete with dogs and cows. In Delhi and Jaipur, I frequently observed them taking advantage of their strengths—mainly troop cohesion and manual and arboreal skills—in order to prevail over their rivals; they were the fastest animals in reaching garbage bins, were adept at overturning them, were highly skilled in opening bottles and untying knotted plastic bags, and so on. Interrupting the constant flow of food from humans to macaques would first of all reduce the amount of contact between the two species, protecting humans from bites and scratches and decreasing the amount of unhealthy food available to macaques. It would also halt the exponential growth of the urban macaque population and their rapid expansion wherever food is available. In fact, as Malik explained to me, monkeys only frequent areas where they find easy access to food. They do not waste their energy in useless raids. Thus securely covered trash barrels and well-guarded houses are strong deterrents to their presence.

Given its crisis proportions and its many far-reaching consequences for public health, the problem of garbage management is already under examination in many Indian towns, thanks in part to the Swachh Bharat Abhiyan (Clean India Mission). Yet when it comes to preventing macaques from raiding homes in search for food, the responsibility is understood to lie with private citizens. The government of the National Capital Territory of Delhi has thus attempted to focus mainly on the widespread practice of feeding monkeys in public spaces, including temples. It was forced to take action in 2001, when the New Friends Colony RWA (in an affluent South Delhi neighborhood), under articles 226–27 of the constitution of India, filed a written petition with the High Court of Delhi demanding that it take "effective and appropriate steps to deal with the continuing menace of monkeys, stray cattle and dogs and provide them shelter and [that] the road and residential areas of Delhi be kept free from monkeys and other animals." It took several years and a lot of negotiation, but in March 2007 the court ordered that "no person shall feed the monkeys or give food to them in public areas, more particularly, around the Western Command, Rashtrapati Bhawan, Connaught Place, Central Secretariat and around Qutab area and other habitat places wherever the monkeys are present in large number as of today." The then MCD and the NDMC were given the power to fine and prosecute people who continued to feed monkeys "for creating [a] public nuisance," while private citizens were encouraged to file complaints "against the persons found feeding monkeys at public places" and were given specially designated phone numbers at which to reach local authorities.

Of course, the judges and policymakers who issued these laws and regulations were aware that the cultural and religious habit of feeding macaques would not be easy to eradicate and would certainly not disappear overnight. To facilitate the transition, they designated two spots—Hanuman Mandir in New Delhi and Yamuna Bazar in Central Delhi—where people could drop food off and allow municipal employees to distribute it to the monkeys in a more controlled way. The food is collected only on Tuesdays and Saturdays, however, and is then transported to macaques in the Asola Bhatti Wildlife Sanctuary. A public notice issued by the Department of Forest and Wildlife titled "Stop Feeding Monkeys at Public Places" was posted on a blue metal sign at the Hanuman Mandir. Unfortunately, it is very hard to spot, being positioned on an isolated corner of the shopping area to the left of the temple frequented by shoppers rather than by monkey feeders. It is also difficult to read owing to the rust that is corroding it. Moreover, it is written only in English. That few people have actually read it became clear when the nearby stall keepers saw me taking pictures of the sign and began asking me about this food-collection system; they were surprised to learn of its existence. Even Jayraj, an old man who has been selling wicker here for decades, said he had never seen this system in practice. Apparently, the plan has been completely botched. The New Friends Colony's petition, with its hope that Delhi could solve its macaque problem in three months, was nothing more than a pipe dream. In the meantime, on the other side of the temple, on the trunk of a magnificent Banyan tree, a benefactor has built a small tiled platform and planted a plaque in front of it with the inscription "*Prasad* area." It overflowed with food every day I visited the Hanuman Mandir.

As for the Asola Bhatti Wildlife Sanctuary, a state park established in 1992 in a protected forest area located in the southern fringe of Delhi, in 2007 it was identified as a suitable shelter for the macaques of the city. Malik led a team of primatologists who recommended that a forest area be designated for this purpose, located far from human settlements, covered with native plants and fruit trees, surrounded by a monkey-proof fence, and equipped with medical facilities, health-screening protocols (particularly in the case of infectious diseases such as rabies), and an effective and reliable system of food distribution. Food supply was planned to come from the offerings made by pious devotees on Tuesdays and Saturdays at the Hanuman Mandir and Yamuna Bazar and on purchases from government rations shops and local vegetable markets on other days. The team also suggested that a temple devoted to Hanuman be constructed in the sanctuary to divert feeders from the other Delhi temples, and to encourage the direct involvement of nearby villagers in the management of the shelter so as to minimize human conflict with macaques. This plan was based on the idea that macaques do not—or no longer can, owing to their increasingly conflictual relationship with humans—belong to the city of Delhi.

Since this project went into effect in 2007, things have not worked out well in the Asola Bhatti Wildlife Sanctuary. When I last met Malik in 2013, she told me that no formal, scientific census had yet been done in the park, and that a lot of rumors about mismanagement were circulating among wildlife experts. According to her, the plan's success had been mainly compromised by the absence of fruit-bearing trees (in spite of government subsidies provided for their planting in 2007) and the city government's failure to provide a regular supply of appropriate food. In 2018, an article in the *Times of India* described an equally dramatic situation. The sanctuary, home to nearly 20,000 monkeys by that time, was already overpopulated yet had to accommodate all the macaques continually relocated there from the city. Every month, 800,000 rupees (US$11,000) was spent on food alone (Gandhiok 2018). Nevertheless, whether because of insufficient food or lack of vital space, macaques have been escaping their bar-less prison. They invade the neighboring human settlements, wreaking havoc and attacking people.

Ten years after the creation of this sanctuary, a study carried out in the southern fringe of Delhi showed a remarkable increase in the incidence of monkey bites in the villages that surround the monkey sanctuary, with ten to twelve incidents happening every week. Epidemiological details are even more worrisome: among the monkey bite victims, 67% are females and 60% are under age fifteen. One-tenth of them had already been bitten by a monkey in the past. Two-thirds of the monkey bites occurred indoors, and almost all of them were unprovoked (Aparnavi et al. 2019, 42). In addition to occupying these adjacent settlements, macaques have been returning to their previous homes in Delhi, where they lived before being caught and relocated to the walled forest of Asola Bhatti. In 2013, Malik estimated that at least 50% of the relocated macaques had already left. Her calculation agrees with the figures from a veterinarian who works for the North MCD and who says that between April 2007 and April 2012, 13,157 macaques were captured and brought to Asola Bhatti; of these, about 6,500 returned to Delhi.

Another factor hindering the success of this relocation project and the overall management of Delhi's macaques, according to Malik, was the method used to capture the monkeys. In February 2015, I spent the day with a man named Saleeq, whose job was to round up these macaques; I was introduced to him by a veterinarian at the North MCD who was in charge of monkey relocation. In the Delhi schoolyard where he had been assigned, he had installed a rectangular metal cage measuring roughly one square meter, with a vertical gate, the lower half of which was raised and tied to a thirty-meter cord. Saleeq's job was to hold on to that cord until a macaque entered the cage, and then drop the gate, locking the monkey in. Fruit, corn, bread, and vegetables had been put inside the cage as bait. Nearby stood a smaller cage, into which captured macaques would be transferred and transported to the sanctuary. I never saw this small cage in use, as ten hours of patient waiting yielded not a single monkey capture.

A man of few words, Saleeq told me that he had received no training in catching monkeys, and he evinced little interest in the job. He was simply a poorly equipped and ill-informed freelancer doing his best to carry out his assignment of capturing as many monkeys as possible. By way of incentive, Saleeq, like his colleagues hired by the North, South, and East MCDs, was paid 650 rupees (US$9) per monkey captured. While this arrangement provided him with motivation, it also undermined the goal of capturing and relocating urban macaques efficiently and humanely. The primatologists who advised on the project emphasized that macaques must be captured with a minimum of chaos and trauma, to avoid bites to humans, injuries to the monkeys themselves, and long-term damage to this already precarious multispecies relationship. Families were not to be separated; the entire group of close relatives was to be captured and relocated together, in order to avoid the potentially devastating consequences that the loss of a troop member could inflict on the monkeys' psychological balance and hence their aggressiveness.

I never saw Saleeq demonstrate concern for this precaution; on two occasions he was ready to shut the door on a lone macaque. He then missed even these opportunities waiting for more monkeys to enter the trap. Just before sunset he finally managed to catch one animal, but it was late and he thought it did not make sense economically to travel across Delhi for just one young individual. Monkey catching is recommended only in cold months, because the summer heat makes macaques irritable and aggressive. Moreover, in March, young macaques start to roam around on their own, and the risk of separating them from their mothers is particularly high. From Saleeq's pragmatic point of view, since the summer months were not lucrative, it was all the more critical that he catch as many monkeys as possible in the fall and winter. Moreover, monkey catchers like Saleeq face the constant risk of being injured by macaques and prevented by animal welfare activists and Hanuman worshippers from doing their job. Most monkey catchers are Muslim, which further aggravates this religiously driven tension (Gandhi 2012, 46). Predictably, this tug of war between the trappers, the monkeys, the brokers who recruit them, and the people who sabotage them does not bode well for peaceful cohabitation among species in Delhi.

The problem is further exacerbated by political issues and bureaucratic setbacks. At issue is the identity of macaques, at present a kind of gray area: if they are considered an urban species, then they are under the jurisdiction of the North, South, and East MCDs, which claim that they are already too busy dealing with dogs and cattle. If they are seen as a wild species, then they must be managed by the Delhi Department of Forest and Wildlife. Moreover, if managed as wild animals, macaques fall under the jurisdiction of single states, and not of the national government. Although in exceptional circumstances their export and relocation to another state is permitted by law (as happened in 2004, when the Supreme Court ordered the relocation of three hundred macaques from Delhi to the Kuno Palpur Wildlife Sanctuary in Madhya Pradesh), the issue must usually be managed internally so as to avoid simply moving the conflict to a new location. Illegal transfers do take place, as Uttarakhand villagers know all too well, plagued as they are by "outsider" monkeys who threaten not only their crops but also their safety and that of their dogs (Govindrajan 2015).

A similar debate on the macaques' identity has occurred in Himachal Pradesh, four hundred kilometers north of Delhi. In May 2016, after a two-month political and legal battle, the then Ministry of Environment and Forests consigned macaques to the status of "vermin" for a period of one year in the urban and agricultural areas of thirty-eight subdistricts of this state, in view of the huge amount of damage they cause to agriculture and farmers' livelihoods. Shifting macaques from schedule II to schedule V of the Wildlife Protection Act of 1972 (where they joined mice, rats, fruit bats, and crows, all nonendangered species that feed on crops) made it legal for anyone—not just the local authorities but also private citizens—to kill them. Yet even though their status as vermin was eventually extended to 2019, from May 2016 to February 2019 only five monkeys were officially killed, owing to religious, political, ethical, and logistical reasons—simply put: who should shoot them, and how? While an official, scientifically grounded plan is eagerly awaited, in late 2019 Himachal farmers turned to poison to exterminate the macaques (Khanna 2019).

Violence at the Human-Macaque Interface

Of course, this close proximity between humans and macaques often results in encounters with harmful consequences. Some are accidental—yet very common—such as the electrocution of monkeys who move around via electrical cables. Some are deliberate, as when people resort to violence to get rid of macaques, pelting them with sticks and stones or throwing acid or boiling water on them. But the most common harm consists of monkey bites. Data on monkey bites suffer from the same unreliability that affects data on rabies cases, making it difficult to compare them in the long run. In March 2016, the then minister for home affairs, Haribhai Parthibhai Chaudhary, informed the Indian Parliament that 1,490 people had been bitten by macaques in Delhi in the previous twelve months. According to the *Times of India*, this was about three hundred more cases than in the previous year (Jain 2015). The Primate Research Centre of Jodhpur claims that more than 1,000 monkey bites are reported every day in India's urban areas (Chakravartty 2015, 28). Thus even if macaques do not account for the highest number of cases of human rabies in India, they are a source of growing concern.

The number of these painful encounters is not the only pressing issue, however. Indeed, the close proximity—even intimacy—between people and macaques when food is involved is a matter of concern in itself, owing to the risk of pathogen transmission. An article on the health implications of feeding and interacting with monkeys in a temple in Kathmandu (Nepal) states, "Macaques climb on the heads and shoulders of visitors, which may bring macaque body fluids into contact with visitors' eyes and nasal and oral mucosa, potential portals of entry for infectious agents" (Jones-Engel et al. 2006, 901). Rabies can be transmitted in the same way, not necessarily through a bite. In Indian temples like the Hanuman Mandir in Delhi and the Galta Mandir in Jaipur, the same type of intimate contact often occurs between people and macaques.

As this chapter has shown, while food plays a primary role in creating this intimacy between macaques and people, it also has the best chance of breaking it. In the Ubud Monkey Forest Temple in Bali (Indonesia), Agustín Fuentes and Scott Gamerl (2005, 201) observed that 73% of the aggressive interactions between temple monkeys and visitors revolved around food. In Shimla, food exchanges were the context for conflict and aggression, particularly in temple areas (Chauhan and Pirta 2010, 12). I remember well how Malik repeatedly stressed that monkeys are not naturally aggressive toward humans; in the forest, they are even shy and try to avoid contact. By contrast, in cities, towns, and other highly anthropogenic settings like temples, the entanglements among people, macaques, and food has had such a detrimental impact on their natural behavior that wildlife scientists now speak of it as "urban wildlife syndrome."

Macaques are intelligent animals and are highly skilled at classifying people along a spectrum that ranges from alliance to open abuse. They do not interact with people at random but know exactly whom to approach and whom to avoid. I observed this behavior at the Kashmiri Gate metro station in Central Delhi, which is surrounded by street vendors who sell food from their stalls. The troop of macaques who live nearby are drawn by the alluring aroma of the fruits and vegetables sold there and patrol the area constantly. The first day I saw the macaques marching on the wall behind the stalls, I felt sorry for the sellers, envisioning their daily struggle to protect their goods. Yet to my surprise, I came to learn from the vendors that the monkeys rarely bother them, aware that the sellers could beat them up badly or shift their business to a safer place, thus depriving them of an easy meal. Instead, they wait for customers to buy food and walk away, and then they attempt to steal and ransack their bags or frighten them into dropping their bags. After these crafty macaques devoured their stolen food, I often saw hopeless customers go back to the stalls for more, this time making sure to hide it and protect it. This kind of mutually beneficial arrangement between the macaques and the sellers left me amazed. It is difficult not to credit these monkeys with what Dario Maestripieri (2007) calls "Macachiavellian intelligence."

Ethnoprimatological studies have shown what people in India already know: that women and children are frequent targets of macaque attacks (Devi and Saikia 2008, 16), with the highest incidence of monkey bites in children under the age of five (Samanta et al. 2016, 59). Women and children are vulnerable mainly owing to their smaller stature and the limited fear they inspire. As Malik wrote in her fieldwork diary, "Monkeys judge the strength of their opponents before approaching them aggressively. If the opponent is stronger and/or outnumbers them, the monkeys would avoid confrontation." It is no accident that Saleeq's colleagues, he told me, often disguise themselves as women so as to increase their odds of catching a macaque. Monkeys target children and women both as harmless sources of food and as scapegoats. In fact, macaques have an efficient tactic for minimizing aggression within the troop and reinforcing its social bonds: they find a scapegoat outsider onto whom to channel violent energies (Maestripieri 2007, 52–54). This scapegoating technique explains why macaque violence toward people can easily spiral in an apparently random way.

Macaque violence toward humans can stem from another misunderstanding between the two species. Certain macaque gestures and facial expressions overlap with those of humans, but they mean different things to monkeys than they do to people. Misled by a false feeling of interspecies understanding, people end up decoding the body language of macaques in an erroneous—and dangerous—way. The most common human mistake is smiling, as macaques see the baring of teeth, especially when the mouth is open, as a threat. For the same reason, laughing, coughing, sneezing, and yawning can be equally risky.

Human cohabitation with urban macaques has become increasingly difficult not only because the macaques' resourcefulness has increased but also because human tolerance for them has diminished. In fact, as is always the case in highly anthropic environments, people's attitude is a key factor in social relations. For years macaques were welcomed into Indian towns and cities, since their population was still low and their religious and cultural value was high. Unlike street dogs, who tend to be considered dangerous, aggressive, and rabid without being given the benefit of the doubt, macaques initially enjoyed considerable human goodwill. "In no time," says Malik, "pets have been converted into pests." This change in attitude has been so destabilizing that even the connection between monkeys and Hanuman has begun to change. Hanuman devotees are well aware that their beloved deity was a naughty child; countless stories describe the tricks he played on meditating hermits. This imagined resemblance to Hanuman increased human tolerance of macaques, at first. But when the balance between forest and urban macaques was lost, so was the balance between respect for Hanuman and disappointment in the macaques. As a visitor to the Hanuman Mandir once told me, "These monkeys are not Hanuman. . . . In this *kali yuga* [cosmic era of darkness and moral degeneration], even they have gone evil." It is interesting to note that Hanuman's star has risen precisely during this "Kali Yuga of spiraling consumerism" (Lutgendorf 2001, 288).

Despite the growing gap between the widespread worship of Hanuman and increasing human impatience with macaques, the Hindu cult of the monkey god, combined with ethical qualms about the treatment of animals, has made implementing rigorous measures of monkey control difficult in India so far. However, this is not to blame the lack of control entirely on religious beliefs. Human-monkey conflict is complex and multifaceted, and it is breaking out now in the heart of the Indian cities, though it actually comes from afar, in terms of both time and place.

CHAPTER 5

COWS

After the umpteenth hot day spent waiting for the monsoon in a village on the edge of the Thar Desert, in Rajasthan, I was enjoying my dinner in the courtyard of the guest house where I was staying in May 2012. Sitting on the floor with my back to the main gate, I suddenly sensed the presence of something approaching me from behind with a clacking rhythm. I had no time to turn around before I found myself face to face with a huge black animal with drooping ears and docked horns, staring at my plate of rice with the patience and the resolution of one who knows it will soon be his. Torn between panic and admiration, I immediately drew back, surrendering my dinner. I started to breathe again only when Sunita, my host, emerged from the kitchen giggling and reassured me that the nine-hundred-pound bull standing in front of me was harmless. She knew him quite well, as he used to walk down the road in front of her house every morning and evening, stopping at every doorstep where he was sure to find some leftovers. At Sunita's house, he was used to finding food in the hole she had dug next to her door, but experience had taught him that knocking at her door with his horns was another way to get some fresh food. Apparently, Sunita observed, her husband had neglected to lock the gate that evening, so the bull had simply sauntered in. Sunita was neither annoyed nor surprised: she merely went back to the kitchen to get some vegetable scraps and, holding them near his mouth, escorted him out the gate. She returned as if nothing unusual had happened.

India is home to about 5.3 million free-roaming cattle, and Rajasthan ranks third in the percentage of this population (Ministry of Agriculture 2012, 117). These street animals represent the tip of a vast and complex iceberg. In the situation of free-roaming Indian cows, we can see the intricate interconnections between devotion and negligence, care and exploitation, poverty and greed, emotion and business, religion and politics, personal choices and structural constraints. This chapter attempts to provide a comprehensive account of the unique entanglements that bring cattle onto the streets of India and contribute to the spread of rabies.

A preliminary word about terminology is necessary. In India, the most common bovines are domestic cattle (*Bos taurus*) and water buffaloes (*Bubalus bubalis*). "Cattle" encompasses both sexes, while "cows" are adult females, "bulls" are intact adult males, "oxen" are castrated adult males, "heifers" are young (female) cows, "steers" are young bulls, and "calves" are male and female youths. The plural feminine form "cows" is used colloquially to refer to cattle collectively, and although bulls have some religious importance in Hindu religion and culture, adult females are actually the main beneficiaries of spiritual affection and practical protection—of social engagement with humans, in other words—and are also the subject of most religious and scientific literature on bovine species in India. In legal, political, and common language, "cow protection" and "cow slaughter" have become widely used expressions that, on the one hand, theoretically encompass cattle of all ages and sexes but, on the other, clearly affirm the prominence of cows. Buffaloes have no comparable religious value.

While many Hindus do not actually revere the cow, her high status in the animal kingdom is considered an axiom of contemporary Hindu culture. Nevertheless, despite the breadth and polymorphism of the Hindu pantheon, cattle are not actually considered proper deities. At most, they appear in Hindu literature and everyday devotion as the companion animals of certain gods or as their mounts or vehicles (*vahanas*). Krishna, one of the most popular Hindu deities, also called Govinda ("one who gives pleasure to the cows") or Gopala ("protector of the cows"), is often depicted as a caring herdsman grazing his cows in the idyllic countryside near the village of Gokula ("the place of cows"). In the Goloka, "the planet of cows" and Krishna's personal abode, he rests peacefully with his cows under the shade of trees and sometimes plays the flute for the cows. Even when he appears with his beloved Radha, Krishna is also often accompanied by a massive, docile cow, the source of the evocative pairing Krishna-cow. With regard to *vahanas*, Nandi ("the joyful one," "the one who pleases") is the bull who faithfully serves as a mount for the god Shiva. In temples devoted to Shiva, a statue of the seated Nandi is commonly found at the main gate, in the courtyard, or at Shiva's feet.

Although the cow lacks true godlike status (for example, there are no temples devoted to her—Basham [1954] 1993, 319), paradoxically, she is considered *more* than divine. In fact, 330 million deities are thought to reside in every atom in her body. In a very common religious image, her silhouette is entirely covered by a constellation of colored miniatures of well-known Hindu gods and goddesses. Worshipping the cow, particularly by means of this visual aid, is tantamount to venerating the entire Hindu pantheon and can save the pious devout twenty-one rotations in the tormenting cycle of death and rebirth (Freed and Freed 1981, 488). On top of this already exceptional physical density, the body of the cow is also said to be a perfect miniature model of the universe (Korom 2000, 190–92). Her udder, for example, is compared to the ocean (Sharma 1980, 4). Her four legs symbolize the four cosmic ages (*yuga*) that make up the temporal cycle to which mankind is painfully tied (Campbell 1974, 142). After an age of flawlessness (the first age of humankind, or *satya yuga*), when the dharma was in perfect balance and the cow stood firmly on her four legs, the second and third ages of humankind (*treta yuga* and *dvapara yuga*), periods of gradual deterioration, opened the way to the *kali yuga* (the fourth and final age of humankind) (Majupuria 1991, 79). This age of suffering and moral corruption, in which the dharma has collapsed and the cow has crumbled to the ground, began on February 18, 3102 B.C.E., on the occasion of Krishna's departure, and is expected to last 1,000 divine years (or 432,000 human years).

Mothers and Milk

Among mythological figures, the cow, known primarily as Kamadhenu, enjoys a prominent position. From *kama* (desire), Kamadhenu is generally translated as "the cow from which every wish is fulfilled" or "the cow of plenty." The level of benevolence that people expect from the cow is evident in the prayer "Let the milk kine that have no calves storm downward, yielding rich nectar, streaming, unexhausted" (*Rig Veda* 3.55.16). In a more earthly context, the Kamadhenu Ati Nirdhan Chikitsa Sahayata Society (an NGO that provides financial assistance to needy patients), launched by the Sanjay Gandhi Postgraduate Institute of Medical Sciences in Lucknow, was named after her because "Kamadhenu . . . nourishes all" (Chandra et al. 2011, 73).

According to the *Adi Parva*, the first book of the *Mahabharata*, Surabhi (another name for Kamadhenu) is the first creature to have emerged from the mythical churning of the milk ocean, when gods and demons fought tenaciously over possession of the *navaratna* (the nine gems, one being Surabhi) lost in this primordial ocean of milk. The *Devi Bhagavata Purana* says that Krishna, growing thirsty while pursuing Radha, created the cow Surabhi—together with her calf Manoratha—with the aim of milking her. While drinking his fill of milk, he inadvertently spilled some of this precious liquid on the ground, which immediately became the primeval ocean of milk, or Kshirasagara. In the meantime, the cows that would later become Krishna's herd emerged from the pores of Surabhi's skin (Mani 1975, 379–81). In addition to her role as producer of milk, ancient literature also describes Kamadhenu as a mother, the mother of many, in fact. In the *Ramayana*, Surabhi is the mother of all cows and of Rohini and Gandharvi, who in turn are the progenitors of all bovines and horses (Sharma 1971, 220). In the *Mahabharata*, Surabhi is the mother of Nandini ("the one who brings joy"), while in the *Harivamsha*, she is the mother of *amrita* (the nectar of immortality) and of Brahmans. In other Vedic texts, she is called Aditi ("infinity," "expansion") and described as the mother of all deities who are *go jata* (born from cows) (Mishra 1985, 61). In the *Vana Parva*, Surabhi is depicted as a caring and protective mother deeply attached to her children, and she is torn by unbearable pain when her son, an ox, is pitilessly exploited during plowing. In hymn 2.17.32 of the *Ramayana*, the image of the cow deprived of her calf becomes the most poignant picture of excruciating suffering.

Kamadhenu is often portrayed with her young calf standing nearby, whom she constantly watches over tenderly. She is in fact the symbol of a pure form of fertility devoid of erotic charge; in other words, more than female, she is mother (Rigopoulos 1998, 231). It is this fertility that associates Kamadhenu so deeply with the earth, so much so that she is also known as Prithivi ("the extended one") and the earth is said to be *gorupini* (cow-shaped) (Iyer 1977, 32). In the *Vishnu Purana*, Prithu (an incarnation of Vishnu) milks Prithivi to ensure a good harvest and put an end to the famine that is decimating humankind. The idea of the cow as the archetypal mother is reflected in the orthodox Hindu custom of referring to this animal as *go mata*, from *go* (cow) and *mata* (mother).

I never really understood the deep attachment that Hindus feel to this animal until I saw it with my eyes on a quiet day at Help In Suffering, the animal hospital in Jaipur where I was working as a volunteer. That day, an elderly couple of farmers brought their ailing cow from the outskirts of the town. She had calved the day before, but during the night she had experienced a severe uterine prolapse. She arrived with her entire uterus hanging out of her vagina inside out, dangling between her hind legs almost to her knees. It broke my heart to imagine the poor cow's discomfort and the fear and worry of her owners, tired from the journey, terrified about her condition, and anxious about how they would survive without her if she died. While the medical staff undertook the long procedure of patiently pushing the uterus back into position, the farmer helped them keep the cow as calm as possible. His wife sat on the ground beside her, rooted to the spot, looking lost. Having no useful role to play in helping the animal, I sat next to the woman to keep her company. All she said every now and then, her eyes filled with tears, was that the cow was their mother.

The idea of motherhood inscribed in the cow is expressed in several ways. The term *vatsalya*, which describes the tenderness and protection of maternal love, comes from *vatsa*, "calf." Children are compared to calves for the unconditional love they receive from their mothers during the Vats Baras festival, which celebrates women and cows who are mothers of males (Lodrick 1980, 161). According to Hindu tradition, each human has seven mothers, and the cow—the *go mata*—is one of them. "To be honest," I was once told by a Hindu woman, a mother of three, "cows are better than [human] mothers, as a mother gives her milk only to her child, while a cow gives it to all the people." As Naisargi Dave puts it, the veneration of the cow as a blessing mother builds on the "native, religio-scientific theory about the impossibility of maternal-fetal conflict" (2017, 40).

Kamadhenu and milk are linked in two ways. First, Kamadhenu is generally depicted as white in color and with a swollen udder and a human breast from which milk pours profusely. Second, the term *dhenu*, from *duhe* (to milk), refers to a milk cow (Walker 1968, 256). In the *Rig Veda*, cows are thought of as *kamadugha*, meaning "milking desires" or "yielding objects of desire, like milk" (Wiley 2014, 57). According to the myth, it was Brahma who compelled the cow to give her milk to all humankind. The Govardhan Puja, the most famous festival in honor of cows, memorializes this event and the incomparable wealth, in the form of nourishing milk, that these animals provide (Lodrick 1987, 107). On social media, pictures of street cows nursing animals of other species, such as macaques and pigs, are regularly circulated by groups like People for Cattle in India. But nothing celebrates milk and butter better than the story of baby Krishna. Raised in a community of cowherds, Krishna soon discovered the sweet taste of cow's milk. He was so fond of milk that he is often depicted interrupting his stepmother while she milks her cows, even suckling the milk directly from the cows' teats, described in the *Bhagavata Purana* as "flowing out of love" (10.20.26). In religious iconography, baby Krishna is often portrayed stealing butter from neighboring houses or dipping his chubby fingers into bowls full of butter. Even today, on Krishna Janmashtami (the anniversary of Krishna's birth), children are dressed in his likeness and are smeared profusely with a butterlike substance on their faces and hands.

In short, the cow is considered the essence of the supreme gift—the gift of life—and milk is the best evidence of this abundance, selflessness, and unconditional love. Apart from the myths and festivals, the significance of milk is especially evident in the everyday life of Indians, and of Hindus in particular. One day I was talking about family with Sakshi, a nine-year-old girl who lives in the Shadipur slum with her mother and stepfather. She explained that she has a father who, she said, "is not my father," but at least a "real mother," and noted sadly that many children no longer have their parents. But she took comfort in the certainty that, "luckily, there are cows who grow them [orphans] with their milk."

When Sakshi sought my approval regarding the importance of cow's milk for infants, I did not have the courage to tell her that I have never drunk it, as I cannot digest it. I did try to explain this several times to many people, particularly cow owners, who wanted me to taste their milk. *Their* milk, they claimed, had nothing in common with the kind I had tasted before. If it was hard to refuse these incessant offers of milky tea or *chhaachh* (a drink made of churned curd, cold water, and spices), it was even harder to make these people believe me when, after finally giving in and tasting their milk, I dared to tell them that it had, predictably, made me sick. They simply refused to believe it, certain that my sickness had been caused by some adulterated food I had consumed. It was impossible that their milk could cause illness, because it comes from *deshi* (indigenous) cows.

Milk and Money

Until the 1960s, when India began importing foreign breeds in massive numbers, the only cattle in India were zebus (*Bos taurus indicus*). The zebu is a subspecies of domestic cattle that originated in south Asia during the Neolithic Age and still bears the evidence of its adaptation, over the course of millennia, to south Asian tropical weather. Zebus are characterized by a large dewlap called a blanket, generally elongated horns, often droopy ears, and, above all, a fatty hump on their shoulders that gives them the colloquial name "humped cattle." About thirty zebu breeds are known, and many of them (e.g., Gir, Sahiwal, Sindhi, Ongole, and Kankrej) can still be found in India. European breeds that have been imported to India in the past sixty years have affected the genetic purity of zebus and pro-duced several hybrids, commonly referred to as Jerseys. As a result, at least 85% of the Indian cattle population today is technically nondescript (i.e., having no recognizable breed characteristics) (Joshi 2000, 33). This hybridization is thought to be a side effect of the White Revolution (Kaur 2010, 27), a large-scale project funded by the World Bank and launched in 1970 by Verghese Kurien. At the core of this revolution was the nationwide dairy cooperative scheme called Operation Flood, which aimed to mod-ernize Indian dairy farming by scientifically improving milk production, increasing rural incomes, and making milk more available and affordable to urban consumers. Interestingly, another of its goals was the removal of dairy cattle from cities. Operation Flood, the world's biggest dairy devel-opment program, sustained poor farmers throughout India by giving them favorable credit terms for purchasing milk cows, preferably high-yield breeds that would generate quick profits (Joshi 2000, 39). Foreign breeds were invariably favored for milk production; when they were not available, crossbreeds were selected.

Operation Flood ended in 1996, but every year on November 26 (Kurien's birthday), India still celebrates National Milk Day. Despite a low yield per animal, with about three hundred million bovines India is, by a good margin, the largest producer of milk (from all mammalian species) in the world, accounting for 18% of global production (Ministry of Agri-culture 2016, 3). In the period from 2016 to 2018, milk production in India rose by a historic 6.6%, reaching 176.3 million tons annually (*Down to Earth* 2019a). While Rajasthan is the second-largest milk producer in India (with Uttar Pradesh leading the way), it ranks first when it comes to the growth in milk production. In fact, its production increased by 308% between 1985 and 2015 (FIAPO 2016, 4). This production depends on about seventy-five million small-scale dairy farms scattered across the country, occasionally organized in cooperative societies at the village level (Sood 2014a, 27).

Just 5% of India's dairy production is exported (Brighter Green 2012, 8); thus the country is also the world's largest consumer of dairy products. In the period from 1998 to 2005, the average annual growth rate was 5%, increasing to more than 8% between 2005 and 2012 (Rajeshwaran and Naik 2016, 9). This rise is visible mainly in urban India, where about 56% of the milk produced in the country is consumed (Lewis 2016), thanks to increased incomes, urbanization, changes in food consumption patterns—particularly among the middle class—and the availability of milk and milk by-products (in Delhi, Mother Dairy stalls and 24/7 vending machines are so popular that they are used as landmarks). While lactose intolerance is found in eastern India, demand for milk has steadily increased in the rest of the country, especially in the northwest (Lewis 2016). Milk's status as a "traditional" food is another reason for its popularity in the rapidly urbanizing Indian population (Wiley 2014, 81). Hindus use milk and its by-products for religious purposes as well, as they are believed to have purifying qualities due to their derivation from the cow. Every day, thousands of liters of milk bathe idols in Hindu temples throughout the country. Sweets made from milk or ghee are used as offerings to the gods (recall that Hanuman is fond of laddus, sweet balls made of chickpeas and flour and fried in butter), and ghee burns in lamps during worship rituals.

Milk production in India comes not only from cows, whether indigenous or crossbred. As of 2014–15, buffaloes contributed 51% of the country's total milk production. The remaining 49% came from exotic (foreign-breed) cows (25%), nondescript cows (20%), and goats (4%) (Ministry of Agriculture 2016, 5). If we consider the per-capita milk yield, crossbred cows provide about seven kilograms (about fifteen pounds) per day, buffaloes seven, and indigenous cows no more than 2.5 (Ministry of Agriculture 2016, 5). In terms of quality, buffalo milk is considerably richer in fat than cow's milk and is thus especially useful in curd, butter, and ghee processing. Since ghee is well suited to India's tropical climate (it does not need refrigeration), is less harmful than milk to lactose-intolerant people, and is thought to have healing properties (it is alleged to facilitate weight loss, cure otitis, stop snoring, relieve constipation, and disinfect wounds), it is very popular. In fact, after milk, ghee is the most preferred dairy product in India (Sood 2014a, 35). The higher fat content of buffalo milk also allows it to be "toned up"—that is, combined with skim milk and water to dilute its fat content and increase the quantity and availability of milk.

Despite the high and increasing production of milk from both cows and buffaloes in India, per-capita consumption data suggest that even Operation Flood had little impact on consumption at the national level, given that it was aimed primarily at urban consumers (Wiley 2014, 76–77). In fact, according to Amrita Patel of the National Dairy Development Board, India still does not produce enough milk to meet even its internal demand (Sood 2014a, 32). Overexploitation of bovines is thus the easiest, quickest, and cheapest way to increase the milk supply, as if the body of the cow was meant to accept whatever violence necessary for the good of her "children." Overexploitation is also the primary way that cattle end up on the streets, where they cross paths with the rabies virus.

Like all mammals, cows and female buffaloes produce milk only when they are feeding their young, so farmers have them artificially inseminated as often as possible. Then, during the lactation period, they are indiscriminately injected with oxytocin (the *dudh ka dava*, or "medicine of milk," as oxytocin is popularly known in Delhi) so that their owners can get more milk out of them. Despite its being banned by the Prevention of Cruelty to Animals Act of 1960 and the Food and Drugs Adulteration Prevention Act of 1954, oxytocin can easily be bought wholesale without a medical prescription. According to data cited by People for the Ethical Treatment of Animals (PETA India 2008, 2), 82% of Delhi cattle farmers use it.

To maximize the benefits of oxytocin, the calf cannot be allowed to consume the milk for which the farmer is waiting. He is allowed to suckle only long enough to stimulate his mother's lactation and is then promptly led away from her udder and tied up. In Kotla Mubarakpur (an urban village in the heart of South East Delhi), where I used to observe the milking at a dairy located on the shore of a *nala* (open ditch), it was common for farmers to tie the calves just taken from their mothers inside the nearby *dalaos* (garbage collection sites), so that they could fill their stomach on rubbish instead of milk. Ironically, in India garbage trucks often have the image of a cow nursing her newborn calf painted on the back. If calves do not survive this forced undernourishment, their bodies are recycled, used as a visual and olfactory stimulus to force their mothers to continue producing milk. On several occasions in Delhi, I saw the *khal bacha*, a calf-shaped dummy made of straw and covered with the skin of the dead calf. It was put before the cow at milking time, to exploit the cow-calf bond and accelerate the lactation process.

A calf's chance of survival largely depends on its sex. Females stand higher in the hierarchy, as they are raised as a long-term investment. Males, who are redundant, for they have no use as draft or breeding animals, come last in the order of preference and are either abandoned or indirectly killed as soon as their mothers' milk production naturally tapers off. In fact, as I learned from the director of the Sanjay Gandhi Animal Care Centre, calves are popularly called *khatra*, "born to be killed." Of the thirty-two dairies surveyed by FIAPO (2016, 7) in Rajasthan, none of the male calves generally survive in twenty-one of them, while the other eight habitually release them into the streets. Sometimes disposing of them is left directly to their mothers: farmers tie a spiked collar around their mouth, so that when the calf approaches his mother to suckle, she feels pain and kicks him away, occasionally to death. More frequently, the calves are simply fastened with ropes so short that they end up strangling themselves, are tethered outside in the elements or, easiest of all, are just abandoned on the streets. In this way, calves are not technically "killed," and this, considered acceptable because it is not directly inflicted *himsa* (violence), allows farmers not to fear bad karma, social contempt, or the rage of cow protectionists. Whether the technique is more or less direct, the final result is evident in the gender imbalance of the cattle and buffalo population: 64% female and 36% male in the former, 85% female and 15% male in the latter (Kasturirangan, Srinivasan, and Rao 2014).

If a male calf manages to reach maturity, he becomes an ox and will be used to pull carts transporting wares, or a bull. If a bull, it is likely that he will roam the streets, owing to his owner's negligence and greed. Until recently, religion also played a role in this matter. The *Garuda Purana* (2.20.42) explains that if funeral rites are not properly performed, the soul of the dead gets dangerously lost. The only way to redeem the deceased is to perform the rite called *vrisotsarga*, in which a bull is let loose. I was told that if the bull is branded with Shiva's symbol, a trident, no one should complain if he invades private property or causes damage; on the contrary, they should take good care of him. This custom has become less common in modern urban India. Religious reasons aside, this system of abandoning male calves has worked well in rural villages by enabling farmers to have their cows impregnated for free by this community bull.

Heifers and nonlactating adult cows are considered an economic burden to farmers. The most convenient solution, again, is to throw them onto the street and let them fend for themselves. This happens most to older cows (the continuous pregnancies that are forced on them can cause them to dry up by the age of five), cows who are barren (usually thanks to botched artificial inseminations), and severely sick animals. Heifers and productive cows are the farmers' priority and thus their neglect is less likely, at least until they become unprofitable—often because, in a vicious cycle, their consumption of garbage has impaired their milk production or reproductive capacity. From the farmer's point of view, in optimal conditions, these animals will become useful again sooner or later. In the meantime, their owners (for these cows remain owned animals) keep an eye on them. They typically know where their cows find food and what streets they roam, because cows tend to be quite methodical under favorable conditions. Unlike the neighborhood dog feeders discussed in chapter 3 (Warden 2015), who refer to particular street dogs as "my dog" even when this implies no actual relationship of possession or ownership, farmers who abandon "their cattle" to the street are quick to claim ownership just when milking time arrives, despite feeling little or no sense of attachment or responsibility for these animals when they need food, water, or shelter. Unfortunately for these animals, their neglectful owners largely rely on their cows' knowledge and desire to return home, because of their supposedly superior intelligence. A farmer in Kotla Mubarakpur told me proudly that when he released his cows, two of them loved to stroll around the Delhi Fort, more than ten kilometers (six miles) from their home. Every evening before nightfall they left the house, successfully navigating traffic lights and busy roads, and every morning they came home along the same route, even routinely begging for their food, he swore.

This blind confidence in the navigational skills of cows stands in inverse relation to that of buffaloes. These animals, a buffalo herder informed me solemnly, are never found on the streets, because "they are so stupid that in the cowshed they even step on their calves." A colleague of his went further, attesting that while a cow could make it home to Delhi from Jaipur in a few days, a buffalo would be lost immediately, rooted to the spot even if left in the neighbor's yard. Buffaloes could never be trusted to wander free in Delhi. According to popular wisdom, buffaloes' stupidity is passed on to people who drink their milk, who will gain impressive physical strength but be hampered by poor memory, slow reasoning, and low powers of concentration. Although dairy farmers generally prefer buffaloes for economic reasons, they are scorned at the cultural and religious level (Narayanan 2018), so much so that it is not uncommon to find, written on water tanks for animals installed on the streets by charitable organizations or private citizens, the words: "It is forbidden to let buffaloes drink this water." It is also not uncommon for traditional households to keep a cow for religious purposes and a buffalo (or crossbred cow) for her milk. In other words, the cow is kept for home, the buffalo for the outside—a phrase used to refer to the existence of both a wife and a mistress in a man's life (Govindrajan 2018). Paradoxically enough, thanks to their economic value, buffaloes are never let loose in the streets.

Another reason why cattle owners are not particularly worried about turning their cows into the streets is that they know the animals will benefit from the devotion of their fellow Hindus. In fact, most of the university students I interviewed cited Hindu devotion as the main reason for the presence of cattle on the streets. In contrast, most of them (60%) did not mention the exploitive dairy industry.

A Give-and-Take Relationship

Having learned a lot by watching macaques at the banana stand near the Ridge, I repeated this kind of observation with cows, following them in their urban wandering. I selected Kotla Mubarakpur in South East Delhi as the site for this activity, as it is one of the so-called urban villages in the city. These villages, founded centuries before the term "Delhi" meant anything, preserve a shred of rural India in the heart of a city of nineteen million citizens. There are about three hundred urban villages in Delhi (Shah 2012), and it has been calculated that they house nearly 3,500 *tabelas* (commercial animal factories) and backyard family farms (Baviskar 2011a, 397). Although historically valuable and socially vibrant, Kotla Mubarakpur is now overcrowded, chaotic, and poorly planned, with sheds arranged at apartment building entrances, cows tied in alleys as if they were motorcycles, and a strong smell of cattle dung in the air. In fact, it was in this village that I found myself making my first *upla*, a dung cake.

Dung is used in rural India as a slow-burning cooking fuel in the kitchen, to fertilize the fields, and to periodically cleanse the house (diluted with water, the dung paste is smeared on the floor and interior and exterior walls and left to dry, also because it is thought to keep mosquitoes away). Preparing dung cakes is a predominantly female job, and I was taught how to do it by a woman in her nineties. As the cowshed had just been cleaned up, the dung was already piled in the middle of the small yard and mixed with chopped straw. She had me squat on the ground and showed me how much dung to pick up. Then she told me how to compress it and, finally, how to stick it on the *upla*-covered exterior wall behind us. When I removed my hand, she had some fun in comparing our handprints. Depending on weather conditions, she would remove the dung cakes from the wall when they were completely dry and store them for future use. When I looked for some water to wash my hands, she invited me to spend some minutes in idleness with her, to allow, she explained, "the dung to make our skin smooth and beautiful." Like all cow by-products, dung is thought to have purifying qualities and to "kill the bad bacteria" on our skin.

On a Saturday in March 2013, I reached Kotla Mubarakpur at 6:30 in the morning. At 7:00 I officially started my first twelve hours of uninterrupted cow shadowing, initially finding hospitality on the steps of a butcher shop conveniently located at a busy crossroad in front of a *dalao*, a covered structure for the disposal of garbage. Indian cities that have free-roaming cattle invariably have designated locations where, at certain times of day, cattle know that food will be available, and this was one such place. From this position I could observe the scene easily and could keep a low profile so as not to annoy the animals—or their owners. Delhi farmers are very alert and they do not like it when their cows receive attention. In fact, that first afternoon, a man brandishing a stick shouted at me vehemently, making it very clear that he did not want me around. I decided to stay anyway, till 7:00 P.M. as scheduled. My intention had been to follow the same cow all day long, but when the various cows were taken back in rotation to the shed for milking, I decided to shift my attention to the animal closest to the one I had been watching up until that point. By evening, I had observed seven young and adult females, and had monitored all of their foraging and interactions with people. From my field notes that day:

Cow 1. At 7:02, a boy passed her and bent to touch her forelegs; at 7:05, a girl in Western clothes with her mother in a sari selected this cow from the herd, fed her a banana (from their hands directly to her mouth), joined their hands in a short prayer, and touched the cow's forehead and her fore hooves; at 7:06, a man stopped his motorcycle to receive a phone call and the cow sniffed insistently at his pockets; at 7:07, she ate some carrot peelings found on the ground; at 7:12, a man on a bike herded her to the milking shed.

Cow 2. At 7:13, a woman arrived carrying a banana on a plate, fed it to her, and touched her forelegs; at 7:17, a woman fed her a roti and touched her forelegs; at 7:31, a man emptied a bag of bean pods onto the ground and she ran to eat them; at 7:32, a man stopped his bike and fed her a roti; at 7:33, she ate some unsorted rubbish from the cart the garbage collector was unloading (he shouted at her, wielding a stick, and she trotted a few meters away); at 7:36, she returned to the cart and ate more garbage; at 7:37, a man in his underwear brushing his teeth fed her three rotis and threw a plastic bag of unsorted garbage onto the cart, which she immediately began to chew; at 7:39, a boy fed her a roti; at 7:40, a girl touched the cow's forehead with her right hand and then touched her own; at 7:44, she ate three rotis found on the ground; at 7:46, a girl was afraid to approach her (the girl's mother tried in vain to convince her); at 7:49, she licked a thick layer of lubricant off the engine of a parked motorcycle; at 7:55, a man placed a newspaper sheet covered with organic waste on the ground and put a plastic bag of unsorted garbage on the cart that she began eating; at 7:56, a man fed her a roti; at 7:58, another man fed her a roti from a bagful; at 8:00, she chewed the electric wires dangling from a control unit on top of a utility pole; at 8:05, a child who was fixing zippers next to the fruit seller threw some pebbles at her to chase her away and warned the man of the potential threat to his fruit; at 8:07, a man gave her a roti in her mouth; at 8:08, a man walking by was scared of her horns and raised his arms to push her away; at 8:10, a man arrived on his bike and fed her seven rotis from a bag; at 8:11, a woman hit her with her son's schoolbag to keep her at a distance; at 8:17, a man fed her two rotis; at 8:20, a boy touched her forehead with both hands and then touched his chest; at 8:30, a man fed her two rotis; at 8:35, a man touched her forehead and then touched his other hand and chest; at 8:37, she went back to the lubricant-covered motorcycle engine; at 8:45, a boy came and took her to the shed.

Cow 3. At 8:50, she ate some bean pods found on the ground; at 8:56, a man stopped his car and gave her two rotis; she then chewed some newspaper sheets found on the ground; at 8:59, she drank from a puddle; at 9:00, another boy took her to the shed.

All of this happened to these three cows in the space of two hours, while I observed seventy-two further interactions, involving four other cows, in the remaining ten hours. Considering the 108 human-cattle relations I registered, cows resorted to eating garbage twenty-five times (mainly in the afternoon) and were given food forty-two times (mostly in the morning, when people leave their homes with food prepared for this purpose). The most frequent food offering was roti (homemade traditional bread), a culturally important food that is given to others as a demonstration of caring attention. On twenty-eight occasions the cows were fed directly hand to mouth, principally when rotis were given. The ritual importance of this gesture is so great that even children and others scared of cattle were insistently encouraged and taught how to approach and feed the cows. Food is not to be put on the dirty, impure ground, and the cow is to be fed only with the right hand, which is traditionally used for auspicious activities, like offering and receiving money and accepting *prasad*.

In a rabies-endemic country like India, feeding cows in this manner is potentially very risky, as it exposes people's hands to saliva that may be infected. Should the hands have wounds or scratches on them, or should they touch the person's mucous membranes (eyeballs or mouth), exposure to rabies may occur. Given the general paucity of reliable data on human rabies deaths, reported cases of cattle-mediated human rabies are statistically negligible. Yet this does not mean that rabies in cattle, and transmission from cattle to humans, should be ignored. Indeed, in 2019 a study carried out in Punjab, based on active surveillance and laboratory testing, indicated that the incidence of rabies in dogs and street cattle is much higher than previously suspected. The authors estimate that "if similar enhanced surveillance for rabies was conducted state-wide," 98 buffalo, 18 horses, 56 farmed cattle, 96 stray cattle, 128 pet dogs, and 62 stray dogs would be expected to be confirmed with rabies in Punjab annually (Gill et al. 2019, 1). Worryingly, only 30% of the owners who noticed a bite wound on their animals requested veterinary consultation (8). Twenty people in this study were exposed to rabies: eleven from a dog and three via a cow, among other animals (13). Again in Punjab, during a two-week rabies outbreak in bovines—in which fourteen cows and one buffalo eventually died—none of the owners observed bite wounds on their animals. Similarly, none of them noticed a possibly rabid dog around their animals. One farmer speculated that rabies may have been transmitted by an unowned, free-roaming puppy (Brookes et al. 2019). Data from southern India show that cows and young cattle of either sex, who are most commonly encountered on the street, are more prone than other cattle to dog attacks (Islam et al. 2016,

254) and thus to catching rabies. These are the animals to whom people make their food offerings.

In Jaipur, Udaipur, Jodhpur, and other cities in the state of Rajasthan, an ad-hoc service is also available for cow feeders. Vendors can usually be found in the markets selling fresh grass for cattle. Customers can simply buy the grass and distribute it wherever they find a roaming animal, though in some cases the vendors keep some cows by their stalls, so that the donor can save time by offering it immediately. *Goshalas* (cattle homes, described in more detail below) offer two additional feeding services for donors. They can visit the *goshala* and pay to feed a certain number of animals, choosing whether to feed the cows themselves or have the staff do it. Or they can have donations collected at their homes by *goshalas* such as the Shri Krishna Gaushala in Bawana or the Kamdhenu Dham Nagar Nigam Gaushala in Carterpuri, both on the outskirts of Delhi, which have a door-to-door collection system. On a rickshaw adapted for the purpose, staff members regularly arrive at their donors' doorsteps to collect kitchen scraps or fresh-baked rotis, or donations of money to buy preferred designated quantity of fodder.

Whatever the method by which food reaches cattle, Hindus do not consider it *prasad*, the sanctified food offered to deities. As a *pandit* (Hindu scholar) I met in the Hanuman Mandir in Delhi told me, "Cows are animals and are alive, so we give them *daan* [food given to the needy]. *Prasad* is for deities, for their *murti* [statue] in temples." *Daan* is traditionally given in an act of charity by a householder to the poor, the sick, people of lower castes, and animals. Because of their religious significance, cows are thought of as particularly appropriate recipients of *daan*, especially those unfortunates who are considered "special" because of prenatal malformations, usually additional legs, often sprouting from their back. In a religion in which deities rarely have only two arms, this genetic anomaly is associated with a divine nature, so much so that the additional leg is often painted as if it was the trunk of the elephantine god Ganesh. It is thus not uncommon to meet people who roam the streets, a portable stereo playing prayers for Krishna, with decorated cows dressed up in wreaths who, for a price, are thought to foresee the future and deliver blessings. I met one such cow in Defence Colony, an affluent neighborhood of South East Delhi, named Lakshmi, a much-loved cow whose namesake is the goddess of material and spiritual prosperity.

The Role of Meat

In most of the world, the value of cows is weighed in beef. Not in India, at least not officially. "Beef cattle" do not technically exist in the country, and cattle eventually appear in the livestock market as a collateral effect of the dairy industry. As noted above, India's biggest investment in livestock—Operation Flood—was meant to increase milk production, not beef. Beef (i.e., cattle meat; I refer to buffalo meat as "carabeef," though this distinction is rarely made in India) is a controversial issue in India, where the economy, religion, and politics all play important roles.

The preamble of the constitution defines India as a "sovereign socialist secular democratic Republic." The term "secular" was added in 1976, thirty years after the Constituent Assembly first discussed banning the slaughter of cows, their place in the constitution, and above all their significance to the country. Finally, article 48, "Organisation of Agriculture and Animal Husbandry," was included in the "Directive Principle of State Policy" (rather than in the more binding "Fundamental Rights," as cow lovers had hoped); religious issues were not mentioned, but "the slaughter of cows and calves and other milch and draught cattle" was prohibited. Article 48 thus contained an apparent contradiction between the sacred value and the economic value of the cow, as if the country could not make up its mind about which was more important and in need of constitutional protection.

The "preservation, protection and improvement of stock" is the exclusive responsibility of individual state legislatures, and the laws governing bovine slaughter, and even the definition of "cow," vary greatly among the states of India. In the northeastern states of West Bengal and Kerala, there are no restrictions; bovines can be slaughtered and beef and carabeef can be consumed. Assam, Andhra Pradesh, and Bihar forbid the slaughter of cattle, but the "fit-for-slaughter" certificate allows exceptions depending on the age (e.g., dairy cows over the age of fourteen), sex, economic value, and health of the animals. In the National Capital Territory of Delhi and Rajasthan, cattle slaughter is illegal (this includes bulls, oxen, heifers, and calves), and Chhattisgarh and Himachal Pradesh ban buffalo slaughter as well. Gujarat has the harshest punishment for those who break the law: people who commit *go hatya* (cow murder) are imprisoned for life or fined 100,000 rupees (US$1,450).

The most restrictive states also ban the export of cattle for the purpose of slaughter, the sale or transport of beef in any form, and the possession of beef, domestic or imported. The Delhi Agricultural Cattle Preservation Act of 1994, for example, permits the export of cattle only on the condition that animals will not be slaughtered, nor can they be exported to a state where slaughter is permitted. In 2016, the Haryana police announced the launch of a twenty-four-hour helpline to report incidents of cow smuggling or slaughter (*Indian Express* 2016a). Given the recent increase in political, religious, and economic attention to cow-related issues, new amendments to these laws are expected. Gujarat strengthened its law in 2017, and Uttar Pradesh, also in 2017, began to comply with the stringent National Security Act and Gangster Act, which give police the power to detain people suspected of slaughtering cattle for a full year (Rashid 2017).

Of course, these bans and other laws have important consequences on economic, environmental, ethical, and health levels. In the long run, they may also involuntarily contribute to the spread of rabies. For one thing, in the states with particularly strict laws, it may be difficult to euthanize rabid cattle. International guidelines for the observation and confinement of possibly rabid animals exist only for dogs, cats, and ferrets. For other species, prompt and humane killing is recommended. In India, cattle affected by an infectious disease (whether it is recognized as notifiable in the state or not) can be euthanized only in a few states, among them Haryana, Goa, and Daman and Diu. In addition, dairy farmers who are stuck between the high demand for dairy products, anti-slaughter laws (and the related fear of raids by police and cow vigilantes), and religious or ethical qualms about illegally sending their animals to slaughterhouses predictably resort to the convenient solution of getting rid of unproductive cattle. The result is a continuous overcrowding of the streets, where the rabies virus already circulates and where there are no more vultures to dispose of cattle carcasses, which greatly benefits the dog population.

Needless to say, when cattle who suffer from infectious diseases are abandoned to the streets, the risk of rabies transmission increases. Predictably, instances of abandonment increase rapidly during tough times such as severe drought. In the Bundelkhand region of Uttar Pradesh, which has a long history of turning loose unmanageable cattle (a practice known as *annapratha*), 91% of the 14,000 cattle owned across three districts were released onto the street in the dry summer of 2016, and some of them were locked up in hospitals and schools for months on end, without care or assistance, to prevent them from devastating crops (Santoshi 2016). Even worse, in the spring of 2018, residents of the Sitapur district resorted to dumping their cattle in Nepal, across the border; they also dumped some of them in the Katarniaghat Wildlife Sanctuary, where infectious diseases like rabies can have devastating consequences (*Down to Earth* 2019b).

The lack of consistency in state laws on cattle slaughter makes it hard to keep accurate records of the Indian cattle population and its health, a situation complicated by the fact that there is a massive nationwide clandestine movement of live animals, as people try to evade local bans on slaughtering cattle. West Bengal, in northern India, and Kerala, in the southern part of the country, are the primary destinations of continual convoys of cattle headed for slaughterhouses. *Beoparis* (animal traders) buy these cattle directly from farmers or, more often, in cattle markets where weekly transactions take place. Forged "fit-for-slaughter" certificates are then used to transport the cattle across state borders. Since they are faked, these certificates do not provide reliable information on the health of the animals. Thus, if they are rabid, the disease moves with them across India. This transfer of potentially sick animals throughout the country is also worrisome because its true extent is difficult to quantify. The documentary film *Their Last Journey: Cattle Trafficking to Kerala*, produced by the Temple Worshippers Society and the Blue Cross of India, quotes the Kerala Department of Animal Husbandry and Dairying as saying that in 2009–10, six million cattle entered Kerala, mainly from Tamil Nadu, through various checkpoints, and two million more are estimated to have entered unchecked. A 2016 law requiring that vehicles transporting livestock be partitioned to provide each bovine with two square meters is routinely violated so as to maximize profits; similar laws are also ignored. I saw more than thirty animals squeezed into the back of a truck meant to hold only a few; there are also reports of tourist buses with their seats removed packed with dozens of sedated animals (Tiwari 2014). Needless to say, this inhumane overcrowding has such a deleterious impact on the animals' health that half of the transported animals die in transit (PETA India 2008, 10). Traffickers who drive cattle to slaughter on foot use secondary roads to evade checkpoints and thus veterinary checking.

The animals who do make it to the slaughterhouse have been deprived of food, water, and proper rest, so they arrive in critical condition. It is illegal to slaughter sick animals (per the Prevention of Cruelty to Animals [Slaughter House] Rules of 2001 and the Food Safety and Standards Regulation of 2011), but medical exams at the destination are cursory—the Idgah slaughterhouse in Delhi, closed in 2010, had no laboratory for proper testing, for example (Jamwal and Dua 2003). It is thus very difficult to detect the presence of serious diseases, such as rabies, that may spread not only among the cattle but also among the people who had contact with them during their final journey and in the slaughterhouses themselves. Handling raw meat without protective gear is perilous if animals are rabid, and given the poor facilities of many improvised slaughterhouses in India, the current risk is potentially very high.

This dire situation also evades all forms of (medical) control when cattle are transported across international borders. Along the 4,000-kilometer border with Bangladesh, thousands of cattle, coming from as far away as Delhi and Rajasthan, have been smuggled every day for decades. Techniques for getting them across the border include putting mashed chili peppers on their genitals, causing them such pain that, in an effort to escape it, they run and eventually break through the barbed wire fence; using underwater snorkelers who, breathing through hollow papaya stems, guide cattle across the rivers and channels that flow into Bangladesh; using a crane made of bamboo to swing animals over the fence; and tying a cow to two pieces of a banana plant and letting her float to the neighboring country. The result is that nearly two-thirds of the cattle slaughtered in Bangladesh are imported from India (Rath 2015). A cow who costs 5,000 rupees (US$72) in India can fetch up to ten times that much just across the border (Karmakar 2017).

On May 23, 2017, the then Ministry of Environment and Forests issued the Prevention of Cruelty to Animals (Regulation of Livestock Market) Rules, which could, theoretically, make a crucial difference in the control of rabies and other infectious diseases in connection with these cattle transfers. Criticized as a fascist measure designed to curb beef consumption, these rules were met with strong and immediate opposition from the millions of Indians who work in the beef industry and from those sections of the population that eat beef. The animal welfare organizations that pushed for these rules deny that this was their intention (Maulekhi 2017), explaining that the real impetus behind them was the need to curb the illegal export of cattle to Bangladesh and Nepal. These rules forbid the sale and purchase of cattle—and also buffaloes—for slaughter at animal markets, while continuing to allow breeders and farmers to sell their animals directly to slaughterhouses. This law actually had a threefold purpose: to curtail the illegal, unfair black market in cattle smuggling, to safeguard the welfare of animals on their way to slaughter (thus protecting the health of human consumers as well), and to keep track of the animals' origin—essential in case of infectious diseases—through proper veterinary supervision. Similarly, FIAPO's most recent guidelines for *goshalas* (cattle homes) recommend that all cattle be vaccinated for hoof-and-mouth disease and rabies (FIAPO 2018b, 59). The Prevention of Cruelty to Animals (Regulation of Livestock Market) Rules were soon withdrawn and replaced by a weaker version that does not mention the interstate transportation of bovines but still prohibits the sale of unfit animals (Sharma 2018). In the meantime, in 2017, the introduction of an identification number to be assigned to cattle at birth was proposed (*Times of India* 2017a).

Because of religious and political sensitivities on the topic of cow slaughter, in India it is generally believed—or at least said for purposes of moral convenience—that most slaughtered bovines are buffaloes rather than domestic cattle (the vagueness of meat labeling does not help clarify this). The Ministry of Agriculture's official data (2016, 7) claim that in 2014–15, 1.4 million tons of meat were produced from buffaloes and 334,000 tons from cattle. However, given that according to the *Report of the National Commission on Cattle*, drafted in 2002 by the same department, there are 4,000 legal slaughterhouses in India but more than 100,000 illegal ones (chap. 6, art. 62), it is difficult to put much stock in these data. It becomes even more challenging if we consider that the top three states for cattle slaughter are Kerala, Bihar, and Maharashtra (Kumar 2017), though it is legal only in Kerala. In fact, the director-general of foreign trade reports much higher numbers: fourteen million buffaloes and twenty million head of cattle slaughtered annually, yielding 1.9 and 2.1 million tons of meat, respectively (Shariff 2015)—and, incidentally, reversing the relative proportions of buffalo and cattle meat that the Ministry of Agriculture claims are produced in India.

According to the U.S. Department of Agriculture, India is the biggest beef exporter in the world (this includes carabeef), supplying mainly Vietnam, Malaysia, the Philippines, and Saudi Arabia (Heinrich Boll Foundation 2014, 8). It also ranks fifth in global beef production and seventh in domestic consumption (Shariff 2015). This clearly clashes with the popular perception of India as a cow-protecting country and of Indians as a vegetarian people. According to Balmurli Natrajan and Suraj Jacob (2018, 55), close to 80% of Indians eat meat and fish. But since, as food historian Pushpesh Pant observes, "India is full of closet meat-eaters because we are a nation of hypocrites," the number of vegetarians may be even lower (Jishnu 2014, 37).

There are several reasons for meat consumption in India. For one thing, although 80% of the population is Hindu, the other 20% comprises primarily Muslims, Christians, and Sikhs, faiths that do not require abstention from meat. Even within Hinduism, Brahmins, particularly in the eastern fish-eating states, are often not vegetarian. In the lactose-intolerant northeastern part of the country, the protein deficit caused by a dairy-free diet is commonly counterbalanced by the consumption of meat. In addition, despite the social stigma attached to it, low-caste Hindus have traditionally eaten meat, forced both by poverty and, historically, by the task of disposing of dead cattle assigned to them by upper castes. In fact, in 1958 the Supreme Court of India openly recognized that beef and carabeef are consumed by the most destitute segment of the population (Rajagopal 2015). In 1993, a study conducted by the Anthropological Survey of India revealed that 88% of the surveyed communities ate meat, from rats to jackals, but also that 5% had become vegetarian to avoid discrimination (Jishnu 2014). More recently, a 2006 survey found that only 43% of Hindus who define themselves as observant are actually vegetarians. The religious foundation of vegetarianism seems to be crumbling under the weight of a growing desire to enjoy meat, particularly among upwardly mobile, cosmopolitan, emancipated urban people (Yadav and Kumar 2006). To meet the growing demand for meat, foreign fast-food chains like Burger King are quickly pushing their way into the market, as in other emerging countries with a booming middle class (Heinrich Boll Foundation 2014, 16). As long ago as the 1990s, researchers were finding that most of India's meat eaters were middle-class Hindus, "without any apparent sense of contradiction of the Hindu faith" (Robbins 1999, 414).

Perspectives on Street Cattle

How is it possible, skeptical readers may ask, that cows are suffering hell on earth in India, of all places? In the opinion of a veterinarian I met at a shelter for street animals in Rajokri (New Delhi), this is due to a profound change "in the mindset, the logic, the culture, the system." "Somewhere," he claimed, "things have gone wrong, and it is especially in the 'holy cows,' or whatever you call them, that you see the egoistic attitude that is emerging now." Arvind, an elderly inhabitant of the Okhla slum, had a different view. "Listen," he said to me sharply, "things are like this. It's good and bad, right and wrong. . . . Animals should stay on the street because this is India, not America. It's the country of cattle and buffaloes. It's the country where the most milk and ghee is produced. And in the Hindu religion, we feed street animals." Arvind's neighbor Rishi, a pragmatic buffalo farmer, puts the blame for the poor treatment of cows squarely on Delhi's overcrowding. In his opinion, it is good for cattle to be released into the streets, where at least they can move around a little bit; it would be worse, Rishi said, if they had to spend their whole life in tiny, dirty sheds, where they are at risk of skin infections and their legs are ruined by prolonged inactivity. Ratan, a former buffalo farmer in the Sarai Kale Khan slum, strongly disagreed. He described street cattle as *avara* (homeless, abandoned, separated from their family). "A cow becomes *avara* when you haven't taken proper care of her, when you haven't treated her as if she was your child, when you haven't taken any interest in her," he claimed. I heard this comparison of free-roaming cattle with children, especially daughters, frequently. My next-door neighbor in Lajpat Nagar believed that "it's not nice to see a cow or a girl going around alone, abandoned, without anybody taking care of them."

Like this woman, many people do not like seeing cattle on the streets, but for very different reasons. In 2002, the Delhi chapter of Common Cause submitted a petition to the High Court on the "menace" of free-roaming cattle: they caused car and motorcycle accidents, clogged traffic, contaminated the environment with their dung, and attacked people (Baviskar 2011a, 398–99). Although it is rare, cattle do charge and gore passersby, sometimes fatally (Aradhak 2012; Ghosal and Aradhak 2013). While animal welfare activists blame increasing traffic, noise, and urbanization, which can bewilder cattle and make them aggressive, I believe that rabies may play a role in some of this abnormal behavior. In fact, in July 2015 in Goa, a cow who had attacked several people was eventually captured and diagnosed with rabies, possibly transmitted by the bite of a street dog (*Times of India* 2015). But human-cattle cohabitation in Indian towns and cities is usually peaceful, or at least less violent than human relations with dogs and macaques. In fact, the university students I interviewed had witnessed fewer cases of human violence toward cows (33% of them had seen it) than toward macaques (50%) or dogs (80%).

Common Cause's petition to the High Court aimed to make Delhi "a cattle-free zone." The High Court responded by directing Delhi authorities to intervene more seriously than ever before. The authorities thus implemented a program of catching both cattle roaming loose in public areas and tethered animals as well, per the Delhi Municipal Corporation Act of 1954, which forbade tethering cattle on public streets. They also began confiscating animals on private property without proper authorization (by law, farmers who keep more than five cattle for profit must obtain permission from the municipality). Since 2002, when these measures went into effect, the owners of most of the 60,000 animals kept in Delhi have risked having their cattle confiscated, being fined, or being arrested and jailed for three months.

The measures were designed primarily to target the roughly 2,400 illegal dairies in Delhi (*Hindu* 2011), and a dozen teams of cattle catchers joined the North, South, and East MCD veterinary services in scouring the streets of the city looking for violations. Traveling in trucks and equipped only with ropes, cattle catchers feign indifference, hiding the ropes behind their backs or beneath their coats until they are within roping range. Cattle are extremely alert and tend to run at the first sign of danger; they are also surprisingly receptive to their owners' commands to evade the would-be wranglers and escape. Predictably, struggles arise when the cattle catchers go after owned animals; the owners resort to using *lathis* (bamboo sticks) and pelting the authorities with stones and bricks. Given that nearly 90% of captured cattle are productive, according to a municipal veterinarian, conflicts of this kind occur on an almost daily basis. In his view, the farmers clearly do not care about the cows' welfare so much as the threat to their source of income. Anil, the overseer of a team of cattle catchers in the affluent residential area of Civil Lines in Central Delhi, cites "the holy reason" for the farmers' resistance as well, though he confesses some perplexity as to people's motives, in that "crowds have so many minds, so many thoughts" when it comes to cows and, he concludes, the "emotional level is high in India."

After witnessing an attempt to catch free-roaming cattle in the Ridge behind the Jhandewalan Hanuman Mandir, I have to agree with Anil on the disorienting multiplicity of perspectives on cattle. When the team left the Ridge empty-handed, I asked one of the cattle catchers why so many cattle were drawn to that seemingly inhospitable place, where there was little fresh vegetation, no artificial sources of water, and a scarcity of the garbage available elsewhere in great quantities. He told me that if I visited during rush hour for temple-goers, I would have my answer: at the temple just across the road, he said, every morning and evening people bring food specifically for this herd. He himself was one of these devotees, he admitted. When I expressed astonishment at his double identity as both a feeder and a catcher of cattle, he smiled proudly and said, "This is just a job, a duty. Dharma is different. That is my life."

According to official data from the MCD, between 2002 and April 2012 (when the MCD was divided into the North, South, and East MCDs), its Veterinary Services Department captured 143,243 bovines. Captures were most zealously pursued at the beginning of the project and again just before the 2010 Commonwealth Games. Some of the seized cattle were moved to Ghogha, a planned dairy colony on the outskirts of Delhi established by the MCD by order of the High Court of Delhi. Cattle owners who agreed to move their animals there were allotted plots free of charge. Because of poor management (Jain 2014) and inadequate facilities (lack of water and of systematic means of transportation to distribute milk in the city), however, most farmers refused to relocate, and those who did soon moved back to Delhi with their animals (Garg 2012a).

Cattle Homes

In addition to Ghogha, auctions where commercially valuable cattle are sold off, the return of seized animals to their owners after microchipping, the payment of fines, and promises not to backslide, Delhi's main policy for the management of captured animals is to send them to *goshalas* and *gosadans*. *Goshalas* (run by private individuals) and *gosadans* (run at a state level and inspired by the guiding principles of the Central Council for the Improvement of Cattle, established in 1952) are vast shelters for cattle—but not buffaloes—that combine Hindu devotion for the cow with the needs of India's agricultural economy, giving protection (*rakhsha*) and service (*seva*) to these animals. The Rajasthan Gaushala Act of 1960 defines a *goshala* as "a charitable institution established for the purpose of reception, protection and treatment of infirm, aged or diseased cattle." In addition to free-roaming cattle, these shelters also accept cattle brought in by farmers who can no longer afford to keep them and animals rescued by NGOs in transit to slaughterhouses.

The origins of these institutions are of ancient pedigree. The *Report of the National Commission on Cattle*, drafted in 2002, the Department of Animal Husbandry and Dairying describes the *goshala* movement as synonymous with the protection of cows and cattle wealth of our country. Being practiced for the last five thousand years or so, its origin can be traced in the Vedic period when social customs and rules laid great emphasis on protection, preservation and development of cows for home, and oxen for agriculture-fields. According to Vedic concepts, cows were considered sacrosanct and constituted material and spiritual assets of the people of the country. ... Thus the entire culture of ancient India was "Go-Sanskriti" or Culture based on cow. ... After Independence, with the impact of the western world and growth of cities and towns, the entire socio-cultural and socio-economic patterns of life got revolutionized solely on the basis of materialistic considerations. ... This led to a situation when the only purpose of cow was milk. ... Now, the cow progeny was burden on the farmer. (Ministry of Agriculture 2002, chap. 6, arts. 1 and 2)

Consequently, in 1994, the Delhi government announced its plan to establish ten *gosadans*, with the aim of ensuring "the wellbeing of cows and [their] progeny," providing "shelter, maintenance and feeding for stray and ownerless animals," offering "health care and treatment of injured and sick animals," and "control[ling] and contain[ing] the problem of stray cattle on the roads and streets in the City." Only seven of these *gosadans* were actually set up, their financial management included in the Five-Year Plans around which the Indian economy is organized. In 2001, the Delhi government spent 4,416 rupees (US$64) on each animal hosted in the shelters, more than it allocated per child enrolled in a government primary school (Singhal n.d., 105). By 2019, the annual government stipend for each sheltered cow had grown to 14,400 rupees (US$205) (Withnall 2019). Today, the AWBI uses about 80% of its government funding to support *gosadans* around the country (Thakur and Nandi 2016). In 2018, shortly after starting an ambulance service for cows, the government of Uttar Pradesh introduced a 0.5% excise tax on certain goods to support cow welfare in *gosadans* and asked its magistrates to seek funding from private companies, as part of their corporate social responsibility, for temporary cow shelters.

Despite these financial measures—whether actually implemented or merely advertised—animal welfare activists have been very critical of most *gosadans* (FIAPO 2018b). Bad management and funding delays (*Hindu* 2012), combined with the increasing need for space to relocate the cattle seized in the city, have turned some of these shelters into compounds where animals are simply left to starve or die from disease (Joshi and Pillai 2016). From April to June 2017, for example, no cattle were admitted to the *goshalas* of Delhi owing to lack of facilities and overcrowding (Pillai 2017). This was true even of the three *goshalas* (the Shri Krishna Gaushala, the Acharya Sushil and Manav Gosadan, and the Dabar Hare Krishna Gaushala) operated, respectively, by Delhi's North, South, and East MCDs. In January 2019, in an effort to rethink and reorganize the overall management of *goshalas*, Delhi's animal husbandry minister, Gopal Rai, announced a plan to modernize a cattle shelter in South West Delhi by combining it with an old-age home (*Economic Times* 2019a). No further details about this pilot project have been released.

But the problem of cattle starving to death in *goshalas* is not limited to Delhi. In early 2016, hundreds of cows died of hunger and neglect at the Hingonia Gaushala, run by the Jaipur Municipal Corporation (*Deccan Chronicle* 2016), to give just one example. By 2018 there were an estimated 5,000 cattle shelters throughout India (FIAPO 2018b, 9), and their number is expected to increase to provide room for the animals saved by anti-slaughter laws—or at least politicians promise as much. But many of these *goshalas* are plagued by lack of funding and mismanagement. In Uttar Pradesh, for example, as of January 2019, only one out of a proposed 104 cow shelters was functional (Sharma 2019).

New Developments for the Human-Cattle Relationship

The logic and operation of *goshalas* provide important insights into how free-roaming cattle and their role in the spread of rabies, among other issues, are managed in India. Although they began in part because of the religious importance of cows in Hinduism, most *goshalas* have always operated at a deficit (Lodrick 1980, 199). In theory, they are supposed to provide cattle with food, water, shelter, and medical care until their natural death. Consequently, cattle in *goshalas* are not meant to be used for material gain of any kind—not for milk, dung, urine, meat, skin, bones, or their physical power as draft animals. Since maintaining such *goshalas* is expensive, the animals are generally not free to mate, in order to avoid overcrowding and additional costs. However, many *goshalas* have recently begun to make use of the urine and dung produced by the sheltered animals, in an attempt to offset expenses. These by-products are sold to local farmers for agricultural purposes or are used in the production of vermicompost, bio-fertilizers, biopesticides, biogas, building materials, and paper. Initiatives of this kind are particularly encouraged at an institutional level, since they can yield badly needed financial support without exploiting cows for their milk. This last point is a crucial one, both for the management of *goshalas* and for India's overall relationship with its cattle, both inside and beyond the walls of these cow shelters.

In 1946, the Animal Husbandry Wing of the Indian Council of Agricultural Research envisioned *goshalas* as "the fountain-heads of milk" in India (Ministry of Agriculture 2002, chap. 6, art. 3). Five years later, in 1951, the country's first Five-Year Plan recommended that *goshalas* be used to supply "plenty of unadulterated milk & milk products to the people" (chap. 6, art. 7). In a comparison with the "*gosadan* concepts" of the Datar Singh Committee (1947), the *Report of the National Commission on Cattle* (2002) shows that *gosadans* were initially considered a total loss; the National Commission on Cattle thus recommended in 2002 that cows in *gosadans* be used to produce milk, and thus income (chap. 6, art. 49). In presenting "cow sanctuaries" as urban alternatives to rural *goshalas*, the 2002 report proposed to convert some of them into "cattle colonies" where milk production would be the primary aim (chap. 6, art. 51).

Yet in light of the appalling conditions in which most dairy cows are kept in India, animal welfare activists have subjected *goshala* dairies to harsh criticism for their blatant hypocrisy in proclaiming themselves safe havens for dairy cows while in fact exploiting cows unscrupulously, all the while subjecting them to abhorrent conditions (Sharma et al. 2019). In 2018, the Federation of Indian Animal Protection Organizations found that 86% of the *goshalas* it surveyed practiced cattle breeding, and in 74% milk was the primary source of income (FIAPO 2018b, 25). The *Standard Operation Procedure* manual drafted in 2013 by the director of the Kamdhenu Dham Nagar Nigam Gaushala in Carterpuri, which—he claimed—was intended as the management guide for *goshalas* nationwide, clearly addresses the issue of milk production. "The Gaushala should be their 'home,'" it says on page 1, "where they are treated with love, respect and compassion. It should be kept in mind that a Gaushala is NOT a Dairy!" (Chohan 2013, 1).

Milk plays a key role in the public relations strategies of *goshalas*. On the wall of a cattle home in Delhi, I read the slogan "By protecting a dry cow double benefits can be obtained" (that is, the benefit to the cow and

the karmic benefit to its protectors). Such rhetoric is undoubtedly beneficial in fundraising appeals, as it plays on the Hindu devotion to the cow,
who will reward those who protect her by, for example, donating money
to the local *goshalas* or *gosadans*. Donations, in fact, are the main source
of income in five of the six *gosadans* surveyed in Delhi in 1999 (GNCTD
2001, 10), and these shelters also sell *gau gullaks* (cow-shaped moneyboxes)
to their visitors, an additional revenue stream. Nevertheless, a conversation with the manager of another famous *goshala* in Delhi persuaded me
that milk-producing cows are actually much better than dry cows at gen-
erating donations. In fact, although his *goshala* does not sell much milk to
the public, its staff members distribute the milk produced by its cows when
they go door to door to collect food for the sheltered cattle. In this way, he
told me, the *goshala* "keeps the donors connected" and "creates an emotional attachment" with its cows. When I asked the manager whether this
attachment might have anything to do with the selling price of their milk,
he replied that their milk was not economically convenient. People buy it,
he specified, "for its meaning, because it comes from their cows. . . . from
a *goseva* [service to the cow]."

Another factor has recently begun to strengthen the bond between
milk lovers and cattle: the revived popularity of indigenous cattle breeds.
Largely owing to the success of Operation Flood, foreign breeds were preferred for decades because of their greater productivity, but both producers
and consumers of milk have lately begun to look at local breeds through
new eyes. For most of India's dairy farmers, foreign breeds are prohibitively
expensive to maintain. They are also vulnerable to diseases to which indigenous cattle are largely immune, they suffer from the heat and drought
that characterize India's weather, and they need constant supervision and
large quantities of high-quality food, unlike native cattle who can subsist
on crop by-products and kitchen scraps.

Another reason for the recent surge in popularity of native cattle has
to do with the increasing success of right-wing political parties that appeal
to people's national pride, as demonstrated by the momentous triumph of
Narendra Modi and his Bharatiya Janata Party over the Indian National
Congress in 2014 and 2019. These conservative parties are making substantial use of the zebu—the *deshi* cow (local cow, sometimes also called
the "humped Vedic cow" to stress her ancient and glorious origin)—as a
symbol, even invoking the names of rare indigenous breeds in their political discourse (Rao 2011, 84). This political agenda includes declaring the

cow to be "Rashtramata" (mother of the nation) (*Outlook* 2015a) or, alternatively, India's new national animal (displacing the Bengal tiger), in order to protect her from slaughter more effectively (Saini 2017).

While many *goshalas* proceed as usual, untouched by political discourse, others are more aligned with this ideology and incorporate it into their policies. It must be said, however, that in spite of the recent jump in popularity, the protection and safeguarding of native Indian cattle breeds is not exactly new. As far back as India's independence from the British in 1947, the first aim of *goshalas* was "to preserve the Indian cow and progeny and to breed and upgrade them" (Ministry of Agriculture 2002). The White Revolution of the 1970s–90s marked a detour in this process, which is now back on track, as it were, and enjoying a new lease on life. In fact, thanks to the encouragement of both politicians and cattle experts (Joshi 2000, 39), many *goshalas* are now retooling their breeding programs in an effort to protect and relaunch local breeds and to demonstrate the superiority of the milk, urine, and dung of Indian cows. One of the leaders in this rediscovered tradition is the Go-Vigyan Anusandhan Kendra (Cow Science Research Center), a registered research and development institute in Nagpur that works in the fields of health, agriculture, and cattle protection—for example, on the development of medicines from cattle products. In praise of Indian cattle, its website explains that "one liter of good medicinal valued creamy milk of indigenous cow is better than 10 liters of white watery milk of exotic cow."

Indian cows are also thought to produce excellent dung and urine. Dung, described as a "gold mine" (Dhama et al. 2005, 2), is said to absorb radioactive waves and purify air, while urine, which contains the sacred water of the Ganges, is seen as a panacea able "to cure even incurable diseases" such as cancer and AIDS (Pathak and Kumar 2003, 57). When I eventually agreed to have a sip of distilled cow urine, I had just concluded a two-hour discussion on its utility in curing diabetes with a man who has been consuming a few glasses of it daily for several years and is fond of calling cows "mobile clinics." Together with milk, curd, and ghee, dung and urine are fundamental ingredients in *panchgavya* (the five by-products of the cow), a concoction prepared by mixing and fermenting these products for use in household rites, agriculture, and cowpathy (a form of therapy, partly included in Ayurveda [a system of medicine with historical roots in the Indian subcontinent], based on the substances obtained from cattle). According to the Holy Cow Foundation, what makes Indian zebus and their products unique is the animal's hump. As one of its leaflets explains, the hump contains the *surya ketu nadi*, a vein connected to the sun that channels the positive cosmic energies radiated by the stars into cow's milk and other bodily fluids, giving them miraculous healing powers. As Jay Mazoomdaar (2013) puts it, "Milk in India is not just a drink, it is an elixir."

Converging Problems, Diverging Answers

The website of the Shri Krishna Gaushala maintains that "there is no other option to cow milk. It is a divine drink. . . . [H]aving cow milk in itself is a service of Gomata [mother cow]. It is so because using its milk encourages cow rearing and it also protects the cow indirectly. Everyone can contribute to the protection of the cow by doing at least this." The message is clear: if not for their milk production, cattle would be endangered. This point is crucial in the debates over how to manage street cattle, for it lies at the intersection of the priorities of the dairy, meat, and leather industries, the farmers, *goshala* managers, cow devotees, milk consumers, politicians, cattle specialists, wildlife advocates, and animal welfare activists.

Animal activism in India—as elsewhere—is not a uniform movement. But animal welfare activists of all stripes tend to have more in common with one another than they do with those who advocate cow protection, which is a very different thing. Cow protection is a quite nebulous concept, in fact, that is inseparable from the cow's prominent place in the Hindu religion and culture. Animal welfare activists, by contrast, see the problem of free-roaming cattle (and free-roaming animals in general) as primarily an ethical issue of cruelty to and disrespect for animals. Thus the approaches of these two camps diverge sharply.

Cow protectors are shocked that people eat beef, and they advocate drinking milk for the practical, symbolic, and emotional satisfaction it provides, whereas animal welfare activists blame vegetarianism for increasing the consumption of dairy products and propose veganism as the only solution to cattle-related problems. Animal welfare activists also hold that vegetarianism in India is motivated more by people's concern about their karma (and in some cases about their cultural identity or caste position) than by an interest in animal welfare (Srinivasan and Rao 2015, 14), and they strongly oppose the so-called *ahimsa* milk as an alternative to the cruelty of the dairy system. In 2016, for example, FIAPO launched the national campaign "Don't Get Milked" "to bust the myths around the Indian dairy industry," like the idea of happy cows giving their surplus milk to humans. In addition to ideological factors, the tension between cow protectionists and animal welfare activists is exacerbated by the fact that many Indian AWOs were founded and are run by foreigners. Cow protectors condemn what they see as outside meddling by neocolonial elites (Dave 2014, 453).

It is worth repeating that the meat and leather industries are by-products of the Indian dairy sector, which in turn is economically sustainable only because it profits from those businesses, as when dairy farmers sell their unproductive cattle to slaughterhouses and tanneries. India's leading animal welfare activists, with their advocacy of a vegan diet and lifestyle, come up against three major obstacles. The first is that India is both young (31% of the population is under age fifteen—Government of India 2011) and malnourished (with only 6% of children under the age of two getting a "minimum acceptable diet"—Ministry of Health and Family Welfare et al. 2019, 61); thus a well-balanced diet is key to the health of Indian children.

The second barrier to veganism is, of course, custom and tradition. Over the past twenty-five centuries, milk has gradually become not only India's leading agricultural commodity (and thus a living for some ninety million dairy farmers) but also an essential ingredient in household kitchens and temple rituals. Interestingly, a 2006 survey on food habits did not even mention veganism, as if it were impossible for Indians to imagine a life free of dairy products (Yadav and Kumar 2006).

The third obstacle that animal welfare activists face is that the cow protection movement revolves around the issue of cattle slaughter, which it opposes, again, for religious and political reasons. At least since the 1890s, the rationale for protecting cows has rested on the supposedly universal Hindu appreciation of the cow, the desire to rescue an allegedly pristine and untainted Hinduism in which cows are not violated, and the preservation of traditional Indian/Hindu values (such as abstention from eating beef) that are under threat from foreign influence. Since the late colonial period, the cow has symbolized a beautiful, strong, prosperous, motherly nation called "Bharat Mata," Mother India (Gupta 2001). Given this historical context, when right-wing parties recently began advocating a total ban on cattle slaughter, their concern was the increasing beef consumption, or what prime minister Narendra Modi calls "the Pink Revolution" (from the color of flesh) (Khandelwal 2014). The current focus on milk is presented as a strategic countermove designed to shift people's economic and dietary interest in cattle away from meat and toward milk instead. Initiatives like the Rashtriya Gokul Mission, which bestows the Kamadhenu Award on breeders of indigenous cattle (Sood 2014b), and the government's challenge to the dairy cooperative Milkfed to launch a premium brand of indigenous cow's milk (*Hindu* 2015), reflect this emphasis on milk rather than beef (*Indian Express* 2017).

While the debate over the bodies of cows continues, cows continue to die in the streets of India with their bellies full of plastic, their limbs broken by speeding cars, and their brains infected by rabies. Institutionally, very little attention is paid to their health and well-being. In April 2019, the government undertook a bureaucratic reorganization allegedly designed to improve and facilitate the regulation of cow shelters and the enforcement of animal cruelty laws. It transferred responsibility for these tasks from the Ministry of Environment, Forest, and Climate Change to the Ministry of Agriculture and Farmers' Welfare—rather than to the Ministry of Animal Husbandry, Dairying, and Fisheries, which would have been more appropriate. Though the government claimed that this would make the administrative process faster and more direct, animal welfare activists charge that in fact it was designed to allow the regulatory body—the Ministry of Agriculture and Farmers' Welfare—to regulate itself (Mohan 2019).

This move poses a further obstacle not only to safeguarding cattle health in general but also to the control of rabies. Being a zoonotic disease, rabies is stuck between the human health sector and the veterinary sector. The odds of its being eliminated depend largely on the collaboration between these branches of government and on the dialogue between the ministries in charge of rabies in India and the international bodies (WHO for the human side of the disease and OIE for the animal side) that are there to provide technical guidance and assistance. With dogs already receiving little or no attention from the Indian veterinary sector, the relocation of cow welfare to the Ministry of Agriculture and Farmers' Welfare is worrisome. Macaques, for their part, being wildlife, are managed by the Ministry of Environment, Forest, and Climate Change.

To make matters even more complicated, the problem of cattle in urban India is also linked to the poor state of cattle management in the countryside. Owing to the decrease in common grazing land (redistributed by the government or usurped by powerful farmers with political connections) (Joshi 2000, 30), landless farmers now must buy the fodder their animals need. Because of climate change, desertification, reduced soil fertility, and growing specialization in cash crops that receive government subsidies, fodder is increasingly expensive and difficult to come by. Before the White Revolution, India went through a Green Revolution in the early 1960s, though the name is a misnomer by today's standards, as it basically industrialized Indian agriculture by adopting modern methods and technologies such as chemical fertilizers and pesticides, high-yield seed varieties, tractors, and irrigation, which dramatically increased the country's agricultural productivity. The draft power of cattle was not completely abandoned, but new machinery started to replace oxen. Now that no more than 30% of Indian farmers can afford tractors, the government still subsidizes them, ignoring the draft power of oxen and consolidating the idea that cattle are worth rearing primarily for their milk (Joshi 2000, 30), a change that Operation Flood made a reality. When livestock animals become unproductive or too expensive to rear, rural farmers are left with no choice but to sell them for next to nothing or set them free in the streets.

Rural Indian farmers suffer from enormous pressures in trying to make a living, a fact reflected in the annual reports of the National Crime Records Bureau, which show that every day from 1995 to 2014, approximately forty farmers committed suicide, mainly for reasons linked to their occupation. In 2017, 150 farmers from Tamil Nadu, wearing human skulls hung around their necks, protested in Delhi for six weeks against the apathy of the government. Poor cattle management subjects dairy farmers to another lethal risk. As the costs of fodder and other necessities rise, forcing farmers to increase the price of milk, it becomes prohibitively expensive for consumers, and families buy less of it. In an effort to make it stretch as far as possible, poor families stop boiling it, as this reduces its quantity (Kaur 2010, 23–24)—but also increases the risk of getting rabies. About 69% of the milk produced in urban backyard dairies is sold—raw—directly to customers, and 56% of these dairies milk their animals even when they are sick (FIAPO 2018a, 10). Alarmingly, a survey of Punjab farmers revealed that only 17% of them know that cows can get and transmit rabies; in the case of buffaloes, only 18% of the farmers surveyed are aware of this (Singh et al. 2019, 18).

Moreover, owing to environmental degradation, human population explosion, and the rising demand for cultivable land, competition between people and cattle over food and space is increasing in the Indian countryside on a daily basis. To alleviate pressure on resources, livestock experts (Verghese Kurien included) and wildlife experts have advocated long-term, economically sustainable, research-based national policies that address agriculture and animal rearing in an inclusive and integrated way (*Down to Earth* 2000a). Some have also suggested the extreme solution of cattle culling to reduce the number of unproductive animals, but because of the religious context and the level of emotion surrounding the idea, this suggestion has gone nowhere (Joshi 2000, 33). As in the case of street dogs and macaques, bitter division over the significance of the cow is one of the main obstacles to a reasoned discussion, let alone rational solutions (Ranade 2015). Once again, the rabies virus is left undisturbed.

CHAPTER 6

LIVING WITH RABIES

At the beginning of this research, when I began to think about how to tackle the subject of rabies with the people I would meet in India, I had no idea that one of the trickiest challenges would be knowing how to refer to this disease, what to call it. Given the long-term prevalence of rabies in India and the heavy burden that this pathology imposes on the country, I expected to find a specific word for rabies in Hindi and the other languages of India. I soon discovered that there was no precise term for the disease. Instead, people generally resorted to expressions like "the disease you catch when a rabid dog bites you."

Puzzled, I decided to investigate the issue more systematically. The vast majority of the university students whom I questioned in Delhi knew that rabies was a disease, but only one-sixth used the equivalent term for "rabies" in Hindi or their native language. Of this one-sixth, three used the English word "rabies" and five *rebij*, which corresponds to the phonetic adaptation of "rabies" in Hindi. *Rebij*, written in Devanagari script, is also the term I almost always encountered in the awareness material in Hindi and Rajasthani prepared by local NGOs and municipal corporations. But eleven students wrote *jalatak* or *jalantak*, Hindi words that link rabies to its most famous and distressing symptom, the fear of water (*jal*). The Sanskrit term *antaka* can be translated as "lethal," "mortal," or "destructive," and it is associated with Yama, the Hindu god of death (Sani 2009). Four of the students used the word(s) for rabies in their local language—namely, the Kashmiri term *halqai/halgai*, the Gujarati *hadkwa/hadkai*, and the Marwari *hirkia/hidkia*. In Jaipur (and also in Jodhpur and its rural surroundings), rabies is widely known as *hirkia*, including among the children I met.

In addition to these direct translations, a handful of students proposed *pagal kutta* and *rakta bij* as loose, nonliteral translations. *Pagal kutta* literally means "mad dog," thus referring not to the disease per se but to the animal most frequently responsible for its transmission in India. Rabies is also spoken of in relation to mad dogs in Andhra Pradesh (in Telugu, *pitchi kukka*), in Maharashtra (in Marathi, *kutra pisalto*), and in Karnataka (in Kannada, *hucchhu nayi*). Some students did not refer to dogs as vectors of rabies but mentioned the pathogen that causes this disease: *rakta bij*. In Hindi, *rakta* means blood, while *bij* can be translated as germ or seed. During my conversations with street and slum children in Delhi, I heard *hirkia* mentioned only once; mad dogs (*pagal kuttas*) and the disease they cause when they bite were the language we used in our talks.

Thus I decided to investigate the literature on rabies in the Indian linguistic milieu. The *Sushruta Samhita*—the first account in the history of human medicine to treat rabies—refers to this disease as *jalatrasa*, from *jala* (water) and *trasa* (fear), emphasizing the anguish that water causes in patients (Bhishagratna 1991, 734). In northern India, several local languages follow this Sanskrit word. In Hindi, we find *jalasantra* (from *asantra*, fear), *jalabhi/jalabhiti* (from *abhi/abhiti*, fear), and *jalantaka* (from *antaka*, mortal/destructive). The Bengali version of *jalantaka* is *jalatanka*, while the Assamese is *jalatonka*. It is interesting to note that in the *Sushruta Samhita*, *atanka* means disease, fever, pain, mental distress, anxiety, and fear, and it is also used to refer to the roll of drums. Although not common, there is also the Hindi term *alark*, which is translated as "a fabulous animal" and, more specifically, "a mad dog." In Sanskrit, *ala* means not only "poison" and the "discharge of poisonous matter from venomous animals" but also "source of pain" (Turner 1999). In the *Mahabharata* (12.3.13), Alarka is a worm with eight feet, pointed canine teeth, and stinging hairs. Willem Bollée (2006, 40) uses the term *eranda* to refer to rabies.

Here is what the *Sushruta Samhita* says about rabies:

> The bodily Vayu in conjunction with the (aggravated) Kapha of a
> jackal, dog, wolf, bear, tiger or of any other such ferocious beast

affects the sensory nerves of these animals and overwhelms their instinct and consciousness. The tails, jaw-bones and shoulders of such infuriated animals naturally droop down, attended with a copious flow of saliva from their mouths. The beasts in such a state of frenzy, blinded and deafened by rage, roam about and bite each other. . . . A person bitten by a rabid animal barks and howls like the animal by which he is bitten, imitates it in many other ways and, bereft of the specific functions and faculties of a human subject, ultimately dies. (Bhishagratna 1991, 733–34)

Infection and Affection

The lethality of rabies in both humans and animals was acknowledged by 86% of the university students I interviewed, but the number who had an accurate understanding of how it is transmitted was considerably lower. They generally believed that rabies is transmitted only by the bite of an infected animal, as other studies in India have also shown (Mrudu, Basha, and Thangaraj 2012, 377). While bites are certainly the most common path of transmission, rabies can also be spread by the lick or—if the claws have saliva on them—the scratch of an infected animal. My experience in Indian animal shelters taught me this lesson quite well. One day I was watering the macaques in a large cage in the garden, when I carelessly turned my back to them. A large male reached through the bars of the cage, grabbed my hair, and pulled me back against the cage, where the other excited monkeys began examining my head and playing with my hair. I received several scratches on my scalp in the process, some of them causing my skin to bleed slightly. I had been observing these monkeys for weeks, and I knew all too well how often they put their fingers in their mouths during the uncountable hours they spent picking fleas off one another. These particular macaques, safely confined in an animal hospital, presented no threat, but the risk of being scratched or bitten by a potentially rabid monkey in the outside world is painfully evident. And when that happens, it is anything but easy to catch the macaque for observation, or even to be sure that you have caught the right one, in the unlikely event that you do succeed.

Most of the students I surveyed knew that the rabies virus affects the brain. But they thought that the second-most affected part of the body, after the brain, was the skin, especially in dogs. Interestingly, many of the street and slum children I talked with shared this misconception about rabies. They often identified rabid dogs primarily by the condition of their skin, pointing to their scabs, patchy loss of fur, incessant scratching, and abraded skin. Given the prevalence of sarcoptic mange among Indian street dogs, it is not difficult to understand this confusion between rabies and mange, owing to the appalling appearance of dogs with mange and the restlessness caused by the severe itchiness it inflicts on them. Sarcoptic mange, or canine scabies, is a very contagious infestation caused by burrowing mites that tunnel into the skin, causing intense itching and irritation that make the dog scratch and bite himself frantically, provoking fur loss, skin damage, and infection. Although mange is not a fatal disease, it is no wonder that children and others not familiar with rabies would confuse the symptoms.

The street children told me of many other features of rabid dogs, which allowed me to compile a rather comprehensive and coherent "thick description" (Geertz 1973) of these animals. What made Geertz's ethnographic account of cockfighting in Bali a milestone in anthropology was the rich, dense portrayal he provided, which enabled him to show how its technical, social, and symbolic aspects combined to become meaningful to those involved, especially in relation to their cultural context. The children of Delhi slums likewise provided descriptive narratives of *pagal kuttas*, mad dogs, drawing on their physical features, behavior, health status, history, and relationships with people, and they expounded on the interconnections among these causal elements. They explained to me that a mad dog is generically ugly, and so dirty that "it seems he has just come out a sluice." He has "long and sticky" hair, "no fur on its back," or "hairs that fall here and there." He has red eyes, his tail is always down, his tongue is always protruding, and he drools saliva, which sometimes bubbles on his lips. His ears are torn, his skin is covered with scratches or is dry and full of wounds, often "with worms in the wounds." While miming a wrinkled and decaying face, a child named Sapna added that a mad dog looks so emaciated that his bones are visible beneath his skin, and his face "looks like the face of an old person."

A rabid dog's behavior follows from his appalling physical appearance. He is obsessed with terrible itchiness, which he tries to alleviate by constantly scratching himself with his nails and teeth, leaving trickles of blood on his body. Everything about him is frightful. "He looks at you with rage in his eyes," said a boy named Sahil, making a wary and menacing expression, while Manoj even claimed that "you die if only he stares at you." Sutirtha shared the same opinion, stating that "the eyes of a mad dog are different from those of a normal dog, so I don't even want to see them. If a mad dog looks at me, I close my eyes." A mad dog is extremely restless and hyperactive: he always "barks or bites, but he is never calm." He is unstoppable. He "sees something and runs there to bite it, then he sees another thing and he runs there as well," and he always runs "even faster than other dogs" and "is able to climb trees." Ushma said that she had seen a mad dog jump on the back of a cow to bite it. Most of the children agreed that mad dogs are senseless and unpredictable in their choice of victim: a *pagal kutta* "enters in whatever house" to "bite anybody," and "if you tell him to bite anybody, he goes there and does it."

They were convinced that a mad dog always and without exception bites people: "If you face him, he bites you; if you pass by, he bites you"; he "walks behind people to bite them when they don't see him," because "he is already enraged, but if you go past he gets even angrier, [and] he follows you and bites you." His blind rage makes him so prone to biting that he not only "bites even other dogs" but "bites his own tail." According to a child named Sureshwari, it is this aggressiveness that unambiguously identifies mad dogs; in fact, she said, "They are those who the police bring to prison or into the forest, where they cannot bite anymore." Two children told me sadly that a mad dog will bite "even if you haven't done anything" to annoy him and, worse still, "even if you love him."

Despite sometimes being afraid of these dogs, whom they described as dangerous and strange, many of these children were generally very sympathetic toward them, and allowed themselves to become close to them both physically and emotionally. This led some of the children even to excuse the dogs' biting behavior, putting their aggressiveness down to the harshness of life on the street. They thought that a mad dog "bites at night because he is afraid, he is alone without a family," that he "bites [because] he thinks people are thieves who want to take him away or kill him," since, being homeless, "he always roams the streets alone," and because he suffers from not being taken care of. The dogs' loneliness and abandonment are the reason why these children were usually reluctant to accept the idea that a *pagal kutta* could be *paltu* (domestic, a pet). Mad dogs by definition are *jangli* (wild) or *avara* or *gumta* (ownerless, wandering), to their way of thinking. Fatima was particularly touched by the thought that mother dogs feared having their puppies taken away, claiming that on the way home from the market with a bag full of fruit she had once been bitten by a dog who thought she had stolen her puppies. Another child attributed these dogs' madness to the fact that "children throw stones at them and annoy them all the time."

At a dog shelter in Jodhpur (three hundred kilometers from Jaipur), I encountered an equally interesting and sympathetic explanation of the cause of rabies in dogs. This shelter runs awareness campaigns in primary schools and, for children who do not go to school, in slums as well. During my stay there, the coordinator of these campaigns was taking a survey of the young students designed to gauge their understanding of rabies. She kindly allowed me to help her process the 365 questionnaires she had collected. With reference to rabies in humans, more than three hundred children had no doubt in identifying the cause as the bite of a rabid dog. When it came to the cause of canine rabies, this number fell to slightly more than two hundred. About one hundred children identified the cause of rabies in dogs as poor diet, thinking primarily, I suppose, of street dogs who survive on rotten garbage, animal carcasses, and feces. Another forty pupils blamed extreme heat.

Both of these views have been held for centuries as possible causes of rabies. In fact, among the first cultures to experience rabies, from the Nile to the Indus, both uneducated and learned people thought that dogs become rabid because of the weather or the ingestion of dangerous substances. Later, in the Victorian era of British history, rabies was closely linked to disorder, dirt, and sin, so much so that a dog eating his own or others' feces was regarded with fear and suspicion. David Johnson, an English military surgeon working in Bengal during British colonization, ascribed the widespread incidence of rabies in India to the large number of decaying human corpses on which dogs fed (Ritvo 1987, 174).

The children's empathy for *pagal kuttas*, which helped me frame the context for interspecies camaraderie, presented in the conclusion, is a very rare finding in infectious disease research, where victim blaming is generally the norm. Victim blaming is the easy and reassuring conviction that victims of crimes, physical and psychological abuses, and infectious diseases (HIV/AIDS is a good example) bring their condition on themselves. It is this mindset that in fractured social contexts such as that of Delhi—where physical, symbolic, and psychological walls are built around class and caste divisions—prompts privileged citizens "to blame the poor for their poverty and the powerless for their powerlessness" (Ryan 2010, back cover).

Where Does the Danger Come From?

The concern and compassion I saw in the children were a welcome contrast to the widespread contempt in which adults in India often hold street dogs. At the same time, their misconceptions about rabies, and their tendency to equate street dogs with rabies as a rule, are worrisome. As discussed in chapter 3, it is very difficult to classify dogs in India vis-à-vis ownership, control, and care. It is thus important to be careful when looking at data on dog bites, unless the terms *street dog, stray dog, ownerless dog, free-roaming dog, unsupervised dog,* and *pet dog* are defined precisely. The most extensive research performed to date on rabies in India imputes a higher number of bites to stray dogs than to pet dogs (63% versus 37%), with a slightly larger disparity in rural India (APCRI 2004, 27). The 2017 APCRI survey confirmed these findings (APCRI 2018, 60). Various studies claim that stray dogs in India account for 90% (Chhabra et al. 2004, 218), 65% (Ichhpujani et al. 2008, 30), or 59% (Lal et al. 2005, 52) of bites. I have no doubt that these surveys were undertaken in good faith, and that the people who responded gave honest answers, but it seems undeniable that public perceptions and personal understandings of dog ecology play an important role in how these questions are answered.

Support for this thesis can be drawn from Alan M. Beck's (1991, 185) work on dog bites in the United States, a country where the number of street dogs and dog-mediated rabies cases is nothing compared to the Indian situation. In the United States, the general public perception is that stray dogs are responsible for more cases of rabies transmission than pet dogs are, both because their bites are more commonly reported and because these animals are thought to be less healthy than pets and thus the cause of more disease, particularly rabies. However, data show that unvaccinated pet dogs—often owned by the neighbors of victims or, though less often, by the victims themselves—are mainly responsible for rabies transmission. In fact, Beck observes that in conditions where reporting of all bites is high, stray dogs account for fewer than one in ten bites. Nevertheless, because street dogs are perceived as ownerless and thus as probably unvaccinated, people are more likely to seek medical care and report the bite than when bitten by a dog whose owner is known (Beck and Jones 1985, 319).

A veterinarian who runs a clinic for dogs and rabies control in Delhi tried to analyze for me the comparison between stray and pet dogs in relation to their bites. Based on her experience of pet ownership in Delhi over the past fifteen years, she explained that pet dogs are more prone to bite because they often have a difficult relationship with their owners, who very often have no prior experience of animal ownership, receive no training or education on dog behavior, fail to train their dogs, and may resort to beating or chaining their dogs in an effort to control them. Street dogs, by contrast, are often self-taught: they learn by observing human behavior, and in case of potential conflict with people their preferred tactic is to avoid it by fleeing the scene. Their freedom, the result of human carelessness and irresponsibility, is the key to avoiding negative interspecies encounters.

Obtaining accurate epidemiological data on the source of rabid bites and helping people—especially pet owners—understand that the danger of rabies may be closer than they think is key not only at a public health level but also, especially, at a psychological and relational one. Chapter 3 examined the high symbolic and emotional value that urban Indians attach to their pet dogs, and the scorn with which they tend to regard street dogs. This bias has serious repercussions for dog registration and vaccination, and shapes the overall cultural significance of dog bites and rabies. Grasping this significance—this cultural fear, as Wang (2019) writes in her history of rabies in New York City—is essential to understanding human-animal relations in all sociocultural settings.

For example, rabies has never represented a serious public health threat in France or England, yet it had appalling meaning for bourgeois society in those countries, especially with respect to ideas about taming and control over animal lives (Kean 1998; Kete 1994). As rabies could turn the beloved family pet into a vector of disease, reminding people of the animal nature that domestication was supposed to govern and restrain, rabies "revealed the beastly nature of the domesticated beast" (Kete 1994, 112). Both practically and symbolically, rabies disrupted the notion of cultural, social, and biological order that the urban bourgeoisie thought they had imposed, both inside and outside the home. Rabies and the fear of it epitomized their unease about "the uncertain conquest of culture over nature" (Kete 1994, 98). Whoever was seen as undermining the orderliness, cleanliness, and discipline that culture was designed to impose on wild nature was feared, abhorred, and blamed for moral contagion. "Stray or rabid dogs, like their human counterparts"—whether the "lazy" poor in nineteenth-century London or the slum dwellers of twenty-first-century Delhi—"epitomized this threatening presence which cried out for regulation—or destruction" (Kean 1998, 91).

A Matter of Vulnerability

My conversation with the experienced veterinarian in Delhi led to another tricky aspect of rabies and rabies research: the human provocation of dog bites. Let me hasten to clarify that I am not blaming Indians for being bitten by a dog every two seconds. My intention here is solely to stress the importance of understanding the relational dynamics of rabies transmission—not only because they are key to the clinical risk assessment of rabies and to a more targeted pre-exposure vaccination strategy, but also because increased knowledge of dog behavior is one of the tools available for reducing dog bites and improving rabies control. WHO suggests that when ascertaining the risk factor of a bite, it is essential to take into account not only the animal's clinical history (e.g., whether it has been vaccinated) but also his behavior when the bite occurred. Of course, the fact that the lyssavirus attacks the brain, causing unsettling behavioral changes, complicates this matter enormously, but it is nevertheless important to try to distinguish a provoked and thus common and predictable biting reaction from an unprovoked and thus possibly pathological one. In the bitten person, making this distinction requires both previous awareness of animal behavior in general and of the biting animal in particular, and a careful analysis of his own behavior, sensitivity, and attitude toward animals. Since we are all inherently subjective, this is a tall order, and it is made even more difficult by the physical pain and psychological stress that follow an animal bite. That said, in a rabies-endemic country like India, every dog bite should be given due attention.

Unfortunately, the concept of provocation is not as intuitive and easy to determine as it may seem. What humans may consider a well-intentioned gesture, dogs may perceive as a threat. For example, the veterinarian at the Delhi shelter told me that when working with street dogs, she and her colleagues usually assume that a bite has been provoked even when the person has approached the dog with a food offering and even when he has not necessarily touched the dog. "If you don't feed that dog regularly and so he doesn't link you to food," she explained, "your approaching him even in good faith is a provocation to him. He can react well or badly, but the act hasn't started from him, so it's provoked, from an ethological point of view."

As in the case of stray and pet dogs, provoked and unprovoked bites are usually not clearly defined in epidemiological surveys on rabies, at least in India. In most of these surveys, most bites are classified as "spontaneous" (though to varying degrees—see Ichhpujani et al. 2008, 30; Samanta et al. 2016, 58). Coupled with the higher proportion of bites from "stray dogs," I wonder whether a hostile attribution bias is affecting the already poor epidemiological data available on rabies in India and reinforcing the idea that, unlike pet dogs, street dogs are unpredictable, untrustworthy, naturally prone to attack, and likely to transmit rabies.

During my conversations with the children, the issue of bite provocation and, more generally, child-dog interaction modalities emerged as an important topic, particularly in relation to two other epidemiologically significant aspects of rabies: the high incidence of the disease among youths and males. This demographic pattern has emerged from research both globally and in India. My small-scale study provided similar results: among the university students I surveyed, of the 66 (out of 185) who had been bitten by a dog, twice as many were male; I got the same figure from my interviews with the 91 (out of 145) street and slum children who had personally experienced a dog bite. The unequal age and sex distribution among victims of animal bites and rabies is due to several factors. The primary one is that while rabies is endemic in India generally, it is more endemic in some sociocultural clusters than in others, thus exposing the people within them to a much higher risk. Specific pathways of infection, and even more the ways in which they overlap, produce this inequality.

With reference to age, children are generally more attracted to and trusting of animals than adults are; at the same time, they are less familiar with them and less prepared to react appropriately to a given animal behavior. According to a survey of dog bite cases in Delhi, children under age fifteen are most likely to provoke dogs (Khokhar, Meena, and Mehra 2003, 157). With reference to the gravity of the bite, a study carried out in Madras in the 1980s found that the older the bite victim, the less serious the wound (Parthasarathy et al. 1984, 550). In short, younger children are less able to prevent a bite or physically fend off an attack. Children may also be less likely to report a bite, afraid of having to submit to injections and suturing or of punishment by their parents. At a government hospital in Yavatmal, the most common reason for delaying the reporting of a dog bite was a child's reluctance to come forward (Patle and Khakse 2014, 153). When children delay reporting a bite, or fail to report it altogether, the rabies virus has a chance to enter the body undisturbed.

Another reason why rabies is more common in children than in adults is their small stature, which makes them more likely to be bitten on the upper part of the body. Since rabies makes its way from the point of entry to the brain, it has less distance to travel in a child bitten on the upper arm, neck, or face than in an adult bitten on the leg. Moreover, in hot countries like India, the arms, neck, and head are generally not covered by clothing, thus increasing the contact area of the skin susceptible to infected saliva. The cultural variable of clothing cover in relation to bites and rabies was critical in a study of human-macaque interactions in Bali and Gibraltar (Fuentes 2006, 894). In poor areas, where families cannot always afford adequate clothes for all their children, skin exposure increases considerably. This is generally a greater factor for males, in that women and female adolescents in India usually keep their bodies well covered for cultural and religious reasons. In cities like Delhi and Jaipur, men usually wear Western-style trousers, but children, farmers, and elderly men who wear traditional clothes, especially in southern India, tend to have bare legs. A survey in Delhi showed that while most bites were to the legs (55%) or torso (30%), twenty-two of the twenty-nine people who were bitten on the head, face, or neck were children under the age of fourteen (Chhabra et al. 2004, 218).

My ethnographic research suggests that three other factors contribute significantly to the children's vulnerability to bites and rabies, especially street and slum children. First, since they have to fend for themselves (street children) or perform domestic duties (slum children), it is common to see even very young kids carrying food, often poorly packaged and therefore enticingly aromatic, on their way home from markets and roadside eateries. This food is easy prey for hungry dogs, who do not fear children as much as they do adults. A child named Kamla was bitten on the way home from the market after inadvertently dropping some naan (bread) on the ground. When she tried to retrieve it, a dog bit her hand.

Second, because they have poor or nonexistent housing, these children often have no alternative to defecating in the open. The children I met preferred open green areas, railway lines, garbage-dumping areas, and open sewers. Two-thirds of the children I spoke with are afraid—and sometimes forbidden—to go alone to relieve themselves. They (and their parents, if they have them) are concerned about snakes, kidnappers, rapists, bhuts (evil spirits who hide in the dark), moving trains, and hungry dogs who are interested in their feces. They generally take along a stick or some stones with which to try to keep dogs at a safe distance. Railroad tracks are a common hangout for starving dogs who, like the children looking for a place to defecate, daily risk life and limb in the hope of finding food (not only feces but also leftovers tossed by train passengers).

Last but not least, rag picking often occupies a substantial part of children's time, especially street children (in Delhi it is their number-one occupation—IHD 2011, 31). In a typical rag-picking scene along Indian streets, garbage collectors, often barefoot, walk among garbage heaps carrying a plastic sack over their shoulder and stirring rubbish with a long stick. When they find something useful, they pick it up and throw it into the sack; when sorting through the garbage is necessary, they simply squat where they are and begin this painstaking job. They are surrounded in this task by street dogs, cats, pigs, rats, cattle, crows, and egrets who are likewise busy rummaging through the garbage, looking for something to eat. Working in such close proximity to street dogs, who see them as competitors for scarce resources, is clearly risky, yet there are, to date, few studies of this situation (Abedi et al. 2017; Bharti 2015).

The risk of being bitten by dogs who see them as competitors is not the only danger these children face. "The dogs see us carrying a sack and they think we want to put them in it and take them away," a child named Suresh explained to me gravely. That these ragpickers need a stick to prod and stir the rubbish further aggravates the situation, since, as these children know all too well, dogs who have been beaten or threatened with sticks are likely to react negatively to the sight of this object alone. (Watchmen in India are almost always armed with sticks as well.) Makeshift measures such as threatening dogs with sticks to keep them at bay may seem effective in the short term, but they are actually counterproductive in the long term. An experienced veterinarian in Delhi told me that, paradoxically, the lessons children receive from adults about dogs make them *more* likely to be bitten. For example, children are taught to run from street dogs whenever they are approached by them—when in fact dogs are programmed to chase a fleeing person, and they are more likely to bite a child who runs from them than one who calmly stays still. Another risk for ragpickers is that they are usually uneducated on the subject of rabies; a study in Aligarh found that fewer than half of them know how rabies is transmitted (Abedi et al. 2017, 1724).

Let us look now at why males are more likely than females to be bitten by dogs, and thus more likely to contract rabies. In countries like India, men and boys spend more time outdoors than girls and women do. This is the same reason why women are more vulnerable to monkey attacks, as these animals often try to raid kitchens and, triggered by physical proximity and limited escape routes, may resort to biting (Dittus, Gunathilake, and Felder 2019, 101). The children I interviewed provided other hints to understanding this gender gap. In fact, a telling difference emerged in our conversations about how boys and girls approach dogs, especially in moments of play. Most of the boys told me that they liked to play with fully grown dogs, because this allowed a wider range of games. With these dogs they played soccer, boxing, *pakram pakrai* (running around and catching others), hide-and-seek, cricket, and "horseback" riding. The cover photo of Lori McFadyen's book about India's street children, *Voices from the Street*, depicts a fierce young boy riding a dog with his full weight, his feet pressed against the dog's flanks in lieu of stirrups, the dog's ears serving as reins. Other interspecies games include throwing stones at dogs, teaching them how to shake hands/paws, making them stand on their hind legs and dance, making them jump into the air for a biscuit, making them fight one another, and challenging them by pinching them until they react.

Girls generally take a diametrically different approach. They prefer puppies, who are small, soft, and chubby and like to be cuddled, dandled, and petted. Almost all the girls I met saw puppies as sweet, cute, and totally innocent. There is no doubt that juvenile and adult dogs cause more severe bites and represent a bigger risk. Puppies grow up fast, and the level of human handling that they accept changes equally quickly. Yet puppies have no inhibitions about nipping and biting and naturally like to explore and play using their mouths. Worryingly, a higher relative incidence of rabies is reported in dogs younger than twelve months in endemic areas, because they are not vaccinated before they are three months old (Abela-Ridder 2015, 149).

I heard plenty of stories from the boys about games with dogs that ended badly. Amir told me about an incident in which he and his friends were annoying a dog; when he eventually reacted, they all ran away. But Amir was the last to run and the dog managed to catch up with him and bite him. Kushroo admitted that while playing with his friends he had inadvertently stepped over a dog's leg and was bitten, while Kallu purposely pulled the tail of the dog he was playing with. Scornful of danger, Alam tried repeatedly to make the dog lose his temper by pretending to be a snarling dog himself. All of these stories ended with a dog bite.

When the Lyssavirus Succeeds

When dogs become infected with rabies, they may bite or snap at any form of stimulus, attacking other animals, humans, and objects such as rocks and sticks or even air. They may constantly lick, bite, and chew the place where they were bitten and hide in dark places because of hypersensitivity to light. Jaw dropping, dyspnea (shortness of breath), ataxia (lack of voluntary muscular coordination), disorientation, choking sounds or motions, and glazed eyes are also reported, particularly in dumb rabies. But even apparently healthy dogs who are behaving normally have been found to be rabid (Abi T. Vanak, personal communication), which makes rabies even more difficult to deal with.

Very little clinical reporting on rabid macaques is available. A rabid macaque imported from India to a British laboratory was observed avoiding food, refusing human contact, and severely biting at his fingers and hands. Before being euthanized, no aggressiveness, hydrophobia, or paralysis was observed (Boulger 1966, 941).

Rabid cattle may tend to isolation and even depression, and even the most docile animals can suddenly attack by tossing, kicking, or head butting. Continuous pawing of the ground, frenzy, mania, anorexia, frequent urination, cramping rectal pain, dysfunctional digestive processes, inability to drink water or to suckle, hypersalivation, and interrupted milk production may also occur. In the late stages of rabies, cows may produce a hoarse bellow, with the tongue hanging out owing to paralysis of the jaw and tongue. In Turkey, actual attempts to bite were observed in a rabid cow under study (Aytekin and Mamak 2009, 2761). Progressive paralysis causes hypersalivation and incoordination in movements that are much the same as those in rabid dogs and humans.

Having described the symptoms of rabies in humans in chapter 1, I would now like to share the perceptions among the children I met in Delhi and Jaipur of the consequences of this disease in people. Most of the children expressed deep concern about the fate of those who have "the disease you catch when a rabid dog bites you," yet their opinions on the actual outcomes of this disease were confused and often contradictory. The wide range of unfortunate consequences they cited included allergy, malaria, dengue, tetanus, typhus, pus-infected buboes at the site of the bite, itching and the longing to scratch the itch, and irritation due to the presence of lice and worms in the wound.

But most of the children agreed that dogs in particular release a poison into the victim through their teeth. They explained that "the teeth of the dog remain inside the body," "the germs [*bij*] that are on them enter it," and "the poison that is in the body of the dog goes into your body." Pradeep was sure that "the poison of the dog spreads inside your body and you become totally blue," while Ravi observed that "the liquid that comes out of the wound is green [*sic*] because it is the combination between your blood, which is red, and the poison of the dog, which is blue." Interestingly, the reference to blue in these last two statements may suggest the influence of these children's Hindu background. One of the most beloved Hindu deities, Shiva, is also known by the epithet Nilakantha ("the blue-throated one") because he heroically keeps in his throat the poison that was meant to destroy humankind. The children I interviewed claimed that the poison in dogs' teeth comes from the dirty food they eat and the fact that "mad dogs eat everything, even chemicals" (a term that in India is generically used to refer to inedible or noxious materials or substances). A child named Savitri told me that the large amount of poison in mad dogs can be seen in the horrific condition of their mangy coats and skin.

The consequences of a dog bite were very clear to the children I talked with during an afternoon of group homework in the Sarai Kale Khan slum. In short, you get fever, sweat more than usual, and have tachycardia. "You turn mad," said one child, and "become like the dog who bit you." "You start going *wo wo wo*," explained Neha, miming a barking dog, adding, "You eventually stop talking as a normal person and your voice becomes as that of dogs. Your tongue comes out of your mouth and your face becomes scary and dangerous." You start eating bones and digging holes, and you roam the streets without knowing where you are going, biting whoever passes by. "You become as black as the dog who bit you because your skin gets the color of his fur," claimed one child, adding that you start losing your hair and your body is gradually covered with wounds and scabs that make you scratch yourself frantically. The more poison the dog has transferred from his body to the victim's, the more "the dog calms down, as his madness decreases while yours increases." When one of the children turned to his grandmother for confirmation, several adults joined our conversation, largely confirming the children's opinions and adding interesting details of their own. Grandmother Vinaya explained that "you become mad, tear your clothes, shout, always laugh [she laughed manically], look around in a menacing way, change your voice.... You aren't a human being anymore, but you turn into a dog and your brain stops working." Saleem, a man in his mid-forties, observed that "you become scared of water, because you feel like drowning whenever you touch it, even if there is just a little. But you are scared anyway and you behave as if you had epilepsy."

In a shelter for runaway street children in South Delhi, Javed remembered vividly a neighbor's agony in his native village in Bihar. One month after a dog bit him, "he became completely mad." In particular, he threw stones at everybody and shouted incomprehensible things; once he even tried to bite his own sister. Javed did not know exactly what had happened to this man, for around that time he escaped from his violent stepmother and traveled with a friend to Delhi, where he was kidnapped by a man who sexually abused him. When I met him, he thought that the neighbor was still living in the mental hospital where, Javed supposed, he must have been moved. In the Shadipur slum where Puja lived with her family as a ragpicker, she told me about the death of her younger sister Pritha just four months earlier. Pritha was bitten on her left arm by a dog while collecting garbage, and after a while she began to experience feelings of suffocation and could not swallow, so she stopped eating and drinking. What still shocked Puja months later was that Pritha knew that she would soon die, and said so. "And also the doctor said the same thing. In fact, after ten days she died," Puja concluded.

Pregnant with Puppies

Most of the children thought that these symptoms of madness are the worst thing rabies victims must bear. But a few told me of the much worse fate that actually befalls those who experience particularly severe dog bites: they become pregnant with the puppies of the dog who bit them. Arun remembered how the stomach of his friend's dad started to grow exactly three days after he was bitten by a dog in his native village in Assam. "The stomach starts to grow, as it happens to a pregnant woman," Arun explained. "And you feel that your body is heavier than usual, because puppies weigh." Siwri shared Arun's view, although she believed that at least three months must pass between the bite and the beginning signs of this unnatural pregnancy.

Several adults joined this conversation on dog bite–induced pregnancy, showing great interest in this topic, and great concern. Sarita, a woman in her forties from Bihar, added important details. "You feel itchy, because they [the puppies] move. And you also feel a lot of pain, because they bite your stomach. Of course you become mad, how cannot you become mad, with this going on in your stomach!" After a physically and psychologically exhausting pregnancy, death is its only possible outcome, according to Sarita. The puppies cannot be delivered; because they are "poisonous" and "toxic," they die in the womb. The expectant person also dies, slowly killed by this toxicity.

Not everyone agreed with Sarita on the fatal outcome for both species involved. Young Jhoti was absolutely sure that "in women they come out as babies do," but in men, "the puppies will die and so [do] the men who have them in their stomach." Amina, a forty-year-old woman who has lived in the Nizamuddin slum half her life, led me to the exact point on the street where, "a long time ago," a woman had given birth to puppies and had eventually died. Amina was not there to witness it, but others had told her that the woman delivered them "as if they were babies." Amina had arrived later, in time to see the woman's dead body on the road, surrounded by her fourteen newborn puppies. Saleeq, another resident of the slum, could not remember this incident, but he claimed he had known a woman who safely delivered her puppies, although she did not keep them. In her case, the delivery took place at Irwin hospital (now the Lok Nayak Jay Prakash Hospital, one of the biggest hospitals in Delhi), he said, and was preceded by an X-ray that clearly revealed the puppies to the medical staff. The puppies were eventually removed through "an operation"—that is, by caesarean section.

In men and boys, this pregnancy is even more unnatural and also much more dangerous to their health. Muhammad explained how puppies eventually exit a male body. He claimed that as a child, he had seen puppies coming out of a man's mouth and nostrils; he whined like a newborn puppy to simulate the sounds he heard them make. He remembered them as being as long and thick as his forefinger, which he said was the maximum size they can be in order to pass through the mouth and nostrils of a human being. If they grew larger than that, they could not be delivered, and would cause excruciating and terrifying pain to the man carrying them. "When they grow up, they have nails in their paws and they start scratching the body from inside," Muhammad claimed, so much so that the expectant man "will have all blood inside and his intestines will be destroyed." Eventually, "he will die. He will die with the puppies in the wound and in his body." Arjun too saw no hope for any man pregnant with puppies; he remembered as a child seeing a dead man with his stomach burst open, two dead puppies lying within it.

The context for this belief about puppy pregnancy is key to understanding it. The people who told me about it are immigrants to Delhi from central-eastern India, in particular Jharkhand and Bihar, two of the most depressed states in India, where socioeconomic indicators such as income, education, social equity, health, and infrastructure are abysmally low (IAMR 2012). A 2014 report by the Parliamentary Standing Committee on Health and Family Welfare found that, on average, India has one doctor for every 1,674 citizens; in this region, the ratio is even higher. To achieve WHO's ideal ratio of 1:1,000, and thus provide health care for all—particularly in the most isolated and deprived areas, where doctors may be more reluctant to work—half a million more doctors, or a 67% increase in the existing number, would be needed. This goal can be achieved only through a massive public investment, which is unlikely given that in 2016 India spent a mere 1.2% of its GDP on health, one of the lowest percentages in the world (the global mean is 5.4%) (WHO 2016a).

Moreover, access to medical education suffers from sharp geographic inequalities—the states that contain nearly half the Indian population award only a fifth of medical degrees—and the exorbitant cost of tuition is made even worse by the need to offer "capitation fees" to get into degree-awarding programs (*Economic Times* 2016). The shortage of medical personnel is felt most keenly in the public health services of India's poorer states, which are understaffed, overburdened, and poorly equipped. In August 2016, a man in Odisha carried his wife's body on his shoulders for a dozen kilometers, after the hospital where she had died denied him an ambulance—a shocking reminder of this poor state of affairs (Mohanty 2016). In this underresourced context, "medical citizenship"—the unequal result of political and economic negotiations over people's health (Nichter 2008, 183)—makes the lives and health of India's poorest citizens expendable.

Medical citizenship also causes poor, uneducated people to resort to self-help and alternative healing systems, which, more than biomedicine, are deeply embedded in the local cultural and religious context. Hinduism has played a significant role in shaping the belief in dog bite–induced pregnancy. As noted above, it is not my intention to depict this belief, or any other local misapprehensions about rabies, as a cultural pathology (Briggs and Mantini-Briggs 2016, 232), for external structural reasons are also clearly at play. But it would be equally misleading, and scientifically naïve, to discount the influence of Hindu beliefs on local understandings and interpretations of rabies. Every global disease exists within a specific, historically situated cultural milieu that shapes the understanding of any given illness. Illnesses invariably pose additional challenges to disease control—comprehending them from the outside and figuring out what they mean, how they are conceptualized by insiders, and how people cope with them (Baer et al. 2016). With reference to delusional convictions, Wen S. Tseng (2001, 178) calls their cultural context "pathoplastic," meaning that it shapes them, rather than "pathogenic," meaning that it creates them. I believe that this is a good way to view the belief about puppy pregnancy.

Among the cultural and religious beliefs that feed negative attitudes toward street dogs in India, many of them discussed in chapter 3, is the view of their sexuality. In ancient Hindu texts, dogs' sexuality is described as unrestrained, polygamous, and exceptionally frequent; the Sanskrit terms *a-rata-trapa*, which translates as "not ashamed of coupling," and *dirgha-su-rata*, "long in coitus," appear not infrequently in the ancient literature with respect to dogs (Bollée 2006, 10). In my conversations about dog-mediated pregnancy in the Delhi slums, the telling term *bij* was used so often that it cannot be ignored here. *Bij* is often translated as germ or seed (as in cause, origin, nucleus), but it can also mean embryo, ovule, or sperm. In Hindu mythology, Raktabij is a powerful demon who is continually reborn by multiplying himself via every drop of blood that leaves his body. At a deeper symbolic level, these drops embody a reproductive potential found only in semen—the poison that is transmitted via the teeth of biting dogs into their victims, fatally impregnating them.

Attempts at Survival

One of the last questions I asked the university students concerned what to do immediately after a dog bite. A third of them recommended visiting the doctor immediately. Another quarter said wash the wound and then seek a doctor. About 42% of the students said they would seek self-help alone, in the form of antibiotics (15%) (which are totally useless in preventing rabies), washing the wound with soap and water (10%), washing the wound with water only (9%), and applying chili powder to the wound (4%); the final 4% said that they would do nothing. Seeking medical advice is essential in case of an animal bite, but washing the wound with water and soap is the first thing to do immediately after the bite, so as to prevent as much of the rabies virus as possible from entering the body. It is unfortunate that 33% of the university students (who can be expected to have more than the average amount of education) would go directly to the doctor, without first performing this live-saving first aid. This lack of awareness about how to treat an animal bite is confirmed by two other studies of rabies in India, which found that the number of people who did not wash their wound before seeking a doctor's care ranged from 63% (Sudarshan et al. 2006, 36) to 97% (Ichhpujani et al. 2006, 358).

There are other reasons why few people wash a dog bite. One, paradoxically, is the belief that water by itself is completely ineffectual. Unable to fully appreciate the ability of water to mechanically remove infected saliva, people think that something more powerful, something containing a healing property, must be more effective. In fact, the street children I met largely preferred chili powder to treat their bites, the resulting pain not being a concern to them. In fact, a boy named Bibek told me that he would use chili "exactly because it burns, as that is the moment when the poison dies. It is because of this that it burns. Then the pain goes away and you feel better." A study in Punjab found that people prefer to use chili powder procured from the house of the dog owner (Agarwal and Reddajah 2004, 77).

The children provided me with a long list of other curative substances, including turmeric, kerosene, tea leaves, ground coffee, mustard seeds, clarified butter, cooking oil, pepper, tobacco, neem leaves, terracotta chips, salt, cattle dung, and mud. Other traditional remedies include burning the wound with "acid," covering it with healing herbs, pouring sacred water (particularly from the Ganges) on it, or applying a coin that has been heated in a flame, which "absorbs the poison." From a medical point of view, while some of these remedies and substances are neutral in effect, the irritating ones are extremely dangerous, as they damage the tissue around the wound and allow the virus to reach the nerves more quickly. Milk, which is also used as a topical remedy for dog bites, carries the additional risk, if it is raw, of transmitting rabies itself if it comes from an infected animal. Half of the farmers surveyed in a 2016 study in Ludhiana were aware that zoonoses can be transmitted through contaminated milk, yet 70% of them drink unpasteurized milk and 37% apply it to cracked skin as an emollient (Hundal et al. 2016, 188).

My conversations with the children yielded other local cures for rabies that arise from the religious and cultural context. A young boy named

Soro told me that as soon as possible after the bite one must go to a Bheru temple and offer alcohol, rice, and lentils to this Hindu god, who is closely associated with dogs. A girl called Madhur also recommended that bite victims "go to a religious place," but she could name only Fatehpur, in Rajasthan, as a pilgrimage destination. When Chintu was bitten by a dog, his father took him to a "famous *pandit*" (Hindu scholar) who put black powder on the wound, though neither Chintu nor his father knew what it was. According to Akshay, the best treatment for a dog bite is to have a dog lick the wound. "Some dogs are very good, very nice," he told me, "and if they lick a wound, nothing bad happens. They lick and lick us until we feel good." Having a dog lick a bite wound is said to be particularly effective on Tuesdays and Saturdays, the days devoted to Bheru (Lodrick 2009, 513). Other means of treating bites and preventing rabies include avoiding certain foods, such as rice and milk in Maharashtra (Patle and Khakse 2014, 153) and meat in Tamil Nadu (Chinnaian et al. 2015, 12). Not bathing for seven days and abstaining from drinking water for one day are also common strategies (Varsharani, Chinte, and Jadhav 2014, 63). Apart from being ineffective against rabies, all of these practices dangerously retard PEP (Salve et al. 2015, 124).

These allegedly curative substances and practices have been handed down for generations, some of them going all the way back to the *Sushruta Samhita*. This text recommends cauterizing the wound with clarified butter, squeezing *Achyranthes aspera* flowers into it, and covering it with a paste of sesame seeds (*Sesamum indicum*), myrrh (*Commiphora mukul*), the grass *Cynodon dactylon*, pomegranate seeds (*Punica granatum*), and cane sugar. It also suggests that the bite victim ingest purgative drugs along with the bitter milky sap of the *Calotropis procera* plant, plenty of giant cane (*Arundo donax*), and pancakes containing the roots of *Tephrosia purpurea* and *Dhatura metel*. Interestingly, the *Sushruta Samhita* also recommends that a bitten person be washed at a crossroad or on a riverbank, while reciting the formula "Oh thou Yaksha, lord of Alarka, who art also the lord of all dogs, speedily makest me free from poison of the rabid dog that has bitten me" (Bhishagratna 1991, 736).

In an article on the Ayurvedic treatment of dog bites and rabies, Sharad M. Porte (2015, 89) lists twenty useful herbs. In the past, one remedy consisted of smearing a mixture of crushed dog bone and water onto the wound (Bollée 2006, 28, 41). Rabies was also thought to be cured by killing and burning a dog and having the victim inhale the smoke from the burning carcass (Crooke 1984, cited in Lodrick 2009, 514). In eastern India, juice from the leaves of devil's trumpet (*Datura metel*) is mixed with sugar and water and given to cattle to prevent rabies (Saikia and Borthakur 2010, 50).

In addition to these traditional remedies, some children showed resourcefulness in their first response to a dog bite. When Rani is bitten, he hides, so that the dog cannot find him and bite him again, while Habib immediately bites the dog back. Dinesh described a precise methodology: "If a normal dog bites me I take a bath, but if a mad dog bites me, I kill him—and then I take a bath." But most of the children I met added that they would also go to a doctor or hospital to get injected with the rabies shots. This is extremely encouraging, as most of their parents would probably not say the same. The reason for their reluctance lies in the troubled story of rabies vaccination in India.

The Indian Story of Rabies Vaccination

After the pioneering achievements of Louis Pasteur in the nineteenth century, two kinds of post-exposure prophylaxis (PEP) have been available for human use: nerve tissue vaccine (NTV) and cell culture vaccine (CCV). CCV is more recent and more efficient and has limited side effects, and its shots are given in the deltoid muscle of the upper arm in three to four doses over four weeks, depending on the vaccine type. It was created to replace NTV, which was discouraged by WHO in 1983 because, in addition to requiring one shot a day for fourteen consecutive days (plus three booster doses in the following weeks) in the abdomen, it is not as effective as CCV and has a high rate of adverse side effects (from abdominal swelling to neuroparalytic complications that can sometimes be life-threatening) (Garg 2014, 139). After 1983, NTV was abandoned in many countries, but in India its use continued for more than two decades, particularly in the public health sector, where it was given free of charge (Chhabra et al. 2004, 219); it was cheap and readily available thanks to its being produced locally. Since 1995, there has been a significant increase in the use of CCV in India, although its cost remains quite high. NTV was officially discontinued and replaced with CCV only in December 2004, and most of the adults I met in the slums of Delhi remember all too well how painful it was, and how many doses were required—*chaudah kuttewali* injections ("fourteen dogs" injections), I heard again and again, the words often uttered in unison. The

LIVING WITH RABIES | 213

fear and anxiety that adults in India still associate with NTV are so palpable that even their children know the saying by heart: "Fourteen, never less, fourteen," said twelve-year-old Jivan with certainty, spreading his hands far apart to show the length of the needle before pretending to plunge it into his stomach with exaggerated expressions of agony.

It is easy to see why the lingering terror of NTV not only magnifies people's fear of rabies but also discourages them from seeking medical treatment in case of a dog bite. A 2006 survey found that refusal to seek medical intervention after a dog bite is attributable more to the fear of NTV injections (32%) than to lack of awareness or negligence (31%), the cost of treatment (15%), or the length of treatment (6%) (Ichhpujani et al. 2006, 359). This research also confirms that people continue to believe that the number of injections is much higher than it actually is (with CCV) long after CCV began to replace NTV. Only a tenth of those surveyed said that five injections were enough, which shows clearly that most of the people surveyed were thinking of NTV rather than CCV. Almost a decade later, studies carried out in rural Pune reveal that 32% of respondents still believe that fourteen injections are required (Valekar et al. 2014, 9) and 84% believe that the shots must be given in the stomach (Kakrani et al. 2013, 307). The same beliefs persist in Punjab (Hundal et al. 2016, 189), Karnataka (Kulkarni et al. 2016, 1269–70), Gujarat (Singh and Choudhary 2005, 82), and Tamil Nadu (Joice, Singh, and Datta 2016, 587). Even most of the first-year students at a medical college in Maharashtra suffer from the same misconception (Gaikwad et al. 2016, 20).

I argue that in addition to the social, cultural, and religious factors outlined above, the abdominal site of NTV injections has played a key role in shaping the belief that rabies victims suffer from pregnancy with puppies. In fact, in India as well as abroad, most vaccinations are administered either orally or through injections in the arm or the gluteal muscles in the buttocks. Rabies was long an exception to this rule. It is possible that because of the unusual site of NTV shots, people have become convinced that rabies lurks in the stomach. Recall that Amina reported seeing fourteen newborn puppies surrounding the dead woman near her slum. A litter of fourteen puppies would be unusually large, and I suspect that it is no coincidence that fourteen is also the number of NTV injections required to kill the rabies virus. I was never given any number but fourteen by the people I interviewed. When I asked why the puppies always numbered exactly fourteen, no one could provide an answer. It was just fourteen.

As noted above, although most of the children I met were aware of the rabies vaccine, they also harbored serious misconceptions about the proper steps to take after an animal bite. Of greater concern is the deficient preparedness of the health-care system in the clinical management of rabies. A 2001–2 survey in Delhi found that 67% of patients who went to a health center after being bitten received no PEP at all, and of those who did, 61% received the outdated NTV injections rather than the CCV recommended since 1983 (Lal et al. 2005, 53). The same research shows that even when doctors used CCV, they often injected it incorrectly into the buttocks rather than the arm, making the vaccine fruitless. A decade later, while two-thirds of the final-year students at the Shri M. P. Shah Government Medical College in Jamnagar identified the arm as the correct site for rabies vaccination, a third still thought that the abdomen was the correct site (Sarkar et al. 2013, 64). In 2019, I received two rabies shots in private clinics in Mumbai and Solapur, and in both cases I had to beg the nurses to inject them in my arm. They instinctively aimed for my buttocks, explaining that vaccination in the arm is too painful. Shocked by what she perceived as my masochism, the first nurse repeatedly excused herself during the procedure, while the second one purposely injected the vaccine not in the deltoid muscle but in the fat zone nearby, despite our having just discussed the difference between the intramuscular and intradermal routes.

Contrary to what we would expect, improper administration of PEP is more common in urban than in rural India (Sudarshan et al. 2006, 36). Research in Delhi in 2005 showed that 99% of bite patients did not receive appropriate PEP when they sought medical help at health centers in the city (Chhabra et al. 2004, 219). Another study, this one from 2010, found that undergraduate medical students in Delhi, though they understood the gravity of rabies, were seriously uninformed about current trends in PEP (Laskar, Singh, and Saha 2010, 289). The same situation was found in 2013 among physicians at animal bite clinics in Bangalore, a medical hub for southern India (Shankaraiah et al. 2013, 239). This is particularly disturbing because there is no single and reliable test that can diagnose rabies before symptoms occur (by which time it is too late), so diagnosis depends on physicians skilled enough to know when PEP is called for, and on their scrupulousness in administering it.

To make matters worse, since NTV was discontinued in 2004, most government hospitals in India have faced acute shortages of modern rabies

CCVs due to budgetary shortfalls, inadequate vaccine production, delays in distribution, and the relatively high cost of intramuscular CCVs. In 2006, in an attempt to make CCVs available to a larger proportion of the population, Indian health professionals began replacing intramuscular CCV with intradermal CCV, as also recommended by WHO. Less vaccine is needed with intradermal administration, so it is useful in poor countries with a history of administering NTV to the poorest segments of the population. But intradermal CCV carries its own challenges (Abbas and Kakkar 2013b, 200). Intramuscular vaccination is easy to administer, whereas intradermal shots require more medical training. Intradermal injections are also more painful than intramuscular shots, a deterrent for patients with high sensitivity to pain. The vials of reconstituted vaccine used in intradermal shots must be used within eight hours if refrigerated—if not refrigerated, within an hour—which means that unused vaccine is wasted on days when demand is low. On days when many patients need PEP and demand is high, administering intradermal CCV is more time-consuming than intramuscular injections. Despite these challenges, the great merit of intradermal CCV is its affordability—it costs 60 to 80% less than intramuscular CCV (Hampson, Cleaveland, and Briggs 2011, 9), which makes it a good choice for low-income countries like India, where rabies disproportionately kills poor people.

Face to Face

In countries like India, with many competing health-care priorities, inadequate health-care infrastructure, and insufficient drug and vaccine provision, staking everything on PEP in the fight against rabies may not be the wisest choice. This is not to minimize the importance of post-bite treatment in saving people's lives, but preventing bites in the first place, through healthier human-animal interactions, is equally important, if not more so. The old adage that an ounce of prevention is worth a pound of cure is nowhere more applicable than in the case of rabies. In fact, this is true in the case of noninfectious bites as well, which are generally not as lethal as rabies but can still cause significant trauma, both physical and psychological, and can drastically undermine good human-animal relations and animal-related issues.

In my encounters with street and slum children, I always asked whether their schoolbooks contained any information about animal bites or rabies, and I usually met with blank expressions. Only in the Tis Hazari slum did two girls in third grade say that they had seen something on this topic in their science book. One pulled from her rucksack a purple book, which she opened to page 219, where there was a diagram titled "Means of Spread of Disease" depicting a sick person on the left and a healthy one on the right. Five red arrows indicated the pathways of disease transmission from the sick to the healthy person: shaking hands, kissing, the aerial spread of germs, shared tableware, and mosquitoes and ticks. A sixth arrow pointed to the healthy individual from a black dog of indiscriminate breed, with the caption "animal infected with rabies." The text above this diagram explained how disease is spread but made no mention of animal bites or rabies. Clearly, school curricula in India need to incorporate information on bites and rabies prevention (Pawar and Bansal 2010). Public awareness is critically important, not only to disseminate the facts about animal bites and rabies but to counterbalance erroneous information such as the statement in the Hindi exam book *Paryavekshak Sanyukt Chayan Pariksha*, in which students are taught that "all the stray dogs should be killed" (Kotwal 2017).

During my time in Delhi and Jaipur, I saw very little awareness material on rabies and how to prevent it (information about mosquito-borne dengue fever, by contrast, was everywhere, especially in Delhi). Only once, in North Delhi, did I come across a brand-new orange roadside billboard, installed by the local Department of Health and Family Welfare. "Protecting Themselves from Rabies Is Easy," read the billboard, "but Dying from This Disease Is Sure." Below these words, three images illustrated a sequence of events. The first showed a Rottweiler-like dog biting someone on the hand—red dots representing blood had been added—while a second dog barked restlessly. The caption told people not to ignore the bites or scratches of dogs, monkeys, cats, mongooses, and wild rats. The second image depicted a child's bleeding foot under running water, with a caption instructing viewers to wash the wound with soap and water immediately. In the final image, a doctor gave a blond woman an injection in her upper arm, and the caption said that if you are bitten, you should go immediately to a doctor or hospital for anti-rabies vaccination and wound treatment.

Even fewer people must have seen the poster on the wall of the humid office of a high-ranking official in the Department of Veterinary Services of the North MCD. Next to the words "Kill Rabies, Not Stray Dogs," a picture on the left showed a menacing-looking dog with red eyes, his canine teeth bared in a growl. On the right, a group of dogs roamed a sandy roadside.

Beneath this image, a blue text box explained animal birth control (ABC), while a red one recommended vaccinating pet and stray dogs and gave instructions for treating dog bite: "Clean and wash the wound with soap for 8–10 minutes under running tap water, apply antiseptic and start post-bite anti rabies vaccination/treatment immediately. Anti Rabies Vaccine is available at Govt./MCD Hospitals." The poster also explained in red lettering that dog bites increase during mating season, when mother dogs become more aggressive after the delivery of their puppies—thus dog sterilization is recommended. At the bottom of the poster were the words "Let us join hands and adopt ABC-AR Programme to make RABIES FREE DELHI," followed by the phone numbers of the zone offices and NGOs responsible for controlling dog population and rabies in Delhi. The official told me that leaflet versions of this poster were regularly distributed in Delhi. I saw the first and only such leaflet two years later, posted in the hallway of an animal shelter.

Useful information on preventing animal bites can be found in the awareness materials of the international organization World Animal Protection (formerly the World Society for the Protection of Animals), translated into Hindi by its Indian branch. All of the WAP material I came across in India targeted children and aimed to teach them how to interact positively with dogs. One humorous chart explained canine body language and how dogs express their state of mind and communicate their intentions to other dogs and to people who know how to read the signs. For example, the chart depicted the wagging tail of a happy, relaxed dog, the tail tucked between the legs of a dog who is frightened or in pain, and the tail held stiff and high in an angry dog.

A similar WAP leaflet used engaging color drawings to explain the basic rules of positive human-dog interaction—do not approach a dog who is eating; do not run next to dogs; do not stare dogs in the eye. In addition, the leaflet explains, if a dog approaches, the child should remain quiet, speak softly, let the animal sniff him, draw back slowly, or, if attacked, assume the form of a tree (standing stiffly with the arms pressed against the body, head down) or a stone (curling up on the ground and protecting the head and stomach with the arms). When facing an aggressive dog, show no fear. This is easier said than done, of course, but it emphasizes the point that quelling fear, on both sides, is the key to a safer and healthier coexistence between dogs and humans. A FIAPO survey conducted following an intensive awareness program in Kerala schools found that when students are shown how to behave around dogs, the percentage who say they would run away from an approaching dog drops significantly (FIAPO 2017a, 12). Yet in my multi-year survey of Indian newspaper articles on rabies, bites, and human-animal relations, I can count on one hand the number of articles providing information on how to prevent a dog bite and what to do if bitten.

In the case of human-macaque conflict, a specific component of the problem is the unique physical resemblance between the two species, which invariably leads us to anthropomorphize them—as long as we find it fun. When it comes to monkeys, in fact, the boundary line between fun and fear is uniquely narrow, from our perspective. Again, the best way to avoid violent confrontation is for people who feel threatened to show no fear, display empty palms, and calmly walk away backward. In extreme situations, people sometimes resort to making sudden loud noises, hitting the ground with a stick, or pretending to pick up a stone, as if preparing to throw it. All of that said, Iqbal Malik taught me that an emotionally well-balanced monkey will almost always try to reach his goals peacefully, resorting to a physical confrontation with a human only when all else fails. Unfortunately, in Delhi, and to a lesser extent in Jaipur, the human-monkey relationship has already been poisoned by fear, suspicion, and violence—and sometimes by rabies as well.

When Malik finished teaching me the precautions to follow in interactions with monkeys, I wondered why I had never seen any guidelines on positive human-monkey interactions (not in the media, not in temples, not at macaque-feeding spots in Delhi and Jaipur), despite my almost maniacal search for them and my constant exposure to animal-related issues. When I asked Malik if she thought the Delhi government should mount awareness campaigns teaching people how to behave with macaques, she replied that she had been advocating such measures for the past decade—for example, in columns in local newspapers explaining "the dos and don'ts" of interaction with monkeys. She even knew people who had pasted her articles on their car windows in an attempt to spread the word. But "that was the last generation of people and monkeys for whom dos and don'ts could work," she admitted. "Now we are in a situation where they are no more. Only don'ts are left now. Monkeys should not be where they are, they are too many by now. At this point there is nothing more we can do, as monkeys are aggressive, have changed their behavior, and have learned to offer resistance for food, for space, for water, for everything. . . . The time for dos and don'ts is over."

Macaques fight not only with people but also with dogs and cattle, especially when food is involved, whether food offerings from humans or garbage. In conflicts between monkeys and dogs, only a clear numerical superiority on one side or the other can forestall physical consequences, except in the case of large, noisy dogs, who may effectively deter monkeys—though they are also potentially dangerous to children when they are trained to attack macaques (Lee and Priston 2005, 14). In Wazirabad Ghat in North Delhi, I once watched a puppy being mistreated by a young macaque half his size: the monkey pulled his ears, jerked his head around, sat and jumped on his muzzle, and obsessively opened his mouth to inspect his teeth and tongue. The reverse is also possible: in February 2016, video footage of a female macaque in Tamil Nadu who adopted a puppy went viral, showing her picking fleas off him, pre-chewing fruit before feeding him, carrying him on tree branches for safety, and defending him from other dogs.

Cattle easily get the better of macaques thanks to their size. Even in a group, monkeys tend to keep a safe distance from cattle and to approach any food the cattle are eating only when the cattle lose interest and abandon it. However, I would not say that macaques are terrified by cattle; they are just cautious, and they take care not to trigger violence. Moreover, unless a cow is particularly aggressive, macaques rarely need to attack; their quickness and agility easily counterbalance her superior size. Malik wrote in her fieldwork diary that "monkeys are more or less on love-hate terms with the cows of Tughlakabad." While I never personally witnessed any actual hatred between the two species, a troop of macaques did kill a cow in Jharkhand in April 2017 (Mishra 2017). In contrast, at the banana stall in Sardar Patel Marg, I did witness the monkeys routinely letting cows eat their leftovers. I wondered whether this was simply because the monkeys were sated or whether, perhaps, they felt sorry for the cows nobody was caring for, though I recognized, of course, that I was anthropomorphizing them.

Physical conflict between cattle and humans is also unusual, primarily because cattle are generally mild-tempered, and, being herbivorous, they do not resort to biting to attack, defend themselves, or procure food. Most of the street and slum children I met described cows as dangerous animals, but the threat lay in goring, kicking, and running after people, and in "defecating everywhere, even when they are next to people." None of the children feared being bitten by a cow. That said, if being bitten by a cow is uncommon, contact with its saliva is not, especially in a country where cultural, religious, and economic factors create favorable conditions for such contact. Let us not forget, moreover, that the number of rabid cows on the streets of India may be far higher than we think (Gill et al. 2019, 1). I saw several cows, calves, and young oxen who had been brought to animal clinics because they were choking on a foreign body—often a mango seed, which is as big as a child's fist. To remove it, the staff member with the thinnest wrist would reach bare hand into the animal's throat and carefully pull it out, thus coming into contact with a profuse quantity of potentially infected saliva. Only rarely did I see veterinarians use a homemade iron slipknot, when the obstructing object was too deep in the throat to be pulled out by hand. I never saw an X-ray or other diagnostic technique used to confirm the presence of the foreign body. The generic symptoms these animals showed on arrival (e.g., anorexia, weakness, hypersalivation, unusual mouth movements) could easily have been due to rabies (Gill et al. 2019, 7). WHO acknowledges that rabid cattle do not usually bite but recommends that precautions be taken when examining their mouths or when they are salivating (2013a, 3).

As discussed in chapter 5, another pathway for rabies transmission from cattle is feeding them by hand, as religious norms require. Most food offered in this way is of small size—some lettuce leaves or slices of bread—and cows seize it with their lips and teeth, so it is very likely that the donor's hand comes into contact with the animal's saliva; if there are any open wounds on the hands, rabies infection may occur. With cattle who are used to being hand-fed by people and thus have established a high degree of intimate interaction with them, rabies transmission is possible with other kinds of contact. For example, especially in the summer, when I let cattle approach me on the street, they invariably licked my hands and arms profusely, probably for the mineral salts in human sweat. Then they invariably started searching me for food, nosing my pockets or my bag with their snouts.

The same curiosity and search for food may expose them to bites from other animals and thus to the risk of rabies. Cattle have a well-developed sense of hearing and of sight, although they need some time to bring things into focus. But they rely primarily on their sense of smell in their interactions with their surroundings. This is why, as several veterinarians told me, they are often bitten or scratched on the snout and face by dogs who are annoyed by their curiosity, are protecting their food, or are rabid.

CONCLUSION
Interspecies Camaraderie

This book narrates part of the story of the coexistence among people, animals, and rabies on the streets of the overcrowded zoöpolises of Delhi and Jaipur. It is a story in continuous evolution, in a constant state of becoming. It is, inevitably, a long and immensely complex one. It could not be otherwise, as it articulates the relationships among four species and one quasi-species, the rabies virus. When companion species—those that share a mingled evolutionary past and present—are the subject of a book, the relationships among them become "the smallest unit of analysis" (Haraway 2003, 20). Focusing on one species alone would be of no use, and this is especially true when an infectious disease has to be understood. In Donna Haraway's view, human-animal interconnections are bidirectional, free from the centripetal force of anthropocentrism, and this is what allows both parts to "co-habit an active story" (2003, 20). This story is created and evolves through what Bruno Latour (2014) calls agency, understood as the dynamism produced in human and animal subjects by their being alive and doing their best to survive, resist conflict, and thrive. A relationship between subjects, and not one in which animals are thought of as objects in connection to people, is thus established.

222 | RABIES IN THE STREETS

I included a chapter on food precisely to emphasize this more-than-human subjectivity—it would be better to say subjectivities, plural, for each of the animal species discussed here has its own subjective experiences of the animal-human bond. I did not discuss in any detail what humans eat, which might seem a notable omission in the current heated debate about the future of human nutrition. Instead, I focused on what *animals* eat: what is available for them to eat, and what they want to eat. In fact, although the human-animal relationship is clearly unequal, animals are not just passive recipients of food. Rather, they are constantly learning how to live together in human-made landscapes and to benefit from human activities, in a fitting blend of intelligence, resilience, and opportunism. As Agustín Fuentes and Kimberley J. Hockings write of monkeys, "Primate behavioral patterns are not just a result of one particular selective pressure or basic ecological constraint, but instead the result of interconnections with humans, changes in foraging, and patterns of individual behavior, all in the context of an anthropogenic environment" (2010, 842).

This process of reciprocal adjustment takes place in what Marcus Baynes-Rock (2013) calls a "multispecies commons," in which the social, biological, historical, and ecological entanglements of human and animal lives become particularly intimate. Crowded, colorful Indian streets, with their constant swarm of life, make ideal multispecies commons. Yet they should not be considered the mere background of these interspecies entanglements. Instead, multispecies commons can probably be best understood as the zone of entanglement itself (Ingold 2008, 1807). In the urban landscapes of Delhi and Jaipur, nature and culture—categories that we continue to think of as mutually exclusive—are fluid and porous, mutually influencing each other all the time, minute by minute. Fuentes (2010, 603) describes the result of their intertwining as a natural-cultural co-constructed niche. Diseases, of course, are part of it.

The story narrated in this book is marked by agonizing deaths, deep fears, bite scars, imagined pregnancies, beaten dogs, displaced macaques, abused cows, a sneaky virus, and, above all, infectious cross-species contacts. All of this is located within a framework, or "connecting pattern" (Bateson 1979, 6–8), of urban poverty, infrastructural constraints, poor sanitation, social inequalities, class discrimination, economic pressures, cultural diversity, religious fragmentation, and health inequality. In this traffic jam of bodies, viruses, urban landscapes, ecological dynamics, and social processes, the four species considered in this book are all equally stuck, each in its own particular ways. Usually slow-moving, occasionally speeding up all of a sudden (during epidemics, for example), we are all in this jam together—though by *all* I am not including animals who are not affected by rabies, for this book, inevitably, is "mammal-centric." Foxes, cats, skunks, raccoons, bats, coyotes, horses, camels, and many other species are also in the same boat with us, for the threat of rabies, like other zoonoses, teaches us inescapably that human health is never disconnected from that of other animals. Rabies can be seen as the standard bearer in this revised, more inclusive perception of disease. In fact, unlike mosquito-borne infections such as dengue fever, malaria, and Zika virus, which do not kill their carriers (mosquitoes flourish when they bite and infect), rabies mercilessly kills both its reservoir and its host. Rabies reminds us that "when studying health knowledges as social phenomena, [we] should, in short, acknowledge that human societies are not composed of human bodies alone" (Rock, Mykhalovskiy, and Schlich 2007, 1973).

But my goal in this book is not to depict people and animals as joined solely by rabies infection. The awful story of rabies is not new; rabies has been with us for thousands of years. What is novel in this work is the concept of "interspecies camaraderie," which points to a longer-term commitment to safeguarding health and life, not just to avoiding suffering and death. The term "camaraderie" has two connotations that are especially pertinent here.

The first echoes the intense feeling of attachment experienced by soldiers toward their fellows in war. I confess that I am not entirely comfortable with the military analogy, but I remember my grandfather's brother, a soldier in the Second World War and eventually a political prisoner in a concentration camp, movingly describing this feeling. For him, camaraderie was different from, and possibly even stronger than, friendship or even biological brotherhood. It was a very rational, logical, pragmatic feeling, where one's sense of attachment, care, and solidarity was strengthened and amplified by the instinct to survive shared by fellow soldiers. This was not a military strategy, though rejecting it would have amounted to collective suicide. Nor was it an individual choice. The kind of camaraderie my uncle described can best be understood as a collectively built ideal that underwrites the overarching goal of getting out of war alive. In a setting of this kind of true camaraderie, there is no room for suspicion, resentment, bias, discrimination, rancor, or abuse—feelings that sometimes permeate friendships and even brotherhood. To the contrary, camaraderie among soldiers is characterized by reciprocal trust and respect. In such a context, survival depends exclusively on being part of a group devoted to a cause that far exceeds the fate of single individuals.

The second connotation of "camaraderie," a term generally understood to mean team spirit based on deep interpersonal closeness, emerges from its etymology. In Latin, the term *camera* means "chamber" or "room," and it is within the intimacy of the four walls of a chamber that the concept of camaraderie developed. In Italian (my native tongue), *camerata* means the large room where soldiers, patients, orphans, or college students sleep together. It is in this context of living together by force of circumstance, sharing space and sacrificing privacy, trusting one's fellows even in the private and vulnerable act of sleeping, and, in many circumstances, facing physical and psychological pain together, that the concept of camaraderie has taken shape. For this reason, it also suggests complicity, empathy, solidarity, and closeness.

When confronting rabies, the best camaraderie one can expect and benefit from is of an interspecies nature. The rabies virus is a master at hiding in its host until it is too late to stop. The centuries-old frustration at not being able to outsmart it, coupled with the fear of its deadliness—especially in countries where it is endemic, like India—understandably leads people to blame animals indiscriminately, especially dogs, and, in their fear and anger, to take measures that turn out to be unproductive or even counterproductive, like indiscriminate dog culling. Culling remains a component of institutional responses to the risks of zoonoses (Degeling, Lederman, and Rock 2016, 244), but in the fight against rabies, it does not work. Interspecies cooperation, by contrast, makes life difficult for the rabies virus, as vaccinated dogs protect people by creating rabies-free zones that benefit the entire multispecies community. The virtuous cycle of interspecies camaraderie reminds us that "to care is to become subject to another, to recognise an obligation to look after another" (Van Dooren 2014, 291). It is precisely when we give in to fear, hostility, and bias, then, that the rabies virus succeeds undisturbed. In fact, WHO encourages people to keep dogs alive, healthy, vaccinated, supervised, and close by. The invariable result is that dogs do not get rabies, which means that neither do humans, monkeys, cattle, and other animals who are exposed to rabies via dog bite. If dogs are viewed as the perfect comrades in the fight against rabies, then "herd immunity" (the indirect protection of a whole species that occurs when a large part of its population is vaccinated) becomes of interspecies nature. Also called "social immunity," herd immunity, when it comes to rabies, can strengthen relationships across species borders.

If dogs are seen not as partners but solely as agents of infection, little progress will be made (Biehler 2013, 27). Rabies scholars and the groundbreaking One Health framework, introduced at the beginning of this book, recommend that we view dogs as integral agents of interconnection. "Health is created by caring for oneself and others," says WHO's website, "and by ensuring that the society one lives in creates conditions that allow the attainment of health by all its members." One need not be a zealous animal welfare activist, or even an animal lover, to grasp the wisdom in these words. "Being alive" means being in relationship with others, and not just human others (Ingold 2011, 68). When we undermine our relationships with dogs, monkeys, cattle, and other animals, we open the door to death.

Research on human-animal entanglements documents "the ways in which disease, instead of alienating humans from other life forms, brings their intimate relationships into sharper relief" (Nading 2013, 60). This kind of scholarship also reminds us that despite our stubborn attempts to force upon animals binary distinctions like domestic/wild, owned/stray, and pet/pest, these are not essential characteristics of any species but historically and contextually specific categories that humans have invented. As such, they are always open to renegotiation. The macaques of Delhi are a good example: the MCD calls them wild animals, while the Wildlife Department calls them semi-domestic, neither institution willing to accept responsibility for them. Initially loved, now barely tolerated, urban macaques and their increasing conflict with humans force us into a more nuanced understanding of interspecies relations and into questioning people's biopolitical control of other-than-human lives (Foucault 2010).

Delhi is a good setting for such an exercise. The city authorities approach the problem of street animals and rabies in pretty much the same way they approach the city's vast number of poor people, those who live on the streets and in the slums. Blaming dogs for spreading rabies is akin to blaming the poor for their poverty, and just as dishonest, on both a moral and a practical level. Delhi's burgeoning middle class looks with disdain and intolerance upon street and slum dwellers, whom they see as encroachers and parasites who menace the development of the city, soil its public image, and eventually hurt the pride of the entire nation. This was nowhere more visible than in the preparation for the 2010 Commonwealth Games, when street animals were rounded up and slums were razed. "This is the city, not the jungle. In Italy and in London [London is often used vaguely as a stand-in for all of Europe] you don't have monkeys, so why should we accept them here in Delhi?" a woman asked me on the metro, getting off at her stop without waiting for an answer. While this is no doubt a legitimate question—just as the desire to improve the quality of life in the city is legitimate—the problems that are blamed on the poor, both human and animal, are actually the responsibility of the city as a whole.

Delhi's desire to become a world-class city has led to unspeakably cruel attempts to purify itself of its less welcome inhabitants, both human and nonhuman, removing these unwanted members of society from what more powerful fellow citizens refuse to acknowledge as their place—no matter that a baby born on a sidewalk, or a bull splattered with acid, have hardly chosen this place for themselves. Delhi's Department of Social Welfare created "no-tolerance zones," where street dwellers are forbidden to enter, that perfectly embody the transformation of the abstract concept of social purification into a concrete reality. A similar attitude has been shown toward animals, especially the "liminal" ones. On the spectrum between domesticated animals and animals used for food, at one end, and wild animals, at the other, liminal animals are those who have adapted to life among people without being under their direct care—and control. Liminal animals, who often have no choice but to live in urban areas, either because their natural habitats have been destroyed or because they are no longer able to survive in the wild—or both—are, according to animal citizenship theory, provided with "denizenship," the core features of which are the right to residency, tolerant coexistence with humans, and accommodation by humans (Donaldson and Kymlicka 2012, 210).

Although denizenship is, it seems to me, a reasonable, practical, and compassionate response to liminal animals, the presence and proximity of these animals remain unsettling, disorienting, confusing, and even frightening for many people (Thomassen 2012, 21). It is thus not uncommon for liminal animals to become "trash animals" (Nagy and Johnson 2013), and thus disposable. In Delhi, dogs who are not the proper pets of proper citizens, and macaques who stray from the human-imposed confines of temples or feeding sites, easily transgress the borders that humans impose on them and fall out of the limited "in-between" space allowed to them. Cattle face the same problem when they are thrown out of dairies and end up scavenging garbage on the street, their stomachs distended with plastic trash, and when they get trapped on traffic islands and railroad tracks, cars and trains whizzing past. People often see liminal animals not only as breakers of human rules—rather than as fugitives from man-made environmental destruction—but also as greedy cheaters who try to get more resources (food, space, and human indulgence) than they are entitled to. Animals continue to be defined by their usefulness (and lack thereof) to humans: unruly macaques are displaced to the fake jungle-cum-prison of the Asola Bhatti Sanctuary, while langurs are captured in the forest and made to patrol strategic areas of Delhi.

A report on the 2010 Commonwealth Games concluded that the process of readying Delhi for the games involved wholescale infractions of the law and of the Indian constitution and "resulted in an irreversible alteration in the social, spatial, economic, and environmental dimensions of the city of Delhi. . . . Much of this has taken place in contravention of democratic governance and planning processes, including the Master Plan for Delhi 2021" (HLRN 2010, 1). The reference to the master plan alludes to the fact that several of Delhi's slums and poor informal settlements—liminal "non-places" (Baviskar 2011b, 45), like the Yamuna riverfront, that had been ignored till then—were suddenly bulldozed to make room for CWG infrastructure and to beautify the city. The street and slum dwellers of Delhi were thus subjected to the leveling power of the "geography of blame" (Farmer 1992), which defines those who inhabit dirty and polluted parts of the city as pathological per se. In the same way that street dogs are a symptom rather than the cause of pathologies like rabies, the urban poor are not the root cause of urban squalor but its first victims in terms of social discrimination, abuse of power, and denial of basic human rights.

Rabies and rabies control demand that we ask ourselves: do humans and animals have the same right to life when both face zoonoses? If there is a difference, how elastic and negotiable is it? Within our own species, how do we negotiate a truce between factions, like the dog lovers and dog haters discussed in chapter 3? Must human rights and animal rights, human lives and animal lives, invariably be seen as mutually exclusive, or can we imagine them as more accommodating of each other? Is this conflict inevitable, and is it really meant to result in only one winner?

To put the question another way, who exactly is the "public" when we speak of "public health" (Akhtar 2012; Rock 2017) in the context of zoonotic diseases? The One Health agenda acknowledges that the interdependence of humans and animals must be understood, accepted, and built upon if we are to have any hope of defeating rabies. This approach requires that we look at other species in a new way, to move "from 'us vs. them' to 'shared risk'" (Rabinowitz, Odofin, and Dein 2008), and to forge a "more-than-human solidarity" (Rock and Degeling 2015). The One Health concept has clearly been conceived as a technical solution, yet it implies, first and foremost, a change in people's mindset. And herein lies the main challenge to effective rabies control in India. The widespread, long-standing attitude that animal welfare and human welfare are necessarily and intrinsically at odds, and that the fight over scarce resources is a battle of all against all, is a foe almost as formidable as the rabies virus itself. Competing factions feel like they are worlds apart. Animal activists are cast as selfish, idealistic, and antidemocratic, caring more about animals than about already disadvantaged people. Dog cullers are seen as cruel and inhumane monsters who arrogate to themselves the right to choose who lives or dies. How do we bridge this divide and see that human welfare and animal welfare are mutually interdependent, that they go together, that when one fails, the other also fails?

One key first step is acknowledging that rabies is a collective threat that requires a collective response, first among humans themselves. Facing the expense of PEP worries the parents of the child who has been bitten; keeping a pet animal concerns the whole family; the presence of street animals affects the entire neighborhood; spending public money to vaccinate street dogs involves the whole citizenry; managing rabies nationally requires large-scale political participation; combatting rabies at the international level demands global communication and collaboration.

Effective collective involvement necessarily builds upon consensus. This, not funding issues or vaccine shortages, is currently the main obstacle to eliminating rabies in India. Despite this major challenge, and the practical issues that derive from it, there are also reasons for hope. I often think of India as a synonym for adaptability. Living in India can be both exhausting and incredibly enriching. Most Indians are accustomed from early childhood to a life of unspeakable challenges and minimum comforts, and they adjust to this. Adaptability is seen as such a valuable quality in India that in 2010 a global survey revealed that it is considered a determining factor in the Indian job market by 76% of those surveyed (as compared to 36% in the Netherlands, for example) (*Times of India* 2010). The Indian aptitude for patience, stamina, flexibility, and resourcefulness can be summed up in the concept of *jugaad*. The Hindi word *jugaad* is hard to translate, but it suggests a solution that looks questionable but eventually solves the problem, a creation that seems precarious but actually works, a scheme that appears ridiculous but is actually brilliant. *Jugaad* also has a dark side—that of illegality and corruption—but Yamini Narayanan (2019, 1517) describes it as "a mix of social and material innovation." Defined by management experts as "frugal engineering," *jugaad* is a cheap yet valuable tool used in underprivileged contexts where more elaborate and expensive interventions are just not possible.

India's centuries-long training in adaptation and mastery of *jugaad* are valuable resources to be exploited in the fight against rabies. In fact, one of my goals in writing this book is to contribute to abstract global health research by focusing on the locally situated dynamics of disease—specifically, in this case, rabies in urban India. The relatively new One Health strategy has already developed—and expanded geographically—into the One World, One Health concept. Yet although efforts undertaken under the One World, One Health umbrella may achieve benefits like a deeper and more productive collaboration between the Global North and Global South, there is a risk in this approach of glossing over the world's diversity and of undervaluing the place-specific engagements that affect health and disease (Hinchliffe 2015, 28). The tendency to focus on the biological circulation of pathogens at the global level can obfuscate the key role played in diseases by their contingent, local, social, cultural, and political dimensions.

While it is undeniable that rabies is a global disease—OIE and WHO thus consider its reduction a global public good—it does not present the same level of threat in all global settings. Likewise, though rabies is technically the same virus regardless of where and whom it strikes, it is not experienced the same way everywhere; the actual experience of suffering is mediated by social and cultural factors. In India, rabies causes people to suffer not just mental confusion, hydrophobia, air hunger, and paralysis, but also the fear that puppies are growing inside them. What makes India a global hotspot for this pathology is evidently something more than the rabies virus itself: it is the unique interconnections between India's people, animals, ecological webs, and cultural and religious fabric. In short, it is India's "landscape of exposure" (Mitman et al. 2004), its web of historically and politically situated physical, structural, and cultural elements. The lyssavirus simply finds its way among them and "becomes—particularly successful—*with* them" (Haraway 2003, 20).

It is within this complex web of factors that the rabies virus can also be contained. Yet as Abigail H. Neely and Alex M. Nading remind us, "Global health projects encounter bodies-in-place" (2017, 57). In other words, while international guidelines are indisputably essential, no single model of rabies control can be successful in all communities (Cleaveland et al. 2014, 192). This is why the "stimulus packages" for eliminating rabies that OIE, WHO, FAO, and GARC have advocated since 2016 are designed to be adaptable to specific needs, circumstances, and experiences of rabies (WHO 2016b, 3).

In suggesting that India's aptitude for adaptability and *jugaad* could be a valuable tool in containing and limiting rabies, I mean that the country has the capacity to be flexible in its understanding of the unique intricacies of rabies within its borders, patient enough to avoid knee-jerk reactions that address the symptoms rather than the disease, and inventive enough to effectively tailor international guidelines to local circumstances. In India, the relationship between people and their nonhuman neighbors is particularly intense, complicated, and multifaceted. People who spend the morning rounding up street cows are sometimes the same people who feed them rotis in the evening. Thanks to this exposure to plurality—at the personal, community, and state levels—people in India are particularly well suited to appreciate the interconnectedness of the lives, suffering, and death of humans, dogs, macaques, and cattle on their streets and to address the issue of rabies with a multipronged strategy that takes this interconnectedness into account.

Indians are rightly proud of their *jugaad*. I never met a Mumbaikar who failed to boast about the amazing service of the city's *dabbawalas*, or lunch deliverymen, who, using only bikes and trains and relying only on a system of codes and individual memory, deliver boxed lunches to millions of people in Mumbai every day, with an error rate of less than one wrong delivery per million. In 1962, the U.S. ambassador to India, John Kenneth Galbraith, called India a "functioning anarchy." More than forty years later, Viswanathan Raghunathan, an academic, author, and CEO who has been called one of the top fifty thinkers in management across India and the Indian diaspora, claims that India has still not become a system-oriented nation (2006, 115). According to him, this is mainly due to what he calls the "canons of Indianness," a dozen problematic characteristics of Indians, himself included, among them "being privately smart and publicly dumb," having a "fatalist outlook" and a "lack of self-regulation," "being too intelligent for our own good," and "mistaking talk for action" (16–17). Thus designing and implementing an efficient system for defeating rabies, and maintaining that system over the long haul, poses a challenge to India and "Indianness." But it is a challenge that the country may be uniquely equipped to meet.

In 2015, the then Ministry of Urban Development launched the Smart Cities Challenge to improve the quality of life in more than one hundred cities and towns across India by "developing the entire urban eco-system" and its "institutional, physical, social and economic infrastructure." To date, the Smart Cities initiative has not acknowledged the importance of what I am calling interspecies camaraderie; in fact, it does not even mention the animals with whom Indian city dwellers share living space, nor does it address the threat of rabies. But it could, and so could similar initiatives, like Clean Delhi, Green Delhi, which can be built upon, expanded, and adapted to include the other species with which humans co-create their world.

Advances in the field of ethics can contribute to developing new social infrastructures designed to promote interspecies camaraderie and, not incidentally, to contain and reduce the risk of rabies. If the One Health strategy is really the key to improving health at the human-animal environmental interface, then it is worth thinking about how its core concept of inclusivity should be applied more broadly outside the medical field. A comprehensive approach would have the advantage of solving several problems at once: for example, banning plastic saves cattle from ingesting it and people from breathing its toxic smoke when garbage dumps are burned. It is myopic and thus counterproductive to ignore the fact that communities are never purely human and that animals always play an important role in them. Delhi and Jaipur are perfect examples of hybrid communities of this kind (Lestel, Brunois, and Gaunet 2006, 156), where interspecies dependency binds people and animals together in their "cooperating and struggling" with wider social, political, historical, and economic processes (Sanders and Arluke 1993, 386).

As the Smart Cities website explains, there is more than one way to define a smart city, and thus no need to emulate the standardized concepts of modernity and development that are imported from the Global North. To the contrary—especially in this unprecedented historical moment, in which the human species in general but developed countries in particular have been presented with an environmental bill that we do not know how to pay—a country like India could potentially make a critical difference in our communal future. Sea level rise, rapid urbanization, overpopulation, heatwaves, pollution, desertification, water depletion, species extinction, deforestation, and many other grave threats of the Anthropocene suggest a dismal outlook for our fragile planet. Yet demographically young, ambitious, and suffused with *jugaad* as it is, India could set an example of how to minimize and mitigate the damage. The country is already leading the way in developing renewable energy. There is no reason why it could not do the same with interspecies relations and controlling rabies. This would require taking a clear moral stand on fundamental issues such as unity, equity, and empathy. If we are to control and manage rabies and other zoonotic diseases, these values must be extended to animals as well as humans, and India could provide real inspiration in this respect. As Natalie Porter puts it, the configuration of zoonoses involves "how humans should conduct themselves in the name of an existence they share with other species" (2013, 133).

India also has a unique resource to draw on: its outstanding cultural heritage in ethics, nonviolence, and environmental respect, which makes this country one of the few in the world to mandate compassion for nonhuman animals in its very constitution. This attitude of tolerance and inclusion is reflected in a saying I heard several times in India that embodies the country's pride in the diversity of its population: "Despite the thumb being the thickest and the most prominent digit, can you imagine how weak and ugly the hand would be with five thumbs? This is why all our fingers are different." Now that many people in India consider intolerance an issue of growing concern (Amnesty International 2017), and given that the country ranks sixtieth in the Inclusive Development Index, an annual assessment of 103 countries' economic performance (World Economic Forum 2017), it has never been more urgent that we find an answer to this question of how, as individuals and as members of the most influential animal species on the planet—for better or worse—we should share it with others, be they humans or animals. India has the potential to lead the way, by modeling the interspecies camaraderie that is our best hope of eliminating the suffering caused by rabies and other zoonotic diseases.

REFERENCES

Abbas, Syed S., and Manish Kakkar. 2013a. "Research and Policy Disconnect: The Case of Rabies Research in India." *Indian Journal of Medical Research* 138:560–61.

———. 2013b. "Systems Thinking Needed for Rabies Control." *Lancet* 381 (9862): 200. https://doi.org/10.1016/S0140-6736(13)60082-3.

Abedi, Ali J., Samreen Khan, Saira Mehnaz, and Athar M. Ansari. 2017. "Open Garbage Dumps and Knowledge of Rabies Among Sanitary Workers." *International Journal of Community Medicine and Public Health* 4 (5): 1722–26.

Abela-Ridder, Bernadette. 2015. "Rabies: 100 Per Cent Fatal, 100 Per Cent Preventable." *Veterinary Record* 177:148–49.

Adak, Baishali. 2019a. "In Injectable Contraceptive, Forest Dept Finds a Solution to Control Monkey Menace." *Hindustan Times*, April 27.

———. 2019b. "Project to Cut Waste Burden on Ghazipur Landfill Begins." *Hindustan Times*, September 20.

Agarwal, Nitish, and V. P. Reddajah. 2004. "Epidemiology of Dog Bites: A Community-Based Study in India." *Tropical Doctor* 34:76–78.

Agarwal, Siddharth, and Shivani Taneja. 2005. "All Slums Are Not Equal: Child Health Conditions Among the Urban Poor." *Indian Paediatrics* 42 (3): 233–44.

Agoramoorthy, Govindasamy. 2007. "Avoid Using Caste Names for India's Beasts." *Down to Earth*, January. https://www.downtoearth.org.in/blog/avoid-using-caste-names-for-indias-beasts-5480.

Ahmad, Sohail, and Mack J. Choi. 2011. "The Context of Uncontrolled Urban Settlements in Delhi." *ASIEN: The German Journal on Contemporary Asia* 118:75–90.

Akhtar, Aysha. 2012. *Animals and Public Health: Why Treating Animals Better Is Critical to Human Welfare.* Basingstoke: Palgrave Macmillan.

Alley, Kelly D. 1998. "Images of Waste and Purification on the Banks of the Ganga." *City and Society* 10 (1): 167–92.

Amnesty International. 2017. *Annual Report.* London: Amnesty International.

Anand, Cinthya. 2017. "Researchers Find Evidence of Rabies Virus in Indian Bats." *Hindu*, April 3.

Anderson, Aaron, and Stephanie Shwiff. 2013. "The Cost of Canine Rabies on Four Continents." *Transboundary and Emerging Diseases* 62:446–52.

Anderson, David C., ed. 2007. *Assessing the Human-Animal Bond: A Compendium of Actual Measures.* West Lafayette: Purdue University Press.

Aparnavi, P., Geeta Pardeshi, Neelam Roy, Anita Verma, Timiresh Das, and Sunil K. Singh. 2019. "Monkey Bite Menace in a Village in South Delhi." *APCRI Journal* 20 (11): 40–45.

APCRI (Association for Prevention and Control of Rabies in India). 2004. *Assessing Burden of Rabies in India.* Bangalore: APCRI.

———. 2018. *Indian Multicentric Rabies Survey—2017.* Bangalore: APCRI.

Aptekar, Lewis. 1994. "Street Children in the Developing World: A Review of Their Condition." *Cross-Cultural Resources* 28 (3): 195–224.

Aradhak, Purusharth. 2012. "Cow Gores 62-Year-Old in Indirapuram." *Times of India*, August 25.

Arora, Honey. 2013. "Study on Street Children in Jaipur City, Rajasthan." PhD diss., IIHMR University, Jaipur.

AWBI (Animal Welfare Board of India). 2009. *Standard Operating Procedures for the Sterilization of Stray Dogs*. Chennai: AWBI.

———. 2016. *Revised Module for Street Dog Population Management, Rabies Eradication, Reducing Man-Dog Conflict*. Chennai: AWBI.

———. N.d. *Animal Birth Control for Dogs*. Chennai: AWBI.

Aytekin, Ismail, and Nuri Mamak. 2009. "A Case of Rabies in a Cow." *Journal of Animal and Veterinary Advances* 8 (12): 2760–62.

Babb, Lawrence A. 1970. "The Food of the Gods in Chhattisgarh: Some Structural Features of Hindu Ritual." *South-Western Journal of Anthropology* 26 (3): 287–304.

Babu, Ramesh. 2016. "Political Party Workers Kill Stray Dogs, Parade Carcasses in Kerala." *Hindustan Times*, September 27.

Baer, Hans A., Merrill Singer, Debbi Long, and Pamela Erickson. 2016. "Rebranding Our Field? Toward an Articulation of Health Anthropology." *Current Anthropology* 57 (4): 494–510.

Bardosh, Kevin L. 2014. "Global Aspirations, Local Realities: The Role of Social Science Research in Controlling Neglected Tropical Diseases." *Infectious Diseases of Poverty* 3 (35). https://doi.org/10.1186/2049-9957-3-35.

Barry, Ellen. 2015. "For Obama's Visit, India Takes a Broom to Stray Monkeys and Cows." *New York Times*, January 23.

Basham, Arthur L. (1954) 1993. *The Wonder That Was India: A Survey of the Culture of the Indian Sub-Continent Before the Coming of the Muslims*. Delhi: Rupa.

Bateson, Gregory. 1979. *Mind and Nature: A Necessary Unity*. New York: E. P. Dutton.

Battaglia, Luisella. 2002. *Alle origini dell'etica ambientale: Uomo, natura, animali in Voltaire, Michelet, Thoreau, Gandhi*. Bari: Dedalo Edizioni.

Baviskar, Amita. 2004. "Between Violence and Desire: Space, Power, and Identity in the Making of Metropolitan Delhi." *International Social Science Journal* 55 (175): 89–98.

———. 2011a. "Cows, Cars, and Cycle-Rickshaws: Bourgeois Environmentalism and the Battle for Delhi's Streets." In *Elite and Everyman: The Cultural Politics of the Indian Middle Classes*, edited by Amita Baviskar and Raka Ray, 391–449. Delhi: Routledge.

———. 2011b. "What the Eye Does Not See: The Yamuna in the Imagination of Delhi." *Economic and Political Weekly* 46 (50): 45–53.

Baynes-Rock, Marcus. 2013. "Life and Death in the Multispecies Commons." *Social Science Information* 52 (2): 210–27.

———. 2015. *Among the Bone Eaters: Encounters with Hyenas in Harar*. University Park: Pennsylvania State University Press.

Beck, Alan M. 1973. *The Ecology of Stray Dogs: A Study of Free-Ranging Urban Animals*. Baltimore: York Press.

———. 1991. "The Epidemiology and Prevention of Animal Bites." *Seminars in Veterinary Medicine and Surgery (Small Animal)* 6:185–91.

Beck, Alan M., and Barbara Jones. 1985. "Unreported Dog Bite in Children." *Public Health Reports* 10:315–21.

Béteille, Andre. 2001. "The Indian Middle Class." *Hindu*, February 5.

———. 2011. "The Social Character of the Indian Middle Class." In *Middle Class Values in India and Western Europe*, edited by Imtiaz Ahmad and Helmut Reifeld, 73–85. Delhi: Social Science Press.

Bhaktivedanta Swami Prabhupada, A. C. 1986. *Bhagavad-Gita as It Is*. Los Angeles: Bhaktivedanta Book Trust.

Bhan, Gautam. 2009. "'This Is No Longer the City I Once Knew': Evictions, the

Urban Poor, and the Right to the City in Millennial Delhi." *Environment and Urbanization* 21 (1): 127–42.

Bharti, Omesh K. 2015. "Immunizing Vulnerable Populations Like Rag Pickers, Garbage Collectors, Municipality Workers, and Newspaper Hawkers Against Rabies in Shimla Municipality, HP, India." *World Journal of Vaccines* 5:19–24.

Bhasin, Ruhi. 2009. "Just 32% of 2.6 Lakh City Dogs Sterilized: Census." *Times of India*, October 11.

Bhatnagar, Gaurav V. 2013. "The Monkey Menace." *Hindu*, January 27.

Bhattacharyya, Narendra N. 2001. *A Dictionary of Indian Mythology*. Delhi: Munshiram Manoharlal.

Bhishagratna, Kaviraj K. L. 1991. *An English Translation of the Sushruta Samhita*. Varanasi: Chowkhamba Sanskrit Series Office.

Biehler, Dawn D. 2013. *Pests in the City: Flies, Bedbugs, Cockroaches, and Rats*. Seattle: University of Washington Press.

Bögel, Konrad, and François-Xavier Meslin. 1990. "Economics for Human and Canine Rabies Elimination: Guidelines for Programme Orientation." *Bulletin of the World Health Organization* 68 (3): 261–91.

Bollée, Willem. 2006. *Gone to the Dogs in Ancient India*. Munich: Verlag der Bayerischen Akademie der Wissenschaften.

Boulger, L. R. 1966. "Natural Rabies in a Laboratory Monkey." *Lancet* 287 (7444): 941–43.

Bradley, Theresa, and Ritchie King. 2012. "The Dog Economy Is Global, but What Is the World's True Canine Capital?" *Atlantic*, November 13.

Briggs, Charles. 2016. "Ecologies of Evidence in a Mysterious Epidemic." *Medicine Anthropology Theory* 3 (2): 149–62.

Briggs, Charles, and Clara Mantini-Briggs. 2016. *Tell Me Why My Children Died: Rabies, Indigenous Knowledge, and Communicative Justice*. Durham: Duke University Press.

Brighter Green. 2012. "Veg or Non-Veg? India at the Crossroads." Brighter Green Food Policy and Equity Program Policy Paper. https://www.brightergreen.org /files/india_bg_pp_2011.pdf.

Brookes, Victoria J., Gurlal S. Gill, Bhupinder S. Sandhu, Navneet K. Dhand, Rabinder S. Aulakh, and Michael P. Ward. 2019. "Challenges to Human Rabies Elimination Highlighted Following a Rabies Outbreak in Bovines and a Human in Punjab, India." *Zoonoses and Public Health* 66:325–36.

Brown, Hannah, and Ann H. Kelly. 2014. "Material Proximities and Hotspots: Toward an Anthropology of Viral Hemorrhagic Fevers." *Medical Anthropology Quarterly* 28:280–303.

Brown, Peter J., Marcia C. Inhorn, and Daniel J. Smith. 1996. "Disease, Ecology, and Human Behavior." In *Medical Anthropology: Contemporary Theory and Method*, edited by Carolyn F. Sargent and Thomas M. Johnson, 183–218. Westport: Praeger.

Bunce, Fredrick W. 2000. *An Encyclopaedia of Hindu Deities, Demi-Gods, Godlings, Demons, and Heroes*. Delhi: D. K. Printworld.

Burgat, Florence. 2004. "Non-Violence Towards Animals in the Thinking of Gandhi: The Problem of Animal Husbandry." *Journal of Agricultural and Environmental Ethics* 14:223–48.

Butler, J. R. A., and Johan T. du Toit. 2002. "Diet of Free-Ranging Dogs (*Canis familiaris*) in Rural Zimbabwe: Implications for Wild Scavengers on the Periphery of Wildlife Reserves." *Animal Conservation* 5 (1): 29–37.

Campbell, Joseph. 1974. *The Mythic Image*. Princeton: Princeton University Press.

Camperio-Ciani, Andrea. 1986. "Intertroop Agonistic Behavior of a Feral Rhesus Macaque Troop Ranging in Town and Forest Areas in India." *Aggressive Behavior* 12 (6): 433–39.

Candea, Matei. 2010. "I Fell in Love with Carlos the Meerkat: Engagement and Detachment in Human-Animal Relations." *American Ethnologist* 37 (2): 241–58.

CDC (Centers for Disease Control). 1988. "Imported Human Rabies—Australia 1987." *Morbidity and Mortality Weekly Report* 37 (22): 351–53. https://www.cdc .gov/mmwr/preview/mmwrhtml /00000037.htm.

Centre for Science and Environment. 2016. *Not in My Backyard: Solid Waste Management in Indian Cities*. Delhi: Centre for Science and Environment.

Chakravartty, Anupam. 2015. "Out of Control: Why Monkeys Are a Menace." *Down to Earth*, August 31, 24–28. https://www.downtoearth.org.in /coverage/wildlife-biodiversity/out -of-control-why-monkeys-are-a -menace-50817.

Chandra, Hem, Arvind V. Rinkoo, Leela Masih, and K. Jamalluddin. 2011. "Government of Uttar Pradesh State of India: Assisted 'Kamadhenu' Project." *Journal of Financial Management and Analysis* 24 (1): 73–83.

Chandran, R., and P. A. Azeez. 2016. "Stray Dog Menace: Implications and Management." *Economic and Political Weekly* 51 (48): 58–65.

Chapple, Christopher Key. 1993. *Nonviolence to Animals, Earth, and Self in Asian Traditions*. New York: SUNY Press.

Chatterjee, Partha. 2004. *The Politics of the Governed: Reflections on Popular Politics in Most of the World*. New York: Columbia University Press.

Chaudhuri, Nirad C. 1951. *The Autobiography of an Unknown Indian*. London: Macmillan.

Chaudhuri, Sumanta R. 2019. "2 Women Suspected of Killing 16 Puppies in Kolkata, Video Sparks Outrage." *Hindustan Times*, January 14.

Chauhan, Anita, and Raghubir S. Pirta. 2010. "Agonistic Interactions Between Humans and Two Species of Monkeys in Shimla, Himachal Pradesh." *Journal of Psychology* 1 (1): 9–14.

Chauhan, Pratibha, and Girdhareelal Saini. 2013. "Study of Profile of Animal Bite Victims Attending Anti-Rabies Clinic at Jodhpur." *International Journal of Medical Science and Public Health* 2 (4): 1088–91.

Chhabra, Mala, Rattan L. Ichhpujani, K. N. Tewari, and Shiv Lal. 2004. "Human Rabies in Delhi." *Indian Journal of Pediatrics* 71 (3): 217–20. https://doi .org/10.1007/BF02724273.

Chigateri, Shraddha. 2011. "Negotiating the 'Sacred' Cow: Cow Slaughter and the Regulation of Difference in India." In *Democracy, Religious Pluralism, and the Liberal Dilemma of Accommodation*, edited by Monica Mookherjee, 137–59. Heidelberg: Springer.

Chinnaian, Sivagurunathan, Gopalakrishnan Sekaran, Umadevi Ramachandran, Rama Ravi, and Mohan K. Pandurangan. 2015. "Taboos Related to Dog Bite in an Urban Area of Kancheepuram District of Tamil Nadu, India." *Journal of Clinical and Diagnostic Research* 9 (7): 11–14.

Chohan, S. S. 2013. *Standard Operating Procedure*. Carterpuri: Kamdhenu Dham Nagar Nigam Gaushala.

Choudhary, Amit A. 2016. "Supreme Court to Fix Harsh Penalty for Killing Strays." *Times of India*, May 13.

Cleaveland, Sarah, Felix Lankester, Sunny E. Townsend, Tiziana Lembo, and Katie Hampson. 2014. "Rabies Control and Elimination: A Test Case for One Health." *Veterinary Record* 175:188–93.

Coffey, Diane, Aashish Gupta, Payal Hathi, Nidhi Khurana, Dean Spears, Nikhil Srivastav, and Sangita Vyas. 2014. "Revealed Preference for Open Defecation: Evidence from a New

Survey in Rural North India." *Economic and Political Weekly* 49 (38): 43–55.

Coffey, Diane, Aashish Gupta, Payal Hathi, Dean Spears, Nikhil Srivastav, and Sangita Vyas. 2017. "Understanding Open Defecation in Rural India: Untouchability, Pollution, and Latrine Pits." *Economic and Political Weekly* 52 (1): 59–66.

CPCB (Central Pollution Control Board). 2006. *Water Quality Status of the Yamuna River.* Delhi: CPCB.

Crooke, William. 1984. *An Introduction to the Popular Religion and Folklore of Northern India.* Agra: Government Press of the North-Western Provinces and Oudh.

Dandona, Lalit, Yegnanarayana S. Sivan, Mukkamala N. Jyothi, V. S. Udaya Bhaskar, and Rakhi Dandona. 2004. "The Lack of Public Health Research Output from India." *BMC Public Health* 4 (55). https://doi.org/10.1186/1471-2458-4-55.

Das, Ayaskant. 2015. "Disabled Boy Dies in Monkey Attack." *Times of India*, May 8.

Das, Debasis, Arnab K. Mandal, Sujash Halder, Jayati Das, Bidyut Bandyopadhyay, and Somnath Naskar. 2015. "Pattern of Injuries Caused by Animal and Management Among Patients Attending at Out-Patient Department of a Rural Medical College, West Bengal, India." *Journal of Dental and Medical Sciences* 14 (4): 55–59.

Das, S. M., and B. D. Sharma. 1980. "Observations on a Remarkable Association of the Rhesus Monkey (*Macaca mulatta villosa*) with the Himalayan Langur (*Presbytis entellus schistaceus*) in the Kumaun Himalayas, India." *Wissenschaftliche Kurzmitteilungen* 45:124–25.

Dave, Naisargi N. 2014. "Witness: Humans, Animals, and the Politics of Becoming." *Cultural Anthropology* 29 (3): 433–56. https://doi.org/10.14506/ca29.3.01.

———. 2017. "Something, Everything, Nothing; or, Cows, Dogs, and Maggots." *Social Text* 35 (1): 37–57. https://doi.org/10.1215/01642472-3727984.

Davis, Mike. 2006. *Planet of Slums.* London: Verso.

Debroy, Bibek. 2008. *Sarama and Her Children: The Dog in Indian Myth.* Delhi: Penguin.

Deccan Chronicle. 2016. "Hundreds of Cows Starve to Death in Rajasthan Shelter as Caretakers on Strike." August 6.

Deccan Herald. 2012. "Monkey Bite Kills Nine-Year-Old Girl." February 19.

Degeling, Chris, Zohar Lederman, and Melanie Rock. 2016. "Culling and the Common Good: Re-Evaluating Harms and Benefits Under the One Health Paradigm." *Public Health Ethics* 9 (3): 244–54.

Delhi Tourism and Transportation Development Corporation. 2010. *CWG Guide to Delhi.* Delhi: Delhi Tourism and Transportation Development Corporation.

Del Rio Vilas, Victor J., Mary J. Freire de Carvalho, Marco A. N. Vigilato, Felipe Rocha, Alexandra Vokaty, Julio A. Pompei, Baldomero Molina Flores, Natael Fenelon, and Ottorino Cosivi. 2017. "Tribulations of the Last Mile: Sides from a Regional Program." *Frontiers in Veterinary Science* 4 (4). https://doi.org/10.3389/fvets.2017.00004.

Deshpande, Satish. 2003. *Contemporary India: A Sociological View.* Delhi: Viking.

Devi, Oinam S., and P. K. Saikia. 2008. "Human-Monkey Conflict: A Case Study at Gauhati University Campus, Jalukbari, Kamrup, Assam." *Zoo's Print: Communicating Science for Conservation* 23 (2): 15–18.

Dey, Sushmi. 2018. "India's Health Spend Just over 1% of GDP." *Times of India*, June 20.

———. 2019. "Acute Shortage of Anti-Rabies Vaccine Could Trigger Ban on Export of Drug." *Times of India*, April 4.

Dhama, Kuldeep, Rajesh Rathore, R. S. Chauhan, and Simmi Tomar. 2005. "Panchgavya (Cowpathy): An Overview." *International Journal of Cow Science* 1 (1): 1–15.

Dickey, Sara. 2000. "Permeable Homes: Domestic Service, Household Space, and the Vulnerability of Class Boundaries in Urban India." *American Ethnologist* 27 (2): 462–89.

Dickman, Amy J. 2010. "Complexities of Conflict: The Importance of Considering Social Factors for Effectively Resolving Human-Wildlife Conflict." *Animal Conservation* 13:458–66.

Dittus, Wolfgang P. J., Sunil Gunathilake, and Melissa Felder. 2019. "Assessing Public Perceptions and Solutions to Human-Monkey Conflict from Fifty Years in Sri Lanka." *Folia Primatologica* 90:89–108.

Dogra, Chander S., and Pramila N. Phatarphekar. 2004. "State in Monkey's Shadow." *Outlook*, September 27. https://www.outlookindia.com/magazine/story/state-in-monkeys-shadow/225254.

Donaldson, Sue, and Will Kymlicka. 2012. *Zoopolis: A Political Theory on Animal Rights*. Oxford: Oxford University Press.

Doniger O'Flaherty, Wendy. 1976. *The Origins of Evil in Hindu Mythology*. Berkeley: University of California Press.

Douglas, Mary. 1966. *Purity and Danger: An Analysis of Concepts of Pollution and Taboo*. London: Routledge.

Down to Earth. 2000a. "The Great Divide." June. https://www.downtoearth.org.in/coverage/the-great-divide-18236.

———. 2000b. "Pollution of Hinduism." February 15. https://www.downtoearth.org.in/coverage/pollution-of-hinduisim-17622.

———. 2016. "Waste Smart Cities." June. https://www.downtoearth.org.in/coverage/waste/waste-smart-cities-54119.

———. 2019a. "Centre Asks NDDB to Estimate India's Milk Demand." January. https://www.downtoearth.org.in/news/agriculture/centre-asks-nddb-to-estimate-india-s-milk-demand-62778.

———. 2019b. "India's Cow Crisis, Part 1: Nepal Bears the Brunt of India's Cow Vigilantism." January. https://www.downtoearth.org.in/news/agriculture/india-s-cow-crisis-part-1-nepal-bears-the-brunt-of-india-s-cow-vigilantism-62703.

Dutta, Himangshu. 2012. "Man Versus Monkey." *Current Science* 103 (7): 760.

Dwivedi, Bhojraj. 2006. *Religious Basis of Hindu Beliefs*. Delhi: Diamond Pocket Books.

Dwivedi, Vikash, Manohar Bhatia, and Ashok Mishra. 2016. "Profile of Patients Attending Anti Rabies Clinic at Madhav Dispensary, JA Group of Hospitals, Gwalior." *Asian Pacific Journal of Health Sciences* 3 (1): 99–103.

Economic Times. 2016. "India Short of 500,000 Doctors, Bodies on Shoulders Reminders of Health Crisis." September 1.

———. 2019a. "Delhi Planning to Club Old Age Home with Cow Shelter." January 10.

———. 2019b. "MP: Two Dalit Kids Beaten to Death for Open Defecation." September 26.

Edamaruku, Sanal. 2001. "The 'Monkey-Man' in Delhi: A First-Hand Report on How the Rationalists Stopped the Mass Mania." *Rationalist International Bulletin* 72 (May 23).

Evans, Martin. 2010. "Trained Monkeys Guard Athletes at Commonwealth Games." *Telegraph* (UK), September 28.

Ex-Commissioner. 1880. *Destruction of Life by Snakes, Hydrophobia, etc. in Western India*. London: W. H. Allen.

Farmer, Paul. 1992. *AIDS and Accusation: Haiti and the Geography of Blame*. Berkeley: University of California Press.

Favero, Paolo. 2005. *India Dreams: Cultural Identity Among Young Middle Class Men in New Delhi*. Stockholm: Stockholm University Press.

Fernandes, Leela. 2000. "Restructuring the New Middle Class in Liberalizing India."

Comparative Studies of South Asia, Africa, and the Middle East 20 (1–2): 88–112.

———. 2004. "The Politics of Forgetting in India: Class Politics, State Power, and the Restructuring of Urban Space in India." *Urban Studies* 41 (12): 2415–30.

———. 2011. "Hegemony and Inequality: Theoretical Reflections on India's 'New' Middle Class." In *Elite and Everyman: The Cultural Politics of the Indian Middle Classes*, edited by Amita Baviskar and Raka Ray, 58–82. Delhi: Routledge.

FIAPO (Federation of Indian Animal Protection Organizations). 2016. *State of Dairy Cattle—Rajasthan.* November 18. Delhi: FIAPO.

———. 2017a. *Rabies Free India—Kerala.* Delhi: FIAPO.

———. 2017b. *Rabies Free Kerala Programme.* Delhi: FIAPO.

———. 2018a. *Cattle-Ogue.* Delhi: FIAPO.

———. 2018b. *Gau Gaatha.* Delhi: FIAPO.

Fitzpatrick, Meagan C., Hiral A. Shah, Abhishek Pandey, Alyssa M. Bilinski, Manish Kakkar, Andrew D. Clark, Jeffrey P. Townsend, Syed S. Abbas, and Alison P. Galvani. 2016. "One Health Approach to Cost-Effective Rabies Control in India." *Proceedings of the National Academy of Sciences* 113 (51): 14574–81.

Foucault, Michel. 2010. *The Birth of Biopolitics: Lectures at the Collège de France, 1978–1979.* New York: Palgrave Macmillan.

Freed, Stanley A., and Ruth S. Freed. 1981. "Sacred Cows and Water Buffalo in India: The Uses of Ethnography." *Current Anthropology* 225 (5): 483–502.

FSSAI (Food Safety and Standards Authority of India). 2011. *National Survey on Milk Adulteration.* Delhi: FSSAI.

Fuentes, Agustín. 2006. "Human Culture and Monkey Behavior: Assessing the Contexts of Potential Pathogen Transmission Between Macaques and Humans." *American Journal of Primatology* 68:880–96.

———. 2009. "Re-Situating Anthropological Approaches to the Evolution of Human Behavior." *Anthropology Today* 25 (3): 12–17.

———. 2010. "Naturalcultural Encounters in Bali: Monkeys, Temples, Tourists, and Ethnoprimatology." *Cultural Anthropology* 25 (4): 600–624.

Fuentes, Agustín, and Marcus Baynes-Rock. 2017. "Anthropogenic Landscapes, Human Action, and the Process of Co-Construction with Other Species: Making Anthromes in the Anthropocene." *Land* 6 (1). https://doi.org/10.3390/land6010015.

Fuentes, Agustín, and Scott Gamerl. 2005. "Disproportionate Participation by Age/Sex Classes in Aggressive Interactions Between Long-Tailed Macaques (*Macaca fascicularis*) and Human Tourists at Padangtegal Monkey Forest, Bali, Indonesia." *American Journal of Primatology* 66:197–204.

Fuentes, Agustín, and Kimberley J. Hockings. 2010. "The Ethnoprimatological Approach in Ethnoprimatology." *American Journal of Primatology* 72 (10): 841–47.

Gaikwad, Bhaskar, Pramod Kulkarni, Anant Takalkar, Mukund Bhise, and Sarita Mantri. 2016. "Dog Bite and Its Management: Awareness Among the First Year Students of a Medical College." *Journal of Basic and Clinical Research* 3 (2): 18–23.

Gandhi, Ajay. 2012. "Catch Me If You Can: Monkey Capture in Delhi." *Ethnography* 13 (1): 43–56.

Gandhi, Ajay, and Lotte Hoek. 2012. "Introduction to Crowds and Conviviality: Ethnographies of the South Asian City." *Ethnography* 13 (1): 3–11.

Gandhi, Mohandas K. 1926a. "Is This Humanity?" *Young India*, November 4.

———. 1926b. "Is This Humanity? V." *Young India*, November 11.

Gandhiok, Jasjeev. 2018. "Asola Sanctuary Spends Rs 8 Lakh/Month to Feed Simians." *Times of India*, January 17.

GARC (Global Alliance for Rabies Control). N.d. "GARC Releases Statement on Dog Culling for Rabies Control." https:// rabiesalliance.org/news/garc-releases -statement-dog-culling-rabies-control.

GARC and RIA (Rabies in Asia). 2012. *Adopt a Village: A Rural Rabies Prevention Project*. Bangalore: Kempegowda Institute of Medical Sciences.

Garg, Abhinav. 2012a. "Check Stray Cattle, Illegal Dairies: HC." *Times of India*, May 11.

———. 2012b. "NDMC Told to Halt Drive Against Mongrels in Lodhi Garden." *Times of India*, August 18.

Garg, Sudhi R. 2014. *Rabies in Man and Animals*. Delhi: Springer.

Gatade, Subhash. 2015. "Silencing Caste, Sanitising Oppression: Understanding Swachh Bharat Abhiyan." *Economic and Political Weekly* 50 (44): 29–35.

Gautret, Philippe, Jesse D. Blanton, Laurent Dacheux, Florence Ribadeau-Dumas, Philippe Brouqui, Philippe Parola, Douglas H. Esposito, and Hervé Bourhy. 2014. "Rabies in Nonhuman Primates and Potential for Transmission to Humans: A Literature Review and Examination of Selected French National Data." *PLOS Neglected Tropical Diseases* 8 (5). https://doi.org/10.1371 /journal.pntd.0002863.

Geertz, Clifford. 1973. "Thick Description: Toward an Interpretive Theory of Culture." In *The Interpretation of Cultures: Selected Essays*, 310–23. New York: Basic Books.

George, Nirmala. 2011. "India Weddings Faulted for Prodigious Food Waste." *Huffington Post*, July 21.

Geruso, Michael, and Dean Spears. 2015. "Neighborhood Sanitation and Infant Mortality." National Bureau of Economic Research, Cambridge, Massachusetts, Working Paper 21184. https://www.nber .org/papers/w21184.pdf.

Ghertner, Asher D. 2008. "Analysis of New Legal Discourse Behind Delhi's Slum Demolitions." *Economic and Political Weekly* 43 (20): 57–66.

Ghosal, Aniruddha. 2012. "Phobia Makes Hospital Spend Third of Budget on Rabies Vaccines." *Times of India*, October 13.

Ghosal, Aniruddha, and Purusharth Aradhak. 2013. "Stray Bull Gores Man to Death." *Times of India*, March 23.

Gibson, Andrew D., Stella Mazeri, Gowri Yale, Santosh Desai, Vilas Naik, Julie Corfmat, Steffen Ortmann, et al. 2019. "Development of a Non-Meat-Based, Mass Producible, and Effective Bait for Oral Vaccination of Dogs Against Rabies in Goa State, India." *Tropical Medicine and Infectious Disease* 4 (3): 118. https:// doi.org/10.3390/tropicalmed4030118.

Gilchrist, Julie, Jeffrey J. Sacks, Dionne White, and Marcie-Jo Kresnow. 2008. "Dog Bites: Still a Problem?" *Injury Prevention* 14:296–301.

Gill, Gurlal S., Balbir B. Singh, Navneet K. Dhand, Rabinder S. Aulakh, Bhupinder S. Sandhu, Michael P. Ward, and Victoria J. Brookes. 2019. "Estimation of the Incidence of Animal Rabies in Punjab, India." *PLOS One* 14 (9). https:// doi.org/10.1371/journal.pone.0222198.

Global Interfaith WASH Alliance. 2014. "The Yamuna River: Life and Death of a Principal Waterway." http://washalli ance.org/wp-content/uploads/2016/08 /Yamuna-River-Lifz-and-Death-of-a -Principal-Waterway.pdf.

GNCTD (Government of the National Capital Territory of Delhi). 2001. "Evaluation Study Report on Seven Gau-Sadans Functioning in Delhi." Delhi: GNCTD.

———. 2014. *Statistical Abstract of Delhi*. Delhi: GNCTD.

———. 2018. "Animal Health and Welfare Policy." Delhi: GNCTD.

Gompper, Matthew E. 2013a. "The Dog-Human-Wildlife Interface: Assessing the Scope of the Problem." In *Free-Ranging*

Dogs and Wildlife Conservation, edited by Matthew E. Gompper, 9–54. Oxford: Oxford University Press.

———, ed. 2013b. *Free-Ranging Dogs and Wildlife Conservation*. Oxford: Oxford University Press.

Government of India. 2011. *Fifteenth Indian Census*. Delhi: Directorate of Census Operations.

Govindrajan, Radhika. 2015. "Monkey Business: Macaque Translocation and the Politics of Belonging in India's Central Himalayas." *Comparative Studies of South Asia, Africa, and the Middle East* 35 (2): 246–62.

———. 2018. *Animal Intimacies: Interspecies Relatedness in India's Central Himalayas*. Chicago: University of Chicago Press.

Greater Kashmir. 2013. "Infant's Killing by Dogs Human Rights Violation: SHRC." September 25.

Grover, Michael, Paul R. Bessel, Anne Conan, Pim Polak, Claude T. Sabeta, Bjorn Reininghaus, and Darryn L. Knobel. 2018. "Spatiotemporal Epidemiology of Rabies at an Interface Between Domestic Dogs and Wildlife in South Africa." *Scientific Reports* 8: 1–8. https://www.nature.com/articles/s41598-018-29045-x.pdf.

Guha, Dina S. 1985. "Food in the Vedic Tradition." *Food Culture* 12 (2): 141–52.

Gupta, Anjali. 2012. "Social Determinants of Health: Street Children at Crossroads." *Health* 4 (9): 634–43.

Gupta, Charu. 2001. "The Icon of Mother in Late Colonial North India: 'Bharat Mata,' 'Matri Bhasha,' and 'Gau Mata.'" *Economic and Political Weekly* 36 (45): 4291–99.

Gupta, Dipankar. 2000. *Mistaken Modernity: India Between Worlds*. Delhi: Harper Collins.

Gupta, Moushumi D. 2016. "Delhi Development Authority Should Be a Facilitator, Not Just Developer." *Hindustan Times*, October 10.

Haidar, Faizan. 2016. "Delhi Govt to Provide 24/7 Toilet Facility in Slums." *Hindustan Times*, October 25.

Halder, Ritam. 2016. "Delhi Dog Census to Rope in Sanitation Workers." *Hindustan Times*, March 22.

Hampson, Katie, Sarah Cleaveland, and Deborah Briggs. 2011. "Evaluation of Cost-Effective Strategies for Rabies Post-Exposure Vaccination in Low-Income Countries." *PLOS Neglected Tropical Diseases* 5 (3). https://doi.org/10.1371/journal.pntd.0000982.

Hampson, Katie, Laurent Coudeville, Tiziana Lembo, Maganga Sambo, Alexia Kieffer, Michaël Attlan, Jacques Barrat, et al. 2015. "Estimating the Global Burden of Endemic Canine Rabies." *PLOS Neglected Tropical Diseases* 9 (4). https://doi.org/10.1371/journal.pntd.0003709.

Haneef, Mahir. 2015. "Stray Dog Issue: 'God's Own Country' Has Become 'Dog's Own Country,' Says Kerala MLA." *Times of India*, September 28.

Hanlon, Cathleen A., Michael Niezgoda, Patricia A. Morrill, and Charles E. Rupprecht. 2001. "The Incurable Wound Revisited: Progress in Human Rabies Prevention?" *Vaccine* 19:2273–79.

Haraway, Donna. 2003. *The Companion Species Manifesto: Dogs, People, and Significant Otherness*. Chicago: Prickly Paradigm Press.

———. 2008. *When Species Meet*. Minneapolis: University of Minnesota Press.

Harper, Edward. 1964. "Ritual Pollution as an Integrator of Caste and Religion." *Journal of Asian Studies* 23:151–97.

Harris, Nancy, Crystal Davis, Elizabeth Dow Goldman, Rachael Petersen, and Samantha Gibbes. 2018. "Comparing Global and National Approaches to Estimating Deforestation Rates in REDD+ Countries." World Resources Institute Working Paper. Washington, D.C.: World Resources Institute.

Heinrich Boll Foundation. 2014. *Meat Atlas: Facts and Figures About the Animals We Eat*. Berlin: Heinrich Boll Foundation.

Hiby, Lex R., Jack F. Reece, Rachel Wright, Rajan Jaisinghani, Baldev Singh, and Elly F. Hiby. 2011. "A Mark-Resight Survey Method to Estimate the Roaming Dog Population in Three Cities in Rajasthan, India." *BMC Veterinary Research* 7 (August 11). https://doi.org/10.1186/1746-6148-7-46.

Hinchliffe, Steven. 1999. "Cities and Natures: Intimate Strangers." In *Unsettling Cities: Movement/Settlement*, edited by John Allen, Doreen Massey, and Michael Pryke, 137–80. London: Routledge.

———. 2015. "More Than One World, More Than One Health: Re-Configuring Interspecies Health." *Social Science and Medicine* 129:28–35.

Hindu. 2009. "Beware! Delhi Has over 50,000 Quacks." October 4.

———. 2011. "Stray Cattle Menace Still Unchecked." March 28.

———. 2012. "23 Cows Die in Gaushalas Within 48 Hours." September 12.

———. 2014. "29 Stray Dogs Caught from East Delhi Hospitals." September 20.

———. 2015. "Verka to Launch Premium Brand of Milk of Indigenous Cows." December 31.

———. 2016. "Ratan Tata Invests in Pet Care Portal." January 4.

Hindustan Times. 2009. "Bamboo Screens for Slums During Games." August 16.

———. 2013. "New Delhi: Siblings Killed, Left for Animals to Eat." March 2.

———. 2015a. "Over 64K Dog Bite Cases in Delhi, North Delhi Most Affected." December 16.

———. 2015b. "Swachh Bharat Abhiyan Should Aim to Stamp out Manual Scavenging." July 13.

———. 2016a. "70-Year-Old Dies While Trying to Fend off Monkey Attack." February 2.

———. 2016b. "3-Yr-Old Falls to Death While Trying to Ward off Monkey Attack." February 16.

Hirschfeld, Lawrence A. 2002. "Why Don't Anthropologists Like Children?" *American Anthropologist* 104 (2): 611–27.

HLRN (Housing and Land Rights Network). 2010. *The 2010 Commonwealth Games: Whose Wealth? Whose Commons?* Delhi: HLRN.

Houston, Donna, Jean Hillier, Diana MacCallum, Wendy Steele, and Jason Byrne. 2017. "Make Kin, Not Cities! Multispecies Entanglements and 'Becoming-World.'" *Planning Theory* 17 (2): 190–212. https://doi.org/10.1177/1473095216688042.

Human Rights Watch. 2014. "Cleaning Human Waste: 'Manual Scavenging,' Caste, and Discrimination in India." August 25. https://www.hrw.org/report/2014/08/25/cleaning-human-waste/manual-scavenging-caste-and-discrimination-india.

Hundal, Jaspal S., Simrinder S. Sodhi, Aparna Gupta, Jaswinder Singh, and Udeybir S. Chahal. 2016. "Awareness, Knowledge, and Risks of Zoonotic Diseases Among Livestock Farmers in Punjab." *Veterinary World* 9 (2): 186–91.

Hunt, Caroline. 1996. "Child Waste Pickers in India: The Occupation and Its Health Risks." *Environment and Urbanization* 8 (2): 111–18.

IAMR (Institute of Applied Manpower Research), Planning Commission, Government of India. 2012. "India Human Development Report 2011: Towards Social Inclusion." http://www.im4change.org/docs/340IHDR_Summary.pdf.

Ichhpujani, Rattan L., Mala Chhabra, Veena Mittal, Dipesh Bhattacharya, J. Singh, and Shiv Lal. 2006. "Knowledge, Attitude, and Practices About Animal Bites and Rabies in General Community—A Multi-Centric Study."

Journal of Communicable Diseases 38 (4): 355–62.

Ichhpujani, Rattan L., Mala Chhabra, Veena Mittal, J. Singh, Mohan Bhardwaj, Dipesh Bhattacharya, S. K. Pattanaik, et al. 2008. "Epidemiology of Animal Bites and Rabies Cases in India—A Multicentric Study." *Journal of Communicable Diseases* 40 (1): 27–36.

IHD (Institute for Human Development) and Save the Children. 2011. *Surviving the Streets: A Census of Street Children.* Delhi: Save the Children. https:// resourcecentre.savethechildren.net /node/5332/pdf/5332.pdf.

IIPTF (India International Pet Trade Fair). 2013. *India Pet Directory.* Noida: L. B. Associates.

Indian Express. 2016a. "After Strict Law, Haryana Gives Cows 24-Hour Helpline." July 4.

———. 2016b. "Over 1.89 Lakh Stray Dogs in South Delhi, Sterilisation Begins at Brijvasan Centre." December 4.

———. 2016c. "Show Compassion, but Don't Allow Stray Dogs to Become Menace: Supreme Court." September 14.

———. 2017. "Cattle Decline: NGT Seeks Policy to Save Indigenous Cattle Breeds." May 19.

Indian Institute of Public Administration, Centre for Consumer Studies. 2011. *Report on Assessment of Wastage of Food and Ostentatious Behaviour During Social Gatherings in National Capital Region Delhi.* Delhi: Indian Institute of Public Administration.

Ingold, Tim. 2008. "Bindings Against Boundaries: Entanglements of Life in an Open World." *Environment and Planning A* 40 (8): 1796–810.

———. 2011. *Being Alive: Essays on Movement, Knowledge, and Description.* New York: Routledge.

Islam, Kazi M. F., Iqbal Hossain, Shah Jalal, Nurul Quader, Saroj Kumar, Kamrul Islam, Ashif I. Shawn, and Ahasanul Hoque. 2016. "Investigation into Dog Bite in Cattle, Goats, and Dog at Selected Veterinary Hospitals in Bangladesh and India." *Journal of Advanced Veterinary and Animal Research* 3 (3): 252–58.

Isloor, Shrikrishna, Wilfred E. Marissen, B. H. Veeresh, Prabhu K. Nithin, Ivan V. Kuzmin, Charles E. Rupprecht, M. L. Satyanarayana, et al. 2014. "First Case Report of Rabies in a Wolf (*Canis lupus pallipes*) from India." *Journal of Veterinary Medicine and Research* 1 (3): 1012.

Iyer, K. Bharatha. 1977. *Animals in Indian Sculpture.* Mumbai: Taraporevala.

Jackman, Jennifer, and Andrew N. Rowan. 2007. "Free-Roaming Dogs in Developing Countries: The Benefits of Capture, Neuter, and Return Programs." In *The State of the Animals IV: 2007,* edited by Deborah J. Salem and Andrew N. Rowan, 55–78. Washington, D.C.: Humane Society Press.

Jacobsen, Knut A. 2009. *Brill's Encyclopedia of Hinduism.* Leiden: Brill.

Jaffrelot, Christophe. 2008. "Hindu Nationalism and the (Not So Easy) Art of Being Outraged: The Ram Setu Controversy." *South Asia Multidisciplinary Academic Journal* 2. https://doi.org/10.4000/samaj.1372.

Jain, Akanksha. 2014. "NGO Moves HC for Inquiry into Stray Cattle Problem in Delhi." *Hindu,* February 28.

Jain, Bharti. 2015. "Delhi Struggles to Cope with Stray Animal Bites." *Times of India,* December 16.

Jamatia, Hamari. 2013. "Dog Bites on the Rise in North Delhi, Canine Lovers Blame Human Apathy." *Hindustan Times,* March 22.

Jamwal, Nidhi, and Neha Dua. 2003. "The Meat You Eat." *Down to Earth,* August. https://www.downtoearth.org.in /indepth/the-meat-you-eat-13283.

Jamwal, Nidhi, and Farouk Tebbal. 2004. "The Market Usually Decides the Fate of Slum-Dwellers." *Down to Earth,* June.

https://www.downtoearth.org.in
/interviews/the-market-usually
-decides-the-fate-of-slumdwellers-11392.

Jaypal, Renuka. 2006. "Going Digital in
India." *Viewpoint*, May.

Jishnu, Latha. 2014. "Meaty Tales of
Vegetarian India." *Down to Earth*,
December, 36–41. https://www.down
toearth.org.in/coverage/meaty-tales
-of-vegetarian-india-47830.

Jitendra, Sayantan Bera, and Alok Gupta.
2014. "Mission Possible." *Down to Earth*,
February, 30–37.

Joice, Suba Y., Zile Singh, and Shib S.
Datta. 2016. "Knowledge, Attitude, and
Practices Regarding Dog Bite and Its
Management Among Adults in Rural
Tamil Nadu." *International Journal of
Scientific Research* 5 (5): 586–89.

Jones-Engel, Lisa, Gregory A. Engel, John
Heidrich, Mukesh Chalise, Narayan
Poudel, Raphael Viscidi, Peter A.
Barry, Jonathan S. Allan, Richard
Grant, and Randy Kyes. 2006. "Temple
Monkeys and Health Implications of
Commensalism, Kathmandu, Nepal."
Emerging Infectious Diseases 12 (6):
900–906.

Joshi, Mallica, and Soumya Pillai. 2016.
"Life of the Bovine: Delhi Has No Time
for 'Holy' Cows Dying in Shelters."
Hindustan Times, August 11.

Joshi, Rajkumar, and Sirajuddin Ahmed.
2016. "Status and Challenges of
Municipal Solid Waste Management in
India: A Review." *Cogent Environmental
Science* 2 (1). https://doi.org/10.1080/2331
1843.2016.1139434.

Joshi, Sopan. 2000. "Murder Most Foul."
Down to Earth, June.

Joshua, Anita. 2001. "To Catch a Phantom."
Hindu, June 10.

Jyoti, Goel M. Kumar, Brij M. Vashisht,
and Pardeep Khanna. 2010. "Pattern
and Burden of Animal Bite Cases in
a Tertiary Care Hospital in Haryana."
Journal of Communicable Diseases 42 (3):
215–18.

Kakkar, Manish, Vidya Venkataramanan,
Sampath Krishnan, Ritu S. Chauhan,
and Syed S. Abbas. 2012. "Moving from
Rabies Research to Rabies Control:
Lessons from India." *PLOS Neglected
Tropical Diseases* 6 (8). https://doi
.org/10.1371/journal.pntd.0001748.

Kakrani, Vandana A., Sumit Jethani, Jitendra
Bhawalkar, Anjali Dhone, and Karuna
Ratwani. 2013. "Awareness About Dog
Bite Management in Rural Population."
Indian Journal of Community Health 25
(3): 304–8.

Kalra, Sunil Y. 2010. *Road to Commonwealth
Games, 2010*. Delhi: Penguin.

Kappeler, Andreas, and Alexander I.
Wandeler. 1991. *Dog Population Studies
Related to a Vaccination Campaign
Against Rabies in Lalitput City, Nepal*.
Geneva: WHO.

Kapur, Devesh, and Milan Vaishnav. 2014.
"Being Middle Class in India." *Hindu*,
December 9.

Karlekar, Hiranmay. 2008. *Savage Humans
and Stray Dogs: A Study in Aggression*.
Delhi: Sage Publications.

———. 2011a. "ABC of Cruelty Towards
Dogs." *Pioneer*, July 15.

———. 2011b. "Betrayal by the Middle
Classes." *Pioneer*, June 22.

———. 2011c. "Neither Middle nor Class nor
Indian." *Pioneer*, June 22.

Karmakar, Rahul. 2017. "Chilli [*sic*] in
Genitals, Pierced with Nails: How
Cattle Is Smuggled into Bangladesh."
Hindustan Times, July 14.

Kasturirangan, Rajesh, Krithika Srinivasan,
and Smitha Rao. 2014. "Dark and Dairy:
The Sorry Tale of the Milch Animals."
Hindu, November 8.

Kathuria, B. K. 1970. "Studies on Rabies: Its
Epizootology and Diagnosis." *Journal of
Communicable Diseases* 2:1–4.

Kaur, Ravleen. 2010. "Fodder Crisis Raises
Milk Prices." *Down to Earth*, June 30.

Kaushik, Himanshu. 2016. "Veterinary
Doctors Find 100 kg of Garbage

in Cow's Stomach." *Times of India*,
September 3.

Kean, Hilda. 1998. *Animal Rights: Political
and Social Change in Britain Since 1800*.
London: Reaktion Books.

Kesavan, Mukul. 2016. "Before the Change:
When Austerity, Simplicity Ruled
Everyday Middle Class Life." *Hindustan
Times*, July 24.

Kete, Kathleen. 1994. *The Beast in the
Boudoir: Petkeeping in Nineteenth-
Century Paris*. Berkeley: University of
California Press.

Khandelwal, Peeyush. 2012. "Girl Runs to
Fourth Floor to Save Self from Monkeys,
Falls." *Hindustan Times*, May 10.

———. 2014. "Modi Rakes up 'Cow
Slaughter' at Ghaziabad Rally."
Hindustan Times, April 3.

Khanna, Rajeev. 2019. "Himachal Farmers
Now Poisoning Monkeys." *Down To
Earth*, August 29. https://www.down
toearth.org.in/news/wildlife-biodiver
sity/himachal-farmers-now-poisoning
-monkeys-66396.

Khokhar, Anita, G. S. Meena, and Malti
Mehra. 2003. "Profile of Dog Bite
Cases Attending M. C. D. Dispensary
at Alipur, Delhi." *Indian Journal of
Community Medicine* 28 (4): 157–60.

Kipling, John L. 1904. *Beast and Man in
India: A Popular Sketch of Indian
Animals in Their Relations with the
People*. New York: Macmillan.

Kirksey, Eben, and Stefan Helmreich.
2010. "The Emergence of Multispecies
Ethnography." *Cultural Anthropology* 25
(4): 545–76.

Knobel, Darryn L., Sarah Cleaveland, Paul
G. Coleman, Eric M. Fèvre, Martin I.
Meltzer, Mary E. G. Miranda, Alexandra
Shaw, Jakob Zinsstag, and François-
Xavier Meslin. 2005. "Re-Evaluating
the Burden of Rabies in Africa and
Asia." *Bulletin of the World Health
Organization* 83 (5): 360–68.

Knobel, Darryn L., Tiziana Lembo, Michelle
K. Morters, Sunny E. Townsend, Sarah

Cleaveland, and Katie Hampson. 2013.
"Dog Rabies and Its Control." In *Rabies:
Scientific Basis of the Disease and Its
Management*, edited by Alan C. Jackson,
591–615. Oxford: Elsevier Academic
Press.

Korom, Frank J. 2000. "Holy Cow! The
Apotheosis of Zebu, or Why the Cow
Is Sacred in Hinduism." *Asian Folklore
Studies* 59 (2): 181–203.

Kothari, Rajni. 1993. *Growing Amnesia:
An Essay on Poverty and Human
Consciousness*. Delhi: Viking.

Kotwal, Karishma. 2017. "Pet Lovers Seek
Action on Schoolbook 'Teaching' Kids to
Behead Dogs." *Times of India*, March 13.

Kukreti, Ishan. 2018. "India Sees 1.75 Million
Dog Bites Every Year, yet We Face up to
80% Shortage of Anti-Rabies Vaccines."
Down to Earth, August 20. https://www
.downtoearth.org.in/news/health/india
-sees-1-75-million-dog-bites-every-year
-yet-we-face-up-to-80-shortage-of
-anti-rabies-vaccines-61298.

———. 2019. "What Aarey Case Means
for Forest Land Classification." *Down
To Earth*, October. https://www.
downtoearth.org.in/news/
forests/what-aarey-case-means-for-for-
est-land-classification-6713.

Kulkarni, Praveen, Sunil Kumar, Hugara
Siddalingappa, and M. Renuka.
2016. "Effectiveness of Educational
Intervention on Perception Regarding
Rabies Among Women Self Help Group
Members in Urban Mysore, Karnataka,
India." *International Journal of
Community Medicine and Public Health*
3 (5): 1268–72.

Kumar, Abhay, Rishabh K. Rana, Sunil
Kumar, Veena Roy, and Christian Roy.
2013. "Factors Influencing Animal
Bite Cases and Practices Among the
Cases Attending the Anti Rabies
Clinic DMCH, Darbhanga (Bihar)."
*International Journal of Recent Trends in
Science and Technology* 6 (2): 94–97.

Kumar, Arvind, and D. Pal. 2010. "Epidemiology of Human Rabies Cases in Kolkata with Its Application to Post Prophylaxis." *Indian Journal of Animal Research* 44 (4): 241–47.

Kumar, Ashwani. 2013. "Existing Situation of Municipal Solid Waste Management in NCT of Delhi, India." *International Journal of Social Sciences* 1 (1): 6–17.

Kumar, Aswin J. 2017. "Kerala Retains Top Slot in Cattle Slaughter; Bihar 2nd." *Times of India*, April 19.

Kumar, Pradeep. 2016. "Civic Body, PFA Slug It Out over ABC Programme." *Deccan Chronicle*, March 13.

Kumar, Sunil, J. K. Bhattacharyya, A. N. Vaidya, Tapan Chakrabarti, Sukumar Devotta, and Avinash B. Akolkar. 2009. "Assessment of the Status of Municipal Solid Waste Management in Metro Cities, State Capitals, Class I Cities, and Class II Towns in India: An Insight." *Waste Management* 29:883–95.

Kurian, Arun, Premanshu Dandapat, Shija Jacob, and Josephine Francis. 2014. "Ranking of Zoonotic Diseases Using Composite Index Method: An Illustration in Indian Context." *Indian Journal of Animal Sciences* 84 (4): 357–63.

Lahiri, Ashok K. 2015. "Green Politics and the Indian Middle Class." *Economic and Political Weekly* 50 (43): 35–42.

Lal, P., A. Rawat, A. Sagar, and K. N. Tiwari. 2005. "Prevalence of Dog-Bites in Delhi: Knowledge and Practices of Residents Regarding Prevention and Control of Rabies." *Health and Population: Perspectives and Issues* 28 (2): 50–57.

Laland, Kevin N., Tobias Uller, Marcus W. Feldman, Kim Sterelny, Gerd B. Müller, Armin Moczek, Eva Jablonka, and John Odling-Smee. 2015. "The Extended Evolutionary Synthesis: Its Structure, Assumptions, and Predictions." *Proceedings of the Royal Society B* 282. https://doi.org/10.1098/rspb.2015.1019.

Lalwani, Vijayta. 2019. "Ground Report: Killing of Two Dalit Children Exposes Failure of India's Swachh Bharat Abhiyan." *Scroll.in*, September 29. https://scroll.in/article/938766/ground-report-killing-of-two-dalit-children-exposes-failure-of-indias-swachh-bharat-abhiyan.

Laskar, Ananya R., Megha C. Singh, and Sweta S. Saha. 2010. "Gaps in the Knowledge About Advancements in Rabies Vaccines Among the Undergraduate Medical Students." *Journal of Communicable Diseases* 42 (4): 287–90.

Latour, Bruno. 2014. "Agency at the Time of the Anthropocene." *New Literary History* 45:1–18.

Lavan, Robert P., Alasdair I. M. King, David J. Sutton, and Kaan Tunceli. 2017. "Rationale and Support for a One Health Program for Canine Vaccination as the Most Cost-Effective Means of Controlling Zoonotic Rabies in Endemic Settings." *Vaccine* 35 (13): 1668–74.

Lee, Phyllis C., and Nancy E. C. Priston. 2005. "Human Attitudes to Primates: Perceptions of Pests, Conflict, and Consequences for Primate Conservation." In *Commensalism and Conflict: The Human-Primate Interface*, edited by James D. Paterson and Janette Willis, 1–23. Seattle: American Society of Primatologists.

Leslie, Julia. 1989. *The Perfect Wife: The Orthodox Hindu Woman According to the Strīdharmapaddhati of Tryambakayajvan.* Delhi: Oxford University Press.

Lestel, Dominique, Florence Brunois, and Florence Gaunet. 2006. "Towards an Etho-Ethnology and an Ethno-Ethology." *Social Sciences Information* 45:155–77.

Levins, Richard, and Richard Lewontin. 1985. *The Dialectical Biologist.* Cambridge, Mass.: Harvard University Press.

Lévi-Strauss, Claude. 1992. *Tristes Tropiques.* Harmondsworth: Penguin.

Lewis, Martin W. 2016. "Mapping the Consumption of Milk and Meat in India." *Wire,* March 8. https://thewire.in/uncategorised/mapping-the-consumption-of-milk-and-meat-in-india.

Lobo, Lancy, and Jayesh Shah, eds. 2015. *The Trajectory of India's Middle Class: Economy, Ethics, and Etiquette.* Cambridge: Cambridge Scholars.

Lodmell, Donald L., Nancy B. Ray, Michael J. Parnell, Larry C. Ewalt, Cathleen A. Hanlon, John H. Shaddock, Dane S. Sanderlin, and Charles E. Rupprecht. 1998. "DNA Immunization Protects Nonhuman Primates Against Rabies Virus." *Nature Medicine* 4:949–52.

Lodrick, Deryck O. 1980. *Sacred Cows, Sacred Places: Origins and Survivals of Animal Homes in India.* Berkeley: University of California Press.

———. 1987. "Gopashtami and Govardhan Puja: Two Krishna Festivals of India." *Journal of Cultural Geography* 7 (2): 101–16.

———. 2009. "The Sacred and the Profane: The Dog in South Asian Culture." *Man in India* 89 (4): 497–523.

Loudon, James E., Michaela E. Howells, and Agustín Fuentes. 2006. "The Importance of Integrative Anthropology: A Preliminary Investigation Employing Primatological and Cultural Anthropological Data Collection Methods in Assessing Human-Monkey Co-Existence in Bali, Indonesia." *Ecological and Environmental Anthropology* 2 (1): 2–13.

Lowe, Celia. 2010. "Viral Clouds: Becoming H5N1 in Indonesia." *Cultural Anthropology* 25 (4): 625–49. https://doi.org/10.1111/j.1548-1360.2010.01072.x.

Luce, Edward. 2011. *In Spite of the Gods: The Strange Rise of Modern India.* London: Abacus.

Lutgendorf, Philip. 1997. "Monkey in the Middle: The Status of Hanuman in Popular Hinduism." *Religion* 27:311–32.

———. 2001. "Five Heads and No Tale: Hanuman and the Popularization of Tantra." *International Journal of Hindu Studies* 5 (3): 269–94.

Lüthi, Damaris. 2010. "Private Cleanliness, Public Mess: Purity, Pollution, and Space in Kottar, South India." In *Urban Pollution: Cultural Meanings, Social Practices,* edited by Eveline Dürr and Rivke Jaffe, 57–85. New York: Berghahn Books.

Maestripieri, Dario. 2007. *Macachiavellian Intelligence: How Rhesus Macaques and Humans Have Conquered the World.* Chicago: University of Chicago Press.

Mahapatra, Dhananjay. 2009. "A Capital Shame: SC Gets Details of Manual Scavenging in Delhi." *Times of India,* May 10.

———. 2012. "Animals Clean 5 Lakh Toilets, Supreme Court Told." *Times of India,* September 4.

———. 2016. "Dog Bites Killed More Than 2 Terror Attacks." *Times of India,* March 10.

Majumdar, Boria, and Nalin Mehta. 2010. *Sellotape Legacy: Delhi and the Commonwealth Games.* Delhi: Harper Collins.

Majupuria, Trilok C. 1991. *Sacred Animals of Nepal and India: With Reference to Gods and Goddesses of Hinduism and Buddhism.* Katmandu: M. Devi.

Malik, Iqbal, and Rodney L. Johnson. 1994. "Commensal Rhesus in India: The Need and Cost of Translocation." *Revue d'Ecologie* 49: 233–43.

Mani, Reeta S., Ashwini M. Anand, and Shampur N. Madhusudana. 2016. "Human Rabies in India: An Audit from a Rabies Diagnostic Laboratory." *Tropical Medicine and International Health* 21 (4): 556-63.

Mani, Vettam. 1975. *Puranic Encyclopaedia: A Comprehensive Dictionary with*

Special Reference to the Epic and Puranic Literature. Delhi: Motilal Banarsidass.

Marcus, George E. 1995. "Ethnography in/ of the World System: The Emergence of Multi-Sited Ethnography." *Annual Review of Anthropology* 24:95–117.

Marcus, Steven. 1974. *Engels, Manchester, and the Working Class*. Piscataway: Transaction.

Markandya, Anil, Tim Taylor, Alberto Longo, M. N. Murty, Sucheta Murty, and Kishore Dhavala. 2008. "Counting the Cost of Vulture Decline: An Appraisal of the Human Health and Other Benefits of Vultures in India." *Ecological Economics* 67 (2): 194–204.

Maulekhi, Gauri. 2017. "Ban on Cattle Sale for Slaughter: Can We Stop Outraging and Focus on Regulating Animal Markets?" *Firstpost*, June 1.

Mauss, Marcel. 1967. *The Gift: The Form and Reason for Exchange in Archaic Societies*. New York: W. W. Norton.

Mawdsley, Emma. 2004. "India's Middle Classes and the Environment." *Development and Change* 35 (1): 79–103.

Mazoomdaar, Jay. 2013. "The Desi Cow: Almost Extinct." *Tehelka*, January 24. http://old.tehelka.com/ the-desi-cow-almost-extinct/.

McFadyen, Lori. 2005. *Voices from the Street: An Ethnography of India's Street Children*. Delhi: Hope India.

Miller, Sam. 2008. *Delhi: Adventures in a Megacity*. Delhi: Penguin.

Ministry of Agriculture, Department of Animal Husbandry, Dairying, and Fisheries. 2002. *Report of the National Commission on Cattle*. Delhi: Department of Animal Husbandry and Dairying. http://dadf.gov.in/related -links/report-national-commission -cattle.

———. 2012. *19th Livestock Census*. Delhi: Department of Animal Husbandry and Dairying. http://dahd.nic.in/documents /statistics/livestock-census.

———. 2016. *Annual Report, 2015–2016*. Delhi: Department of Animal Husbandry, Dairying, and Fisheries. http://www.dahd.nic.in/documents/ reports.

Ministry of Drinking Water and Sanitation. 2014. *Swachh Bharat by 2019*. Delhi: Ministry of Drinking Water and Sanitation.

Ministry of Environment, Forest, and Climate Change. 2017. *State of Forest Report 2017*. Delhi: Forest Survey of India.

Ministry of Health and Family Welfare, UNICEF, and Population Council. 2019. *Comprehensive National Nutrition Survey National Report*. Delhi: Ministry of Health and Family Welfare.

Mir, Shakir. 2017. "Monkeys Let Loose Reign of Terror in South City, Target Autistic Girl." *Times of India*, March 8.

Mishra, Om P. 1985. *Mother Goddess in Central India*. Delhi: Agam Kala Prakashan.

Mishra, Pankaj. 1995. *Butter Chicken in Ludhiana*. Delhi: Penguin.

Mishra, Subhash. 2017. "Monkeys Allegedly Kill a Cow, Terrorise People in Jharkhand Villages." *Hindustan Times*, April 28.

Mitman, Gregg, Michelle Murphy, and Christopher Sellers, eds. 2004. *Landscapes of Exposure: Knowledge and Illness in Modern Environments*. Chicago: University of Chicago Press.

Mohan, Vishwa. 2019. "Animal Cruelty Issues Now Under Farm Ministry." *Times of India*, April 11.

Mohanty, K. 2016. "More Misery for Odisha Man Who Carried Wife's Body, Govt Apathy Stalls Funeral." *Hindustan Times*, August 27.

Morters, Michelle K., Olivier Restif, Katie Hampson, Sarah Cleaveland, James L. N. Wood, Andrew J. K. Conlan, and M. Boots. 2013. "Evidence-Based Control of Canine Rabies: A Critical Review of

Population Density Reduction." *Journal of Animal Ecology* 82 (1): 6–14.

Mrudu, Herbert, Riyaz Basha, and Selvi Thangaraj. 2012. "Community Perception Regarding Rabies Prevention and Stray Dog Control in Urban Slums in India." *Journal of Infection and Public Health* 5 (6): 374–80.

Nading, Alex M. 2012. "'Dengue Mosquitoes Are Single Mothers': Biopolitics Meets Ecological Aesthetics in Nicaraguan Community Health Work." *Cultural Anthropology* 27 (4): 572–96.

———. 2013. "Humans, Animals, and Health: From Ecology to Entanglement." *Environment and Society: Advances in Research* 4 (1): 60–78. https://doi.org/10.3167/ares.2013.040105.

———. 2014a. "Local Biologies and the Chemical Infrastructures of Global Health." Fondation Maison des Sciences de l'Homme, Working Paper 79.

———. 2014b. *Mosquito Trails: Ecology, Health, and the Politics of Entanglement.* Berkeley: University of California Press.

Nagy, Kelsi, and Phillip D. Johnson II, eds. 2013. *Trash Animals: How We Live with Nature's Filthy, Feral, Invasive, and Unwanted Species.* Minneapolis: University of Minnesota Press.

Naik, Bijaya N., Swaroop K. Sahu, and Ganesh Kumar. 2015. "Wound Management and Vaccination Following Animal Bite: A Study on Knowledge and Practice Among People in an Urban Area of Pondicherry, India." *International Journal of Community Medicine and Public Health* 2 (4): 501–5.

Nair, Harish V. 2009. "Beggars to Be Banished from Prime Locations." *Hindustan Times*, May 5.

Narayanan, Yamini. 2018. "Cow Protection as 'Casteised Speciesism': Sacralisation, Commercialisation, and Politicisation." *South Asia: Journal of South Asian Studies* 41 (2): 331–51. https://doi.org/10.1080/00856401.2018.1419794.

———. 2019. "Jugaad and Informality as Drivers of India's Cow Slaughter Economy." *Economy and Space* 51 (7): 1516–35.

Narula, Joginder. 2005. *Hanuman: God and Epic Hero.* Delhi: Manohar.

Nath, Damini. 2014a. "After Fatal Attack, Civic Body Mulls Passive Killing of Dogs." *Hindu*, July 3.

———. 2014b. "Citizens Divided on 'Passive Killing,' Reveals the Hindu Poll." *Hindu*, July 14.

———. 2014c. "North Delhi Corporation's Dog Sterilisation Programme Fails to Make Impact." *Hindu*, June 19.

———. 2015a. "Monkey Menace Continues to Haunt Municipal Body." *Hindu*, March 3.

———. 2015b. "NDMC Forced to End 'Illegal' Survey on Relocating Dogs." *Hindu*, November 5.

———. 2015c. "Only 300 Pet Dogs Registered This Year." *Hindu*, August 8.

Natrajan, Balmurli, and Suraj Jacob. 2018. "'Provincialising' Vegetarianism: Putting Indian Food Habits in Their Place." *Economic and Political Weekly* 53 (9): 54–64.

Neely, Abigail H., and Alex M. Nading. 2017. "Global Health from the Outside: The Promise of Place-Based Research." *Health and Place* 45:55–63.

Neha, Sinha. 2013. "Dog Bites Tiger." *Economic and Political Weekly* 48 (44): 78–79.

Nelson, Lance. 2006. "Cows, Elephants, Dogs, and Other Lesser Embodiments of Atman: Reflections on Hindu Attitudes Toward Nonhuman Animals." In *A Communion of Subjects: Animals in Religion, Science, and Ethics*, edited by Paul Waldau, 179–93. New York: Columbia University Press.

New Indian Express. 2015a. "Chittilappilly's 24-Hour Hunger Strike Today." October 25.

———. 2015b. "No Dog Census in Delhi for 6 Years, SDMC Fails to Get Bidders." August 16.

———. 2019. "Woman Killed by Pack of Stray Dogs in Odisha." June 1.

Nichter, Mark. 2008. *Global Health: Why Cultural Representations, Social Relations, and Biopolitics Matter.* Tucson: University of Arizona Press.

NIUA (National Institute of Urban Affairs), Ministry of Urban Development. 2011. *India's Urban Demographic Transition: The 2011 Census Results (Provisional).* Delhi: NIUA. http://www.indiagovernance.gov.in/files/urbandemographictransition.pdf.

Ohri, Puneet, Kajal Jain, Rashmi Kumari, and Sudhir K. Gupta. 2016. "A Study About Perception of People Regarding Animal Bite in Urban Area of Dehradun." *Journal of Evolution of Medical and Dental Sciences* 5 (17): 846–49.

OIE (Office International des Épizooties). 2018. *World Animal Health Information Database (WAHIS) Interface.* http://www.oie.int/wahis_2/public/wahid.php/Wahidhome/Home.

Olivelle, Patrick. 2005. *Manu's Code of Law: A Critical Edition and Translation of the Manava-Dharmasastra.* Oxford: Oxford University Press.

Oppili, P. 2017. "Cow Dies of Rabies Near Chennai: Villagers Advised to Take Anti-Rabies Vaccination." *Times of India*, February 3.

Outlook. 2012. "Protests in Kashmir over Stray Dog Menace." February 18. https://www.outlookindia.com/newswire/story/protests-in-kashmir-over-stray-dog-menace/751855.

———. 2014. "Street Dog Menace: NHRC Sends Notices to Centre, Delhi Govt." August 14. https://www.outlookindia.com/newswire/story/street-dog-menace-nhrc-sends-notices-to-centre-delhi-govt/909972.

———. 2015a. "Declare Cow the 'Mother of the Nation': Shiv Sena MP." December 22. https://www.outlookindia.com/newswire/story/declare-cow-the-mother-of-the-nation-shiv-sena-mp/924677.

———. 2015b. "Human or Animal, Everyone's Life Is Important: HC." August 26. https://www.outlookindia.com/newswire/story/human-or-animal-everyones-life-is-important-hc/910955.

———. 2015c. "Kerala: Gram Panchayats Seek to 'Export' Stray Dogs to China, S. Korea." July 31. https://www.outlookindia.com/newswire/story/kerala-gram-panchayats-seek-to-export-stray-dogs-to-china-s-korea/908461.

———. 2015d. "Stray Dogs Defiling PM's Swachh Bharat Abhiyan, Remove Them: HC." July 22. https://www.outlookindia.com/newswire/story/stray-dogs-defiling-pms-swachh-bharat-abhiyan-remove-them-hc/907547.

Pal, Sunil K. 2001. "Population Ecology of Free-Ranging Urban Dogs in West Bengal, India." *Acta Theriologica* 46 (1): 69–78.

Palsetia, Jesse S. 2001. "Mad Dogs and Parsis: The Bombay Dog Riots of 1832." *Journal of the Royal Asiatic Society* 11 (1): 13–30.

Pandey, Kundan. 2018. "Building Toilets Won't Make India Open Defecation Free: World Bank Study." *Down to Earth*, December 26. https://www.downtoearth.org.in/news/waste/building-toilets-won-t-make-india-open-defecation-free-world-bank-study-62594.

Pandit, Ambika. 2012. "32.2% of Households Have Just a Room to Call Home." *Times of India*, November 21.

Pankaj, Jain. 2011. *Dharma and Ecology of Hindu Communities: Sustenance and Sustainability.* Farnham: Ashgate.

Pant, Shubhra. 2018. "If You Have a Pet, You Now Need a Licence from MCG." *Times of India*, November 3.

Parker, John. 2009. "Burgeoning Bourgeoisie." *Economist*, February 14. https://www.economist.com/special-report/2009/02/14/burgeoning-bourgeoisie.

Parry, Jonathan P. 1994. *Death in Banaras.* Cambridge: Cambridge University Press.

Parthasarathy, A., Lucy Joseph, R. Narmada, C. Vaidyanathan, B. R. Santhanakrishnan, and C. Thirugnanasambandham. 1984. "Study of Dog Bite in Children." *Indian Pediatrics* 21 (7): 549–54.

Pathak, Bindeshwar. 1991. *Road to Freedom: A Sociological Study on the Abolition of Scavenging in India.* Delhi: Motilal Banarsidass.

Pathak, M. L., and A. Kumar. 2003. "Cow Praising and Importance of Panchyagavya as Medicine." *Sachitra Ayurveda* 5:56–59.

Patle, Rupali A., and Gautam M. Khakse. 2014. "Clinico-Demographic and Treatment Seeking Profile of Children Below 15 Years Attending the Anti-Rabies Clinic." *International Journal of Medicine and Public Health* 4 (2): 151–54.

Patranobis, Sutirtho. 2018. "China Tight-Lipped About Recall of Fake Rabies Vaccines Exported to India." *Hindustan Times,* August 8.

Pawar, A. B., and R. K. Bansal. 2010. "Need for Incorporating Anticipatory Guidance on Animal Bites and Prevention of Rabies in School Curriculum." *National Journal of Community Medicine* 1 (1): 57.

Perappadan, Bindu S. 2013. "Dog Bites Go Down, but Problem Persists." *Hindu,* July 28.

PETA (People for the Ethical Treatment of Animals) India. 2008. *Inside the Indian Dairy Industry: A Report on the Abuse of Cows and Buffaloes Exploited for Milk.* Mumbai: PETA.

Pew Research Center. 2007. *Pew Global Attitude 47-Nation Survey.* Washington, D.C.: Pew Research Center.

PHFI (Public Health Foundation of India) and WHO (World Health Organization). 2008. "Roadmap for Combating Zoonoses in India." Delhi: PHFI.

PICT (Peace Institute Charitable Trust). 2009a. *Attitude and Practice of Delhiites Towards the River Yamuna.* Delhi: PICT.

———. 2009b. *Sick Yamuna, Sick Delhi.* Delhi: PICT.

———. 2009c. *The Unquiet River.* Delhi: PICT.

Pietkiewicz-Pareek, Beata. 2012. "Common Social Problems Among Street Children in India." *Advanced Research in Scientific Areas* 1 (1): 981–85.

Pillai, Soumya. 2017. "Dogged by Overcrowding, City Shelters Close Doors to Cattle." *Hindu,* June 22.

Podberscek, Anthony L. 1994. "Dog on a Tightrope: The Position of the Dog in British Society as Influenced by Press Reports on Dog Attacks (1988 to 1992)." *Anthrozoös* 7 (4): 232–41.

Porte, Sharad M. 2015. "Ayurvedic Aspect of Rabies and Its Management." *Ayushdhara: An International Journal of Research in AYUSH and Allied Systems* 2 (2): 86–93.

Porter, Natalie. 2012. "Risky Zoographies: The Limits of Place in Avian Influenza Management." *Environmental Humanities* 1 (1): 103–21.

———. 2013. "Bird Flu Biopower: Strategies for Multispecies Coexistence in Việt Nam." *American Ethnologist* 40 (1): 132–48. https://doi.org/10.1111/amet.12010.

Prakash, Vibhu, Toby H. Galligan, Soumya S. Chakraborty, Ruchi Dave, Mandar D. Kulkarni, Nikita Prakash, Rohan N. Shringarpure, Sachin P. Ranade, and Rhys E. Green. 2019. "Recent Changes in Populations of Critically Endangered *Gyps* Vultures in India." *Bird Conservation International* 29:55–70.

Prakash, Vibhu, Rhys E. Green, Deborah J. Pain, Sachin P. Ranade, S. Saravanan, Nithin Prakash, R. Venkitachalam, Richard Cuthbert, Asad R. Rahmani, and Andrew A. Cunningham. 2007. "Recent Changes in Populations of

Resident *Gyps* Vultures in India." *Journal of the Bombay Natural History Society* 104:129–35.

Prakash, Vibhu, Deborah J. Pain, Andrew A. Cunningham, P. F. Donald, Nithin Prakash, Ajay Verma, R. Gargi, S. Sivakumar, and Asad R. Rahmani. 2003. "Catastrophic Collapse of Indian White-Backed *Gyps bengalensis* and Long-Billed *Gyps indicus* Vulture Population." *Biological Conservation* 109:381–90.

Prasad, Sharada C. S., and Isha Ray. 2018. "'It Has to Be Done Only at Night': Human Waste Disposal in Bengaluru." *Economic and Political Weekly* 53 (21): 13–16.

Puppala, Anusha. 2017. "Hyderabad GES: Stray Dogs 'Poisoned' for Ivanka Trump Visit." *Deccan Chronicle*, November 22.

Rabinowitz, Peter M., Lynda Odofin, and F. Joshua Dein. 2008. "From 'Us vs. Them' to 'Shared Risk': Can Animals Help Link Environmental Factors to Human Health?" *EcoHealth* 5 (2): 224–29.

Raghunathan, Viswanathan. 2006. *Games Indians Play: Why We Are the Way We Are*. Delhi: Penguin.

Raghunathan, Viswanathan, and M. A. Eswaran. 2012. *Ganesha on the Dashboard*. Delhi: Penguin.

Raheja, Gloria Goodwin. 1988. *The Poison in the Gift: Ritual Prestation and the Dominant Caste in a North Indian Village*. Chicago: University of Chicago Press.

Rajagopal, Krishnadas. 2009. "Dog Lovers Fear Man-Bite, Move High Court for Protection." *Indian Express*, August 13.

———. 2015. "SC Verdicts Differ on Beef Being a Poor Man's Food." *Hindu*, March 4.

Rajagopal, Shyama. 2014. "Dog Bites on the Rise in District." *Hindu*, June 27.

Rajeshwaran, S., and Gopal Naik. 2016. "Milk Production in India Rises by a Historic 6.25% in 2014–15: A Boon or a Bane?" Indian Institute of Management Bangalore, Working Paper 518.

https://papers.ssrn.com/sol3/papers .cfm?abstract_id=2803149.

Ramani, Shyama V. 2016. "Why It's Easier for India to Get to Mars Than to Tackle Its Toilet Challenge." *Down to Earth*, November. https://www.downtoearth .org.in/news/governance/why-it-s-easier -for-india-to-get-to-mars-than-to-tackle -its-toilet-challenge-56367.

Ramanna, B. C., Guddeti S. Reddy, and Villuppanoor A. Srinivasan. 1991. "An Outbreak of Rabies in Cattle and Use of Tissue Culture Rabies Vaccine During the Outbreak." *Journal of Communicable Diseases* 23 (4): 283–85.

Ramanujan, Anuradha. 2015. "Violent Encounters: 'Stray' Dogs in Indian Cities." In *Cosmopolitan Animals*, edited by Kaori Nagai, Karen Jones, Donna Landry, Monica Mattfeld, Caroline Rooney, and Charlotte Sleigh, 216–32. Basingstoke: Palgrave Macmillan.

Ranade, Chandrashekhar G. 2015. "Livestock Sector Neglected." *Economic and Political Weekly* 50 (50): 5.

Rani, Puteri A. M. A., Peter J. Irwin, Mulukesh Gatne, Glen T. Coleman, and Rebecca J. Traub. 2010. "Canine Vector-Borne Diseases in India: A Review of the Literature and Identification of Existing Knowledge Gaps." *Parasites and Vectors* 3:28. https://www.ncbi.nlm.nih.gov/pubmed /20377862.

Rao, Smitha. 2011. "Saffronisation of the Holy Cow: Unearthing Silent Communalism." *Economic and Political Weekly* 46 (15): 80–87.

Rashid, Omar. 2017. "Invoke NSA for Cow Slaughter: U. P. DGP." *Hindu*, June 6.

Rashtriya Garima Abhiyan. 2011. "Eradication of Inhuman Practice of Manual Scavenging and Comprehensive Rehabilitation of Manual Scavengers in India." https://www.indiawaterportal .org/sites/indiawaterportal.org/files /Eradication_Inhuman_Practice

_Manual_Scavenging_India_Rashtriya
_Garima_Abhiyaan_2011.pdf.

Rath, Nilakantha. 2015. "Declining Cattle Population." *Economic and Political Weekly* 50 (28): 12–14.

Reece, Jack F. 2005. "Dog and Dog Control in Developing Counties." In *The State of the Animals III: 2005*, edited by Deborah J. Salem and Andrew N. Rowan, 55–64. Washington, D.C.: Humane Society Press.

Reece, Jack F., and S. K. Chawla. 2006. "Control of Rabies in Jaipur, India, by the Sterilisation and Vaccination of Neighbourhood Dogs." *Veterinary Record* 159 (12): 379–83.

RIA (Rabies in Asia). 2011. *Proceedings of the RIA-SAARC Inter-Country Meet on Rabies*. Bangalore: Kempegowda Institute of Medical Sciences.

Richard, A. F., S. J. Goldstein, and R. E. Dewar. 1989. "Weed Macaques: The Evolutionary Implications of Macaque Feeding Ecology." *International Journal of Primatology* 10 (6): 569–94.

Rigopoulos, Antonio. 1998. *Dattatreya: The Immortal Guru, Yogin, and Avatara.* Albany: SUNY Press.

Riser-Kositsky, Sasha. 2009. "The Political Intensification of Caste: India Under the Raj." *Penn History Review* 17 (1): 31–53.

Ritvo, Harriet. 1987. *The Animal Estate: The English and Other Creatures in the Victorian Age.* London: Penguin.

Robbins, Paul. 1999. "Meat Matters: Cultural Politics Along the Commodity Chain in India." *Ecumene* 6 (4): 399–423.

Rock, Melanie. 2017. "Who or What Is 'the Public' in Critical Public Health? Reflections on Posthumanism and Anthropological Engagements with One Health." *Critical Public Health* 27 (3): 314–24.

Rock, Melanie, and Chris Degeling. 2013. "Public Health Ethics and a Status for Pets as Person-Things: Revisiting the Place of Animals in Urbanized

Societies." *Journal of Bioethical Inquiry* 10 (4): 485–95.

———. 2015. "Public Health Ethics and More-Than-Human Solidarity." *Social Science and Medicine* 129:61–67.

———. 2016. "Toward 'One Health' Promotion." In *A Companion to Environmental Health: Anthropological Perspectives*, edited by Merrill Singer, 68–82. Chichester: Wiley Blackwell.

Rock, Melanie, Eric Mykhalovskiy, and Thomas Schlich. 2007. "People, Other Animals, and Health Knowledges: Towards a Research Agenda." *Social Science and Medicine* 64:1970–76.

Rohilla, Suresh K., Bhitush Luthra, Shantanu K. Padhi, Anil Yadav, Jigyasa Watwani, and Rahul S. Varma. 2016. "Urban Shit: Where Does It All Go?" *Down to Earth*, April. https://www.downtoearth.org.in /coverage/waste/urban-shit-53422.

Rosen, Steven J. 2006. *Essential Hinduism.* New York: Praeger.

Roy, K. B. 1962. "Problem of Stray Dogs in India." *Indian Journal of Public Health* 6:141–42.

Rupprecht, Charles E., Ivan V. Kuzmin, and François-Xavier Meslin. 2017. "Lyssaviruses and Rabies: Current Conundrums, Concerns, Contradictions, and Controversies." *F1000 Research* 6:184. https://doi .org/10.12688/f1000research.10416.1.

Ryan, William. 2010. *Blaming the Victim.* New York: Knopf Doubleday.

Sahu, Geetanjoy. 2019. "Whither the National Green Tribunal?" *Down to Earth*, September 24. https://www .downtoearth.org.in/blog/environment /whither-the-national-green-tribunal --66879.

Saikia, Bipul, and Sashin K. Borthakur. 2010. "Use of Medicinal Plants in Animal Healthcare: A Case Study from Gohpur, Assam." *Indian Journal of Traditional Knowledge* 9 (1): 49–51.

Saini, Sachin. 2017. "Rajasthan HC Judge Wants Cow as National Animal, Life

Term for Slaughter." *Hindustan Times*, June 19.

Salve, Harshal, S. A. Rizwan, Shashi Kant, Sanjay K. Rai, Pradip Kharya, and Sanjeev Kumar. 2015. "Pre-Treatment Practices Among Patients Attending an Animal Bite Management Clinic at a Primary Health Centre in Haryana, North India." *Tropical Doctor* 45 (2): 123–25.

Samanta, Moumita, Rakesh Mondal, Ankit Shah, Avijit Hazra, Somosri Ray, Goutam Dhar, Rupa Biswas, et al. 2016. "Animal Bites and Rabies Prophylaxis in Rural Children: Indian Perspective." *Journal of Tropical Pediatrics* 62:55–62.

Sambyal, Swati S. 2014. "A Review of the Draft Plastic Waste Management Rules, 2015." *Down to Earth*, November. https://www.downtoearth.org.in/blog /a-review-of-the-draft-plastic-waste -management-rules-2015-49568.

———. 2016a. "Government Notifies New Solid Waste Management Rules." *Down to Earth*, April. https://www.downto earth.org.in/news/waste/solid-waste -management-rules-2016-53443.

———. 2016b. "Trashing the Ragpicker." *Down to Earth*, April, 16–17.

Sanders, Clinton R., and Arnold Arluke. 1993. "If Lions Could Speak: Investigating the Animal-Human Relationship and the Perspectives of Nonhuman Others." *Sociological Quarterly* 34 (3): 377–90.

Sani, Saverio. 2009. *Dizionario sanscrito-italiano*. Pisa: ETS.

Santoshi, Neeraj. 2016. "Over 12,000 Cattle Left to Fend for Themselves in Parched Bundelkhand." *Hindustan Times*, June 8.

———. 2018. "Uttarakhand HC Declares Animal Kingdom a Legal Entity with Rights of a 'Living Person.'" *Hindustan Times*, August 5.

Sarkar, Amrita, Sudip Bhavsar, Chintan Bundela, Aniruddha Gohel, Naresh Makwana, and Dipesh Parmar. 2013. "An Assessment of Knowledge of Prevention and Management of Rabies in Interns and Final Year Students of Shri M. P. Shah Government Medical College, Jamnagar, Gujarat." *Journal of Research in Medical and Dental Science* 1 (2): 62–66.

Sathasivam, P. 2014. "Writ Petition (Civil) No. 583 of 2003," Supreme Court of India, *Safai Karmachari Andolan and Ors vs Union of India and Ors on 27 March 2014*. https://indiankanoon.org /doc/6155772/.

Scott, Terence P., Andre Coetzer, Anna S. Fahrion, and Louis H. Nel. 2017. "Addressing the Disconnect Between the Estimated, Reported, and True Rabies Data: The Development of a Regional African Rabies Bulletin." *Frontiers in Veterinary Science* 4 (18). https://doi .org/10.3389/fvets.2017.00018.

Seabrook, Jeremy. 1996. *In the Cities of the South: Scenes from a Developing World*. London: Verso.

Sekar, Nitin, Naman K. Shah, Syed S. Abbas, and Manish Kakkar. 2011. "Research Options for Controlling Zoonotic Disease in India, 2010–2015." *PLOS One* 6 (2). https://doi.org/10.1371 /journal.pone.0017120.

Senacha, Kalu R., Mark A. Taggart, Asad R. Rahmani, Yadvendradev V. Jhala, Richard Cuthbert, Deborah J. Pain, and Rhys E. Green. 2008. "Diclofenac Levels in Livestock Carcasses in India Before the 2006 'Ban.'" *Journal of the Bombay Natural History Society* 105 (2): 148–61.

Sengupta, Ranjana. 2007. *Delhi Metropolitan: The Making of an Unlikely City*. Delhi: Penguin.

Sengupta, Sushmita. 2015. "NGT Orders Strict Action Against Delhi's Yamuna-Polluting Industries." *Down to Earth*, February. https://www.downtoearth.org .in/news/ngt-orders-strict-action-against -delhis-yamunapolluting-industries -48492.

Shadomy, Sean V. 2019. "One Health Zoonotic Disease Prioritization Process."

Paper presented at the United Against Rabies Webinar, Bangkok, September 27.

Shah, Arvind M. 2012. "The Village in the City, the City in the Village." *Economic and Political Weekly* 47 (52): 17–19.

Shankaraiah, Ravish H., Gangaboraiah Bilagumba, Doddabele Hanumanthappa, Ashwath D. H. Narayana, Rachana Annadani, and Veena Vijayashankar. 2013. "Knowledge, Attitude, and Practice of Rabies Prophylaxis Among Physicians at Indian Animal Bite Clinics." *Asian Biomedicine* 7 (2): 237–42.

Shariff, Abusaleh. 2015. "Why India Must Not Disrupt Its Balanced Bovine Economy with a Ban on Beef." *Wire*, June 22.

Sharma, Aman. 2019. "Ahead of 2019 Elections, Yogi Rushes to Build Shelters for Stray Cattle." *Economic Times*, January 4.

Sharma, Arvind, Uttara Kennedy, Catherine Schuetze, and Clive J. C. Phillips. 2019. "The Welfare of Cows in Indian Shelters." *Animals* 9 (4). https://doi:10.3390/ani9040172.

Sharma, B. V. V. S. R. 1980. *The Study of Cow in Sanskrit Literature.* Delhi: G. D. K. Publications.

Sharma, Mohit. 2016a. "1 Dog Bite Every 6 Minutes: Capital Faces Canine Crisis." *Hindustan Times*, January 20.

———. 2016b. "Stray Dogs Are Terror Threat to Delhi Airport, Says DIAL." *Hindustan Times*, February 24.

Sharma, Nidhi. 2018. "Government Dilutes Rules on Cattle Sale in Animal Market." *Economic Times*, April 10.

Sharma, Ramashraya. 1971. *Socio-Political Study of the Valmiki Ramayana.* Delhi: Motilal Banarsidass.

Sharma, Shantanu, Anurag Agarwal, Amir M. Khan, and Gopal K. Ingle. 2016. "Prevalence of Dog Bites in Rural and Urban Slums of Delhi: A Community Based Study." *Annals of Medical and Health Sciences Research* 6:115–19.

Sharma, Vibha. 2017. "More Than 225 Dog Bite Cases in Delhi Every Day, Civic Bodies Struggle to Count Canines." *Hindustan Times*, June 19.

Sheikh, Shanana. 2008. "Public Toilets in Delhi: An Emphasis on the Facilities for Women in Slum/Resettlement Areas." CCS Working Paper 192. Delhi: Centre for Civil Society. https://ccs.in /internship_papers/2008/Public-toilets -in-Delh-192.pdf.

Sheikh, Shahana, and Subhadra Banda. 2014. "Whose Flat Is It Anyway?" *Down to Earth*, April, 52–53.

Shekhar, Shashank. 2016. "Beware of the Dog-Snatchers! How Delhi Gangs Are Stealing 'Exotic' Puppies Like Huskies to Sell or Use for Breeding." *Daily Mail* (UK), June 8.

———. 2017. "Delhi: Business of Renting out Langurs, Punishable Under IPC, Flourishes amid Growing Monkey Menace." *India Today*, March 15.

Sherikar, Adagonda, and V. S. Waskar. 2005. "Emerging Zoonoses and Social-Economic Impact in India: A Review." *Indian Journal of Animal Sciences* 75 (6): 700–705.

Shiva, Vandana. 2016. *Stolen Harvest: The Hijacking of the Global Food Supply.* Lexington: University Press of Kentucky.

Shrivastava, Kumar S. 2016. "Scientists Say a Vulture's Services Worth over Rs 5 Lakh." *Hindustan Times*, February 15.

Shwiff, Stephanie, Katie Hampson, and Aaron Anderson. 2013. "Potential Economic Benefits of Eliminating Canine Rabies." *Antiviral Research* 98:352–56.

Sibley, David. 1988. "Survey 13: Purification of Space." *Environment and Planning D: Society and Space* 6 (4): 409–21.

Sikdar, Shubhomoy. 2014. "Baby Mauled to Death by Dog in Delhi." *Hindu*, June 28.

Singh, Apula, and Viral Shah. 2016. "No More N-I-M-B-Y." *Down to Earth*, September. https://www.downtoearth

.org.in/blog/waste/no-more-n-i-m-b-y -55596.

Singh, Balbir B., and Alvin A. Gajadhar. 2014. "Role of India's Wildlife in the Emergence and Re-Emergence of Zoonotic Pathogens, Risk Factors, and Public Health Implications." *Acta Tropica* 138:67–77.

Singh, Balbir B., Rattanpreet Kaur, Gurlal S. Gill, J. P. S. Gill, Ravinder K. Soni, and Rabinder S. Aulakh. 2019. "Knowledge, Attitude, and Practices Relating to Zoonotic Diseases Among Livestock Farmers in Punjab, India." *Acta Tropica* 189:15–21.

Singh, Darpan. 2012. "Govt to Probe Why Trees Don't Survive." *Hindustan Times*, November 11.

———. 2013. "Planting More Trees Cannot Be an Excuse to Axe Trees for Widening Roads." *Hindustan Times*, November 11.

Singh, Indu P. 2006. "Capital Punishment: Recipe for the Homeless in Delhi." In *Dimensions of Urban Poverty*, edited by Sabir Ali, 218–54. Jaipur: Rawat.

Singh, Jyotsna. 2015. "Urban Children in Slums More Vulnerable to Health Risks, Says Report." *Down to Earth*, August 18. https://www.downtoearth.org.in/news /health/urban-children-in-slums-more -vulnerable-to-health-risks-says-report -50539.

Singh, Mini P., Kapil Goyal, Manasi Majumdar, and Radha K. Ratho. 2011. "Prevalence of Rabies Antibodies in Street and Household Dogs in Chandigarh, India." *Tropical Animal Health and Production* 43:111–14.

Singh, Nagendra K. R. 1997. *Indian Legends*. Delhi: A. P. H.

Singh, Saptal. 2006. *Solid Waste Management in Resettlement Colonies in Delhi: A Study of People's Participation and Urban Policy*. Belfast: Bookwell.

Singh, U. S., and S. K. Choudhary. 2005. "Knowledge, Attitude, Behavior, and Practice Study on Dog-Bites and Its Management in the Context of Prevention of Rabies in a Rural Community of Gujarat." *Indian Journal of Community Medicine* 30 (3): 81–83.

Singh, Vijay. 2019. "Five Held for Death of 90 Dogs in Buldhana." *Times of India*, September 13.

Singhal, Anupriya. N.d. *Gau Sadans: A Scheme of Delhi Government*. Delhi: Centre for Civil Society.

Sinha, Neha. 2010. "Delhi Colonies to Have Demarcated Areas for Feeding Dogs." *Indian Express*, July 6.

Society for Nutrition, Education, and Health Action for Women and Children. 2008. *Making Health Care Accessible to Street Children: The "Hospital on Wheels" Project*. Mumbai: Society for Nutrition, Education, and Health Action for Women and Children.

Sood, Jyotika. 2014a. "Mission to Conserve Indigenous Cow Breeds Kicked Off." *Down to Earth*, July 4. https://www .downtoearth.org.in/news/mission-to -conserve-indigenous-cow-breeds-kick ed-off-45535.

———. 2014b. "Reinventing Dairy." *Down to Earth*, February.

Southwick, Charles H., Mirza A. Beg, and Rafiq M. Siddiqi. 1961. "A Population Survey of Rhesus Monkeys in Villages, Towns, and Temples of Northern India." *Ecology* 42 (3): 538–47.

Southwick, Charles H., and Donald G. Lindburg. 1986. "The Primates of India: Status, Trends, and Conservation." In *Primates: The Road to Self-Sustaining Populations*, edited by Kurt Benirschke, 171–87. New York: Springer.

Southwick, Charles H., and Farooq Siddiqi. 1994. "Primate Commensalism: The Rhesus Monkey in India." *Revue d'Ecologie* 49 (3): 223–3l.

Spears, Dean, and Amit Thorat. 2016. "The Puzzle of Open Defecation in Rural India: Evidence from a Novel Measure of Caste Attitudes in a Nationally-Representative Survey." Research

Institute for Compassionate Economics Working Paper.

Srinivasan, Krithika. 2012. "The Biopolitics of Animal Being and Welfare: Dog Control and Care in the UK and India." *Transactions of the Institute of British Geographers* 38 (1): 106–19. https://doi .org/10.1111/j.1475-5661.2012.00501.x.

Srinivasan, Krithika, and Vijay K. Nagaraj. 2007. "Deconstructing the Human Gaze: Stray Dogs, Indifferent Governance, and Prejudiced Reactions." *Economic and Political Weekly* 42 (13): 1085–86.

Srinivasan, Krithika, and Smitha Rao. 2015. "'Will Eat Anything That Moves': Meat Cultures in Globalising India." *Economic and Political Weekly* 50 (39): 13–15.

Srivastava, Pushker, and Gyanendra Bartaria. 2010. *Commonwealth Games: An Extravaganza*. Delhi: Pitambar.

Srivastava, Sanjay. 2009. "Urban Spaces, Disney-Divinity, and Moral Middle Classes in Delhi." *Economic and Political Weekly* 44 (26–27): 338–45.

Sudarshan, Mysore K., Bangalore J. Mahendra, Shampur N. Madhusudana, Ashwath D. H. Narayana, Abdul S. Rahman, Natesh S. N. Rao, François-Xavier Meslin, Derek Lobo, Kaliamoorthy Ravikumar, and Gangaboraiah. 2006. "An Epidemiological Study of Animal Bites in India: Results of a WHO Sponsored National Multi-Centric Rabies Survey." *Journal of Communicable Diseases* 28 (1): 32–39.

Summer, Rudolf, Stefan Ross, and Wolfgang Kiehl. 2004. "Imported Case of Rabies in Germany from India." *Eurosurveillance* 8 (46): 2585.

Suraksha, P. 2016. "South Corpn to Take Monkey Issue to SC." *Times of India*, March 23.

Taylor, Louise H., Katie Hampson, Anna S. Fahrion, Bernadette Abela-Ridder, and Louis H. Nel. 2017. "Difficulties in Estimating the Human Burden of Canine Rabies." *Acta Tropica* 165:133–40.

Thakur, Atul, and Jayashree Nandi. 2016. "Cry for Holy Cows Fails to Draw Funds for Gaushalas." *Times of India*, June 26.

Thomassen, Bjørn. 2012. "Revisiting Liminality: The Danger of Empty Spaces." In *Liminal Landscapes: Travel, Experience, and Spaces In-Between*, edited by Hazel Andrews and Les Roberts, 21–35. London: Routledge.

Times of India. 2004. "Monkey Kills Sleeping Baby." January 26.

———. 2007. "Monkey Menace: Delhi Deputy Mayor SS Bajwa Dies." October 21.

———. 2010. "2010: A Global Survey." March 22.

———. 2011. "34,000 Tortoises Released into Ganga." May 24.

———. 2012a. "Stray Dogs Drag Body of Newborn in People's Hospital." November 6.

———. 2012b. "Stray Dogs Kill 4-Year-Old Boy, Consume Vital Organs." December 17.

———. 2012c. "Stray Dogs Mutilate Infant's Body." November 4.

———. 2013a. "Dog Carries Man's Head, Shocks Bangalore University Campus." February 22.

———. 2013b. "No Full Stops to Monkey Menace." February 14.

———. 2013c. "Stray Dog Attacks 6-Year-Old Girl in Bangalore." January 26.

———. 2013d. "Stray Dogs Ravage Abandoned Just-Born Girl's Body." March 17.

———. 2013e. "Want to Make Delhi a Place That Everybody Loves: Sheila Dikshit." March 3.

———. 2015. "Cow Suffering from Rabies Caught at Valpoi." July 15.

———. 2016. "City to Get First Dog Pound." April 3.

———. 2017a. "Aadhaar-Like Unique Identification Numbers for Cows?" April 24.

———. 2017b. "80 Ill After Consuming Milk of Cows Bitten by Rabies Infected Dog." January 21.

———. 2017c. "Stray Dogs Mutilate Stillborn's Body Outside KGMU." June 3.

———. 2018. "Jaipur Municipal Corporation Turns Blind Eye to Menace of Stray Dogs." March 26.

———. 2019a. "Over 50 Stray Dogs Shot Dead in Bikaner Village." March 13.

———. 2019b. "6-Year-Old Boy Mauled to Death by Half a Dozen Stray Dogs in Bhopal." May 10.

Tiwari, Harish K., Ian D. Robertson, Mark O'Dea, and Abi T. Vanak. 2019. "Knowledge, Attitudes, and Practices (KAP) Towards Rabies and Free Roaming Dogs (FRD) in Panchkula District of North India: A Cross-Sectional Study of Urban Residents." *PLOS Neglected Tropical Diseases* 13 (4). https://doi.org/10.1371/journal.pntd.0007384.

Tiwari, Mrigank. 2014. "Tourist Bus Used to Smuggle Cattle." *Times of India*, August 31.

Tomar, Shruti, and Ranjeet Gupta. 2019. "2 Minors Defecating in Open, Filmed and Then Beaten to Death in MP." *Hindustan Times*, September 25.

Trivedi, Saurabh. 2019. "In U.P. Village, Dog Menace Keeps Farmers off the Fields." *Hindu*, May 16.

Tseng, Wen S. 2001. *Handbook of Cultural Psychiatry*. San Diego: Academic Press.

Tsing, Anna L. 2005. *Friction: An Ethnography of Global Connection.* Princeton: Princeton University Press.

Tulpule, Shankar G. 1991. "The Dog as a Symbol of Bhakti." In *Devotion Divine: Bhakti Traditions from the Regions of India; Studies in Honour of Charlotte Vaudeville*, edited by Diana L. Eck and Françoise Mallison, 273–85. Groningen: Egbert Forsten.

Turner, Ralph L. 1999. *A Comparative Dictionary of Indo-Aryan Languages.* Delhi: Motilal Banarsidass.

UN (United Nations). 2015. *Human Development Report 2015.* New York: United Nations.

UNICEF (United Nations Children's Fund). 2012. *Sanitation and Hygiene Strategy Framework.* New York: UNICEF.

———. 2015. *Progress on Sanitation and Drinking Water.* New York: UNICEF.

Uniyal, Meghna. 2019. "Who Let the Dogs Out?" *Down to Earth*, June 4. https://www.downtoearth.org.in/blog/governance/who-let-the-dogs-out-64908.

Uniyal, Meghna, and Abi T. Vanak. 2016. "Barking up the Wrong Tree: The Agency in Charge of Controlling Street Dogs Is Completely Ineffective." *Scroll. in*, October 29. https://scroll.in/article/819565/why-the-animal-welfare-board-of-india-must-be-disbanded.

Valekar, Smita S., Maya V. Kshirsagar, Madura D. Ashturkar, Mayavati Mhaske, Parvinder S. Chawla, and Kevin Fernandez. 2014. "A Cross-Sectional Study of Awareness Regarding Dog Bite and Its Management in Rural Community of Maharashtra." *International Journal of Community Medicine and Public Health* 1 (1): 8–11.

Vanak, Abi T. 2017. "Why Does Rabies Still Plague India in the Twenty-First Century?" Ashoka Trust for Research in Ecology and the Environment. https://www.atree.org/news/why-does-rabies-still-plague-india-21st-century.

Vanak, Abi T., Aniruddha V. Belsare, and Matthew E. Gompper. 2007. "Survey of Disease Prevalence in Free-Ranging Domestic Dogs and Possible Spill-Over Risk for Wildlife: A Case Study from the Great Indian Bustard Sanctuary, Maharashtra, India." Final report submitted to the Rufford Small Grants Foundation, UK.

Vanak, Abi T., Aniruddha V. Belsare, and Meghna Uniyal. 2016. "The Street Is No Place for Dogs." *Hindu*, October 3.

Van Dooren, Thom. 2014. "Care." *Environmental Humanities* 5:291–94.

Varikas, Eleni. 2010. "The Outcasts of the World: Images of the Pariahs." *Estudos Avançados* 24 (69): 31–60.

Varma, Pavan K. 2004. *Being Indian*. Delhi: Penguin.

———. 2007. *The Great Indian Middle Class*. Delhi: Penguin.

Varsharani, Kendre V., L. T. Chinte, and Y. U. Jadhav. 2014. "Cultural Practices Among Animal Bite Cases of Government Medical College, Latur." *International Medical Journal* 1 (2): 61–64.

Venkateshwarlu, K. 2015. "India Takes Major Step to Save the Vulture." *Hindu*, September 3.

Verma, Satish K., and D. K. Srivastava. 2003. "A Study on Mass Hysteria (Monkey Men?) Victims in East Delhi." *Indian Journal of Medical Sciences* 57 (8): 355–60.

Vishwanathan, Chettiyappan, and J. Tränkler. 2003. "Municipal Solid Waste Management in Asia: A Comparative Analysis." http://citeseerx.ist.psu.edu /viewdoc/download?doi=10.1.1.572.6735 &rep=rep1&type=pdf.

Voice of Street Dogs. 2011. "Hell for Stray Dogs Is the Greater Hyderabad Municipal Corporation (GHMC) Autonagar Dog Pound." August 19. https://strays.in/index.php/2011/08 /stray-dogs-greater-hyderabad-munici pal-corporation-ghmc-dog-pound -autonagar.

Waldrop, Anne. 2004. "Gating and Class Relations: The Case of a New Delhi 'Colony.'" *City and Society* 16 (2): 93–116.

Walker, Benjamin. 1968. *The Hindu World: An Encyclopaedic Survey of Hinduism*. New York: Praeger.

Walk Free Foundation. 2016. *Global Slavery Index*. https://www.globalslaveryindex. org.

Wang, Jessica. 2019. *Mad Dogs and Other New Yorkers: Rabies, Medicine, and Society in an American Metropolis, 1840–1920*. Baltimore: Johns Hopkins University Press.

Warden, Lisa. 2015. "City of Gods, City of Dogs: Interspecies Communities in Delhi, India." Paper presented at the International Companion Animal Management Coalition's Dog Population Management Conference, Istanbul, March 3–5, 2015.

Wasik, Bill, and Monica Murphy. 2012. *Rabid: A Cultural History of the World's Most Diabolical Virus*. New York: Penguin.

Webb, Eugene J., Donald T. Campbell, Richard D. Schwartz, and Lee Sechrest. (1966) 2000. *Unobtrusive Measures: Nonreactive Research in the Social Sciences*. Thousand Oaks, Calif.: Sage Publications.

Whatmore, Sarah. 2002. *Hybrid Geographies: Natures, Cultures, Spaces*. London: Sage Publications.

White, David G. 1991. *Myths of the Dog-Man*. Chicago: University of Chicago Press.

WHO (World Health Organization). 1986. *Ottawa Charter for Health Promotion*. Geneva: WHO.

———. 1988. *Report of a WHO Consultation on Dog Ecology Studies Related to Dog Rabies Control*. Geneva: WHO.

———. 1992. *WHO Expert Consultation on Rabies*. WHO Technical Report Series 824. Geneva: WHO.

———. 2013a. *Frequently Asked Questions on Rabies*. Geneva: WHO.

———. 2013b. WHO Expert Consultation on Rabies. WHO Technical Report Series 982. Geneva: WHO.

———. 2014. *A Brief Guide to Emerging Infectious Diseases and Zoonoses*. Geneva: WHO.

———. 2015. *Investing to Overcome the Global Impact of Neglected Tropical Diseases*. Geneva: WHO.

———. 2016a. *Country Report: India*. Geneva: WHO.

———. 2016b. *Stimulus Package for Eliminating Dog-Mediated Human Rabies*. Geneva: WHO.

———. 2017. "Human Rabies: 2016 Updates and Call for Data." *Weekly Epidemiological Record* 7 (92): 77–88.

———. 2018a. "Rabies Vaccines: WHO Position Paper—April 2018." *Weekly Epidemiological Record* 16 (93): 201–220.

———. 2018b. *WHO Expert Consultation on Rabies. WHO Technical Report Series 1012.* Geneva: WHO.

WHO and OIE (Office International des Épizooties). 2015. *Global Elimination of Dog-Mediated Human Rabies.* Geneva: WHO and OIE.

WHO and WSPA (World Society for the Protection of Animals). 1990. *Guidelines for Dog Population Management.* Geneva: WHO and WSPA.

Wiley, Andrea S. 2014. *Cultures of Milk: The Biology and Meaning of Dairy Products in the United States and India.* Cambridge, Mass.: Harvard University Press.

Williams, George M. 2008. *Handbook of Hindu Mythology.* Oxford: Oxford University Press.

Withnall, Adam. 2019. "Inside India's Plastic Cows: How Sacred Animals Are Left to Line Their Stomachs with Polythene." *Independent* (UK), February 24.

Wolch, Jennifer. 1998. "Zoöpolis." In *Animal Geographies: Place, Politics, and Identity in the Nature-Culture Borderlands,* edited by Jennifer Wolch and Jodie Emel, 119–38. London: Verso.

Wolcott, Leonard T. 1978. "Hanuman: The Power Dispensing Monkey in North Indian Folk Religion." *Journal of Asian Studies* 37 (4): 653–61.

Wolf, Meike. 2015. "Is There Really Such a Thing as 'One Health'? Thinking About a More Than Human World from the Perspective of Cultural Anthropology." *Social Science and Medicine* 129:5–11.

World Economic Forum. 2017. *The Inclusive Growth and Development Report.* Cologny, Switzerland: World Economic Forum.

Yadav, Yogedra, and Sanjay Kumar. 2006. "The Food Habits of a Nation." *Hindu,* August 14.

CPSIA information can be obtained
at www.ICGtesting.com
Printed in the USA
BVHW072248180421
605193BV00001B/64

9 780271 085968